NEEDLESS SUFFERING

DAVID NAGEL, MD

Needless Suffering

HOW SOCIETY FAILS

THOSE WITH CHRONIC PAIN

ForeEdge

ForeEdge

An imprint of University Press of New England

www.upne.com

© 2016 University Press of New England

All rights reserved

Manufactured in the United States of America

Designed by Mindy Basinger Hill

Typeset in Fresco Plus Pro

For permission to reproduce any of the material in this book,
contact Permissions, University Press of New England,
One Court Street, Suite 250, Lebanon NH 03766; or visit
www.upne.com

Library of Congress Cataloging-in-Publication Data

Names: Nagel, David, 1959– author.

Title: Needless suffering : how society fails those with
chronic pain / David Nagel, MD.

Description: Lebanon, NH : ForeEdge, an imprint of University
Press of New England, [2016] | Includes bibliographical references
and index.

Identifiers: LCCN 2015047540 (print) | LCCN 2016005187 (ebook) |
ISBN 9781611689624 (cloth) | ISBN 9781611688894 (pbk.) |
ISBN 9781611689631 (epub, mobi & pdf)

Subjects: LCSH: Chronic pain—Social aspects. |
Chronic pain—Health aspects.

Classification: LCC RB127 .N34 2016 (print) | LCC RB127 (ebook) |
DDC 616/.0472—dc23

LC record available at http://lccn.loc.gov/2015047540

5 4 3 2 1

This work is dedicated to the many

people who suffer from the ravages of chronic pain,

especially my mother, Florence Nagel,

and also to my father, Richard Nagel,

who was always there for her.

The lessons you have taught me have

enriched my life beyond words.

Thank you!

CONTENTS

FOREWORD

David Nagel is the physician all of us would yearn for to care for ourselves and our families if we were in unrelenting pain—smart, compassionate, tenacious, and funny. He also happens to be a whale of a storyteller who, by his own admission, has become a social activist. Thank goodness!

Needless Suffering: How Society Fails Those with Chronic Pain is a self-help book for society. From the get-go, Dr. Nagel's book grabs the reader with the story of Jane, her son, and himself. By talking about the struggles of patients he has served—Mr. Smith, Ray, Viola, and others—Dr. Nagel affirms the Institute of Medicine's call for "a cultural transformation in the way pain is perceived, judged, and treated."

Nagel is absolutely right—"pain management (in the us) is a travesty." However, with the body of literature on chronic pain that is emerging, including *Needless Suffering: How Society Fails Those with Chronic Pain*, and the resulting awareness of the American public, I believe change is inevitable. The status quo simply is no longer acceptable.

Myra Christopher

Kathleen M. Foley Chair | Director, pains | Center for Practical Bioethics
Kansas City, Missouri | September 10, 2015

ACKNOWLEDGMENTS

I would like to take this opportunity to thank all those who made this project possible.

I would like to begin by thanking Dr. Richard and Florence Nagel, my mom and dad. In addition to being wonderful parents, they also showed me how to live a dignified life despite pain and disability.

I would like to thank my wife, Mary, and my sons, Tommy and Andrew. Their never-ending support for all I do is inspirational. I also would like to thank Anjali Shah and her family, our extended family in Kolkata, India, who has made the example of Mother Teresa, and so many others who minister to the poorest of the poor, real for me.

I am indebted to all those who have mentored me throughout my personal and professional life; oftentimes the two were enmeshed. It would be challenging to name them all, but many are mentioned in the book. I am most indebted to my patients. In working together to help them overcome their barriers, I have learned much more than I ever could in a classroom. Those lessons have enriched all aspects of my life. Thank you!

I was honored to have attended medical school at the University of Rochester, the only medical school in the United States with a four-year curriculum dedicated to teaching doctor-patient communication, a skill invaluable in my work in pain management. I would like to thank all my mentors, patients, fellow students, and faculty alike, who have helped me become who I am. I would especially like to thank my special mentor, Dr. David Rosen. I learned so much from him. He taught me to use writing as a tool to deal with strong emotion. I took his advice, and I have been writing ever since. It was strong emotion that led me to start writing this book. Thank you, David!

This book, like many of the other stories I have written, began as an emotional catharsis intended for my eyes only. After I had completed what became the prologue and much of part 1, I shared it with Mary Ashcliffe, an author and a chronic pain sufferer. She told me that what I had written was too important not to be shared. She told me I was giving people like her a voice. Thank you, Mary, for the inspiration!

Writing is easy, getting published is not. I would like to thank the folks at the New Hampshire Writer's Project, especially Linda Chestney, for your guidance on that step of my journey. I would have been lost without your support. Linda referred me to Jeremy Townsend, who did a wonderful job with the first edit of the manuscript. Thanks, Jeremy!

With an edited version in hand and no clear direction, I fortuitously bumped into Dr. John Butterly. He asked me to send a summary of the book to him, which he shared with Phyllis Deutsch at University Press of New England. I would like to thank both of you for your support. What you have done means the world to me and so many others.

Phyllis referred me to Stephanie Golden to edit and prepare the final manuscript. Stephanie did a wonderful job, and I will greatly miss our weekly, sometimes daily e-mails, which helped keep me concise and focused, two skills I am lacking. I am forever indebted to her.

I would like to thank my friends Pat D'Ambrosio, Gail Petterson, and Cindy Steinberg for reviewing the manuscript. I would especially like to thank Myra Christopher, the director of the Pain Action Alliance to Implement a National Strategy (PAINS), for her friendship and support. Throughout this project, I felt like a meek voice crying out in the wilderness on behalf of the patients with whom I work. Myra truly believes that all voices, big and small, have value and should be listened to. Thank you, Myra, for reviewing my work, listening to me, and supporting me!

NEEDLESS SUFFERING

The Forest for the Trees

Love the poor. Do you know the poor of your place, of your city?
Find them. Maybe they are right in your own family.

Mother Teresa, *Love: The Words and Inspiration of Mother Teresa*

It was a morning in fall 2003, a typical day in the office. There was more to do than time allowed. Still, I did my best to keep up with the demands of my comprehensive pain management practice. I offered soup-to-nuts care for as many pain patients as I could see. I had long since stopped taking on new patients. In a world where so many suffer, sometimes needlessly, I had learned that I am only one person and I could only do what I could do. My goal was to do the best I could for the person in the room with me.

While most would consider my job stressful, I found joy in doing it. One of my role models is Mother Teresa, who found satisfaction in ministering to the "poorest of the poor," those abandoned by most of society. I see parallels between the poor and those in chronic pain, and I have worked hard medically in my clinic, and also socially at the local, state, and sometimes national levels, to help raise awareness of the plight of these individuals—the "poorest of the poor" of the medical world.

It seems ironic that in a profession where we strive to keep people alive, death is a constant companion, often just around the corner. In my years as a physician, I've come to feel that life is a gift, a temporary one. It is our job to do the best with the gift we are fortunate enough to be given. Death is inevitable. The only aspect of death I feared was the possibility that I might someday be responsible for causing the death of another, a very real possibility in medicine. That particular day, I marveled at having been able to do my work solo for over fifteen years. Others had told me there would be days when bad things would happen. So far I had been fortunate—nothing really bad had ever happened to any of my patients, and I was very proud of that record. But on that typical day, something did happen, which changed everything for me.

As I drove to work, I tuned in to the local news on the radio and heard that a twenty-eight-year-old male had succumbed to an accidental overdose the night before. His name was not familiar to me. Shortly after arriving at work, I received a message that a longtime patient needed to see me right away. She wouldn't give my secretary a reason, only insisted it was urgent. Given the stress of the day, I was reluctant to oblige. Jane (not her actual name) suffered valiantly from a very difficult pain syndrome. While many would resort to large doses to treat the problem she faced, she relied on a minimum of pain medication. Her life had been in as much order as it could be until the insurance company changed its posture toward her.

Long before I met her, Jane suffered from a complicated spine problem, a herniated (ruptured) disc in her low back. Three operations failed to resolve the problem, and she developed a condition called reflex sympathetic dystrophy, which did not respond to therapies. She complained of a burning pain in her leg and severe pain in her back. She refused a fourth operation, a fusion to stabilize her back, and did her best to live with her pain.

When things seemed to be going as well as could be expected, she reherniated and developed weakness in her legs and urinary incontinence (a condition known as *cauda equina* syndrome). She so feared another operation that she kept her symptoms to herself, only reluctantly informing me of them several weeks later. An MRI confirmed the new disc herniation, which substantially narrowed her spinal canal. I told her she really needed to see a surgeon, but she wished to see how the "tincture of time" worked. She was lucky. She regained bladder function, and her legs got stronger. However, her pain increased substantially, and her ability to walk decreased. To help her get around, I requested that her insurance company provide her a motorized scooter. The company assigned a rehabilitation nurse to verify the need for this device. It was not clear what this individual's agenda was, but she launched an investigation that changed Jane's life.

With virtually no compassion, the nurse questioned every service we provided for Jane. She hired private investigators to follow her every move. They found little, but what little they found, they embellished. Jane became quite aware that she was being followed, and she lived in fear. Without the insurance, she could not afford what little support she was receiving. Though I advised her to stay as active as she could, she became a recluse, fearing that anything she did would be misinterpreted. The insurance company challenged her disability; and she was called before the state labor board, where the private investigator showed a short video of her mowing the lawn on a riding mower. What had been a half-hour outlet for my patient became an albatross. The insurance company used the video to claim Jane was faking her injuries and could do much more than she claimed. Despite the facts, which verified her complaints, the insurance company still refused to accept her symptoms and her limitations as "real."

I was livid and wrote letter after letter angrily supporting my patient. To counter, the insurance company hired a well-respected expert who, while lauding my efforts, stated that I had lost my objectivity, and was "mired in the woods, seeing only the forest from [sic] the trees." He also stated that Jane was addicted to the six Percocet she took each day, a stable dose that she had not changed in years. His impressions were derived merely from a chart review. He did take the time to chat with me on the phone, but he never met with me or my patient.

The day of the labor board hearing eventually arrived. While I hoped to help Jane, I also saw this as a pivotal moment. If the insurance company won, I feared that pain management specialists and their patients would lose everything we had worked for in achieving acceptance of compassionate prescription of opiates for all pain patients in New Hampshire who needed them.

In the hearing, Jane's attorney patiently addressed all the issues. What fascinated me was that my comments attracted attention not only from the three members of the panel, but also from the opposing counsel, who took me aside after the hearing and shared a number of personal stories of friends in pain and the lack of care they received. He asked me questions about how they could receive adequate care. I left satisfied, feeling I had done my job.

Several weeks later, we found that Jane had won her case. Although I was convinced we had won a major victory for the pain community, Jane herself was not a winner. The insurance company's failure to listen to her, believe her, and treat her compassionately had a lasting effect. A pain syndrome that had been easy to control became impossible. She required repeated hospital admissions in a vain effort to control her pain. Pain was not her problem—fear was. She suffered from a very real posttraumatic stress disorder and became afraid of modern medicine. She feared repercussions from the insurance company and the legal system if she did any of the things that made life worthwhile, worrying that someone might be watching. In effect, she had lost her life. The medications did little to quell her growing pain and anxiety. Having to wait ninety days for the labor board decision did not help. Even after she heard the good news, her pain was not relieved. Never again could we control it.

I lost too. I lost faith in our system, a faith I still have not regained.

Now, several years later, she was begging to see me. Quite distraught, she told me she had come to warn me. That morning, she had found her son dead. He was the person I had heard about on the radio. He had been out partying the night before, and apparently had taken a cocktail of drugs, possibly including some of Jane's medications. The police had cleared the family from the house and searched it. They found all her medicines. She asked for them to be returned but was told they were "evidence," and the investigating officer informed her that they were going to take a long hard look at me.

Several weeks later, a sheriff arrived at our office representing the medical board, with subpoenas for the medical records of several of my patients. This development shattered my sense of immunity, my shield, and I was laid bare. Someone I had never met was dead, and someone else was blaming me. That is a terrible cross to bear. While I took consolation in the facts that I was a founding member of the New Hampshire State Pain Management Task Force, had served on two state boards overseeing physical therapists and occupational therapists, and had a very good reputation in the community, I still realized that my life, my career, and everything I had worked so hard to attain was now in the hands of others. At the same time, I struggled to keep things in their proper perspective and grieve the unnecessary loss of a young life.

My practice manager notified our attorney, who immediately made things worse by suggesting we consult a criminal attorney to see if I was at any risk for criminal prosecution. As I saw it, my only crime was to do my best to relieve Jane's suffering. The thought that someone would even consider charging me with a crime was unbearable. Fortunately, the lawyers quickly concluded it was unlikely that I would be charged, but the damage to my psyche was done.

It took a full year for the medical board to render a decision favorable to me. The wait was torture, compounded every few months when another sheriff arrived with yet another subpoena requesting yet another chart. I learned of physicians in other states who had endured similar trials. I heard of two who were arrested—one set up by a sting operation, convicted of drug dealing, and sentenced to jail. As I reviewed their stories, it seemed obvious that the only thing they were guilty of was caring too much, enough to be vulnerable to the indiscretions of others. I heard of friends in the pain community who also had been investigated.

I went into medicine because I wanted to make a difference in other people's lives. I never saw myself as a social activist, but I suddenly realized that was what I had become. I had come to see pain management in America as the travesty it was, and I longed to change that, to bring attention to the plight of my patients.

I suddenly began to live in fear. I feared for my family. What if I were arrested, tried, and found guilty? What would happen to my patients if I were sent to jail? Although my attorney told me this would not happen, I still did not feel safe. Every time I saw a police car or heard the doorbell ring, I feared they were coming for me.

I began to fear my patients even as I feared for them. To the police, I was not a compassionate doctor; I had become a "prescriber." For the first time in years, I feared that one of my patients would accuse me of leading him astray, and began to question whether, in prescribing opiates, I was really doing the right thing for them. I analyzed the trials and tribulations of the great social activists. Knowing that they suffered and questioned their own actions as I was questioning mine, I realized that we grow from introspection. Still, I wondered if my passion for helping my patients warranted the potential punishment I saw looming. I wondered if it was fair for my family to suffer the repercussions of my crusade. I recalled a newspaper photo of a child of one of the convicted doctors, crying as her father was led off to prison. In my mind, I saw that child as my own.

In order to bolster our position, my attorney proposed that we get a supportive opinion from an expert. Over the course of Jane's treatment, I had already obtained several supportive second opinions, but he felt we needed one from a disinterested party. We searched for such a person, and based on the recommendations of a friend, we contacted someone who agreed to review the voluminous chart.

Again, this expert never met me or my patient, nor did he make any attempt to do so, something I consider an egregious error. He made no comment on my management of the patient, but said that he would not endorse my care of her because he felt I had lost my objectivity and was, again, not seeing the forest "from" the trees. It was no coincidence that he used the same incorrect phrase that the independent evaluator had used, since we had given him that report to review. He went a step further and said that I saw myself as a "hero, on a campaign to serve the interests of my patients, not amenable to the suggestions of others."

To the second charge, I plead "not guilty." When I questioned my actions, which I frequently did, I sought the advice of others.

To the charge of not seeing the forest for the trees, I do plead guilty and offer no apologies. As a medical student, I was taught to value the thoughts and concerns of the patient. Dr. Robert Joynt taught me to "listen to your patients, they might be trying to tell you something." Dr. Henry Herrara taught me that each patient is an individual, and we need to learn to appreciate each one for his or her uniqueness. I contend that to have the courage to listen to the patient, you have to enter into the forest; you cannot appreciate the individuality of each patient from the outside. You do risk losing objectivity by doing so, but it is a risk that must be taken.

Entering into the forest generates strong feelings. Dr. George Engel taught me that a doctor can examine those feelings and use them diagnostically to better understand the patient and himself. He taught me that my feelings are a very important piece of data, which must be studied and understood. To do this, I must venture into the forest and summon the courage to talk to the patient, listen, and accept his or her individuality. The physician must be aware that preconceived notions can be erroneous, dangerous, and sometimes harmful. When you stare at the trees from the outside, you inevitably rely on those preconceived notions, and that is more problematic than venturing inside. Unfortunately, that is how many doctors usually approach the pain patient.

I have spent the past twenty-eight years studying pain from every perspective possible. I have sought counsel from as many sages as I could. Some advice I valued and some I discounted, but I always felt the "house of pain management" had many rooms and a place for everyone. An individual physician, if he or she tries, can learn something from everyone. There is no greater source of wisdom, however, than the patient.

My travels into the forest of the pain patient have created an uncomfortable cynicism within me. I have come to appreciate that the way the pain patient is treated is not just a medical issue. The treatment of any disability is a bio-psycho-social phenomenon that involves every aspect of our society.

I have also come to understand how society feels about the pain patient, best summed up in an episode of the *Brady Bunch*. Marcia, shortly after learning how to drive, rear-ends another driver. The driver sues her and appears in court with a cane, a collar, and a pitiful look—a societal stereotype of the pain patient as a fraud who embellishes his symptoms for personal gain or as a slacker who uses pain to avoid the responsibilities of life. It is amazing how this stereotype changes when we are the ones in pain. Too often I hear the words: "I never believed anyone's pain until it happened to me"—including from the mouths of two law enforcement officers and an insurance adjustor.

This book is about a social problem: undertreated pain in America and its social causes and ramifications. It is written from two perspectives: it takes a step back "out of the forest" in order to examine how our society manages the problem of pain in America, while also offering the view from inside the forest and the pain patient's individual experience. My goal is to change the way people and society perceive and treat those who suffer from chronic pain.

Therefore, this book is not merely a critique of how health-care providers address these issues. It is a critique of society as a whole.

What are the unintended effects of well-intentioned health-care reforms on those who suffer?

How do the bottom-line mentality in medicine, the legal system, insurance companies, and business harm pain patients unnecessarily?

How do the use of computer medical records and practitioner productivity incentives adversely affect doctor-patient communication?

How does the intellectual dishonesty of health-care providers harm pain patients?

How do our system of entitlements and the structure of our labor force conspire to keep pain patients from being as productive as they can be?

In addition to pointing out problems, for each one I offer specific, practical policy recommendations.

This book is for chronic pain patients, family members, health-care providers, businessmen and women, attorneys, insurance company representatives, and the public at large. We all can learn a lot from each other, and each of us has an important role to play in minimizing the needless suffering of those in pain.

What I say here is based on my twenty-eight-year experience as a pain specialist. My current specialty is chronic spine pain management. Thus many examples I provide are spine related. However, throughout my career I have managed pain along its entire continuum, and I grew up in a home where pain was no stranger. My examples generalize well to other types of pain.

I intend this book to be provocative. I do not expect the reader to agree with everything I say, and I will be disappointed if that proves to be the case. I do hope to make the reader think, though; to think about a costly problem that is too often ignored and creates too much needless suffering.

Throughout I cite scriptural and other philosophical writings. While I am a practicing Roman Catholic, I see value in all inspired writings, no matter the faith. I am most inspired by Mother Teresa. My family has been fortunate enough to support a family in Kolkata, India, that was touched directly by Mother Teresa. In visiting them, I have come to appreciate Mother's actions and see how one person, armed only with faith, through her ministrations to the poorest of the poor can change a whole city, a whole country, and the whole world. I long to be merely a shadow of the person she was.

Finally, I frequently refer to the Golden Rule first taught me by my mother: "Do unto others as you would have them do unto you." In various forms, this credo is shared by all major religions and all cultures. It is the basis for most professional codes of ethics. This book explores the gap between what we say we will do for those in need and what we actually do—myself included—because of ignorance, laziness, and greed. I hope to challenge all of us to do better, not for ourselves, but for those who suffer.

PART ONE

Poor Man, Pained Man

The biggest disease today is not leprosy or tuberculosis (or pain), but rather the feeling of being unwanted, uncared for, and deserted by everybody. The greatest evil is the lack of love and charity, the terrible indifference toward one's neighbor.

Mother Teresa, *Love: The Words and Inspirations of Mother Teresa*

According to a report from the Institute of Medicine, *Relieving Pain in America: A Blueprint for Transforming Prevention, Care, Education, and Research,* published in 2011,[1] one hundred million people in the United States suffer from chronic pain. Some are calling this a public health crisis, which it is; however, that is not the biggest problem that intractable pain poses. The real problem is that most of us are unaware the problem exists at all. If we are aware, too often we trivialize it. Even those burdened with pain are often unaware. Too many are convinced they are the only ones, and so they suffer in isolation. That is the problem.

It would be easy for me to condemn others for failing to appreciate this crisis. That would be hypocritical for me to do, for in the not-too-distant past, I too was ignorant. That seems so strange for a doctor and the son of someone suffering from chronic pain to say, but it is true; therefore, I will hold my judgment. However, as if guided by fate or destiny or my mother, I came to understand the problem chronic pain creates for all of us. This transformation did not occur overnight, but by trial and error over several years. In this section, I would like to share the process of my transformation with you. In doing so, I will share what I have learned about pain from a biological, psychological, and social perspective. In doing so, I hope I can help begin to transform your thoughts as well.

ONE

A Young Doctor Transformed
by a Man in Pain

Pain is the most terrible of all the lords of mankind.
Albert Schweitzer, *On the Edge of the Primeval Forest*

The year was 1986. I was a resident in physical medicine and re-habilitation and had been asked to see a man who had recently had back surgery.

"Have fun," my colleagues joked. "Nothing like wasting time on a chronic painer!" Those back patients were all the same, weren't they? Just lazy people looking for a ticket out of their responsibilities. X-rays all negative. No "objective" explanation for their pain. If they only got off their butts and lost some weight, they would be fine. Why did they have to waste my time? I had more important things to do than treat people who weren't going to get better no matter what I did. All they wanted were drugs. At least, that's what my professor said.

I hardly thought that my encounter with Mr. Smith would change my life.

The Veteran's Administration hospital where I was training was very large, and it was a long walk to this man's room. I purposely made the walk longer, for I dreaded what was at the end of it. But eventually, I arrived at his room and reluctantly entered. It was one of the old VA four-bed rooms with flimsy yellow curtains separating the beds. I looked for bed "B," saw the patient, "Mr. Smith," and watched him for several moments.

Mr. Smith lay uncomfortably in his bed. Every few minutes he shifted in agony. Then he was still, the grimace on his face replaced by a look of fear. What did he fear, I wondered? Several minutes later, the agony reappeared; his face contorted in a manner only pain can produce.

At first, I was suckered into this performance. Who could fake such an act? But the doctors who had operated on him told me nothing was wrong, and it was my job to get him off his butt and out of the hospital.

They couldn't be wrong, could they? I didn't know it, but I was caught in a battle. Whom should I believe, patient or doctor?

I sat down next to the man, coldly introduced myself, and dutifully began to take a history. "Hello, Mr. Smith. I am Dr. Nagel, and I am here to help get you back on your feet," I said with no enthusiasm. Mr. Smith showed little acknowledgment of me. He continued to alternate between expressions of fear and agony. But as we talked, his story unfolded.

Mr. Smith was forty-seven. He had been born in the same city and with the same hopes as me, maybe even at the same hospital. His parents didn't have a lot of money, so he had to work after school. Up at 5:00 AM to do homework, off to school, then to work, and back home by 10:00 PM five days a week. He worked on Saturdays too. His job was physical, and pain was a part of his life. School didn't offer him much, so he left to work full-time. When he turned eighteen, he joined the army. He served in Korea and returned with medals. He was a hero, but he didn't have time to relish his accomplishments. Medals look good on shelves, but they don't pay the bills.

He returned to work. The best jobs were at the steel plants. They were physically demanding, but the pay was good. At twenty, he was a war veteran and a work veteran. At twenty-one he had his first back injury. He ignored it. Pain was part of life, and a hard worker had back pain. It was a medal, an award for his labors. Over the years, though, the pain increased. At first, it was just in his back. Then it started to go down his leg. First it was just a little numbness, but then an electrical fire shot through him that tore at his soul.

He had never been to a doctor in his life. "Pain is part of life," he kept telling himself, but over time he believed this less and less. He decided his pain was one medal he wanted to send back. Disabled by pain at twenty-five, he wanted to see if the doctors could help him.

The doctor he saw was very supportive. After an examination and tests, he told Mr. Smith he had a "ruptured disc." All he needed was a simple operation, and he'd be back to his old self in no time. He was told he had a 99 percent chance of being cured. Mr. Smith thought those were pretty good odds. He told his boss he needed an operation, and he'd be back soon.

One of Mr. Smith's buddies drove him to the hospital. Back then, the early 1970s, patients typically stayed in the hospital for a few weeks after such an operation. As he limped slowly in, he wasn't scared. The words "99 percent chance" rang in his ears.

A nurse showed Mr. Smith to his room, handed him a roll of cloth that she informed him was his "ensemble" for the next few weeks, instructed him to change his clothes, and then announced the schedule for the next few days. Blood tests, EKG, meals, and so on. She handed him a menu card and left.

On the day of the surgery, as two orderlies rolled him to the operating room on a gurney, he kept telling himself, "Ninety-nine percent . . ."

He awoke several hours later. He was not better. His pain was horrible, much worse than anything he had ever had before. It seared down his leg like a hot burning poker. Before the surgery it had let up sometimes; now it didn't. He begged the nurse for help, but she told him it wasn't time for his pain medication. As she left the room, he did something he had never done before. He cried.

His doctor reassured him that his pain was normal and would get better, but with each passing day, that prophecy failed to materialize. Each day, the doctor spent less time in the room, and stood farther and farther away, afraid to confront his failure.

Two weeks passed, two weeks of agony. The surgeon entered the room and announced it was time for Mr. Smith to go home.

"I cannot go home like this!" Mr. Smith cried. "I can't walk or take care of myself, or go to work. What am I to do?"

"I am sorry, Mr. Smith," the surgeon said. "The surgery was a success. There must be some problem with you. I have someone I would like you to see. You will be leaving us tomorrow. I will see you in my office in two months. Good-bye."

The surgeon turned and left before Mr. Smith could respond. The nurse handed him an appointment card that said: Dr. Wilfred Kröninger, Practice of Psychiatry. Mr. Smith started to doubt himself. The surgery was a success. This doctor feels it is all in my head. Is it? What is the matter with me? I will overcome this.

He tried to pretend there was no pain, but with each movement came that terrible burning that told him otherwise. He felt lost and, much worse, dependent. As he left the hospital, he greeted the self he had left behind three weeks before. The difference was that he had walked calmly into the hospital. Now he limped out, a beaten man. He had lost his confidence. The doctor himself had told him all this was in his head. Why couldn't he control this pain? He looked at the prescriptions he had been given. None were for pain.

Over the next several weeks, Mr. Smith struggled to convince himself he had no pain. He saw Dr. Kröninger, who examined every crevice of his psyche. After several weeks, Mr. Smith was told that his whole problem was some internal conflict over the way his mother had treated him at an early age. If he could give up that conflict, he could give up his pain.

That was too much for Mr. Smith. He stormed out of the room and returned to his apartment. Now what to do? He was convinced that there was someone, somewhere, who could help him. The problem was that there was no clear guidance to help him find that person. Over the next twenty years, he searched for that person in doctor after doctor. He couldn't accept a life like this. He wanted his old life back.

Over that time, he had three more operations, saw dozens of therapists, and took all sorts of medications. At times, he grew despondent, and the pain got the best of him. At such times, he drank. The whiskey calmed the pain, and he could walk more comfortably. The problem was that he was sick without it.

He never worked again. He tried, but he couldn't last more than a few days at a job before the pain got the best of him. Some employers shooed him out the door. Others compassionately offered him a couch or whatever they could and tried to find something he could do. He wanted to work more than anything, and they wanted to help him; but they had a business to run, and eventually they gave up on him too.

His family grew estranged from him. He had never married. His brothers and sisters tired of seeing him in pain. At times they blamed him: "If you only had done this or that, you wouldn't have pain," they seemed to say, as if blaming him eased their discomfort. Like the surgeon, they couldn't handle seeing him in pain. Being with him was more agony than they could bear. They didn't need to take a pill to get rid of this agony. All they had to do was run to the safety of their own homes.

Mr. Smith was left to suffer on his own, a broken man. Somehow, though, he held out a hope that the future would be better. God wouldn't leave him like this. He prayed each and every night. That hope alone kept him on the side of existence. But it really wasn't life, because what he lived was based totally on the future. There was no present, and life is the present. He was, in fact, dead and awaiting rebirth.

It was at this point that I met Mr. Smith. He had just had his fifth operation. The previous four had destroyed his spine by leaving it unstable. One vertebra had slid half its width to the side of the vertebra below. His whole lumbar spine was curved to the side at a grotesque angle. He had seen a surgeon at our hospital who announced that he would fix the problem. Put a little metal here and there, slide this bone here or there, fix it all with a few screws, and he would be fine.

The surgery hadn't worked. If Mr. Smith had pain before, he had no idea what to call what he was experiencing now. The burning was constant. No position relieved it. He truly was in hell.

The surgeon had given him Percocet: one to two pills every four hours for pain as needed. When he took one, he was still in agony; but when he took two, he could move. The pain, although still there, was tolerable. That was the first relief he had felt in over twenty years. He became addicted, not to pain medicine, but rather to *pain relief.* He longed for it. As the weeks passed, though, the nurses and surgeons became more reluctant to provide the medicine, the first thing that had ever helped him.

One day, one of the surgeons announced to Mr. Smith that he was addicted to the medication, and "for his own good," it must be stopped. Mr. Smith begged them not to. He had escaped the vortex that had drawn him into hell and now they were threatening to throw him back.

The surgeons backed off, but only for a time. They decided to prove he was addicted and didn't need the medicine by administering a placebo. They congratulated themselves when the patient did not immediately report an increase in pain. They actually did not know that the previous dose still needed an hour or two more to filter out of his system. While the surgeons celebrated the apparent success of their ruse, the level of medicine in Mr. Smith's system continued to decline, and his pain began to return. He called the nurse and told her he needed something for it. She told him he wasn't due. Two hours later, he was given another dose of placebo. By now the pain was intolerable, and he was back in the vortex.

Listening to this saga, I stared at Mr. Smith. My head was about to explode. His story threatened everything my sages had taught me. I had the power to help this man. I longed to simply write the order and relieve his suffering. And mine. Yet in the back of my mind, I could hear my teachers telling me not to do it.

"Don't open Pandora's box. He will only want more, and he will become a burden to his doctors, forever addicted to medicine, powerless to come off it."

I thought about that. Then I wondered, isn't the hypertensive patient equally addicted to blood pressure medication? Isn't the depressed patient "addicted" to antidepressants? Isn't the infected patient addicted to antibiotics? I thought of all the medicines my mother took for her rheumatoid arthritis: antiinflammatories, Cytoxan, methotrexate, prednisone—all much more toxic than the pain medication that would ease this man's suffering.

"You'll only hide the pain," the sages said.

Maybe so, but what purpose was this man's pain serving? Pain is a signal the body uses to tell us something is wrong and encourage us to do something about it. Pain shouldn't be a means of interminably taunting us, destroying us, tearing us apart. This man's pain was not serving any useful purpose, yet it couldn't be ignored. Fire, too, serves a useful purpose. However, like the fire that burns out of control, this pain needed to be extinguished.

My head throbbed from the mental effort. I looked into Mr. Smith's eyes. I could see the suffering. I could see the sincerity. With a strength born of anger at the actions of those who would ignore this man's plight, I did something I never had done in my life. I questioned my sages and then defied them.

"Mr. Smith, your surgeons have given you a placebo and that is why your pain is returning. While they needed to know whether your pain was real, it quite clearly is, and we are going to do something about it. What dose worked best for you?" I asked him calmly. I put my hand gently on his shoulder and said: "I won't let you suffer."

I could see conflicting emotions arise in him. His eyes flared with anger when he learned of the placebo. He was incredulous that anyone could willingly do something so callous to a person who was suffering so. Yet as I told him what I was going to do, his eyes softened and showed both hope and relief.

I left his room, went to the nurse's station, and found his chart. With a firmness born of conviction, I took the chart, and wrote the order: *Percocet po 2 tabs q 4° around the clock.*

A nurse came over and touched me on the shoulder.

"Thank you, Doctor. We couldn't handle his suffering anymore."

I was surprised to find the nurses felt the same way I did. I collapsed into a chair, exhausted from the mental effort and the experience of being in the presence of such suffering.

As it turned out, I was not alone, nor was Mr. Smith. This happened in 1986. I didn't know it, but other doctors around the country were doing the same thing I did that day.

I returned the next day to see Mr. Smith. His look of agony was replaced by a smile. His movements, his attitudes were totally different. He got up and walked to the bathroom. He sat on the toilet. He stood up. He did all those little things that we take for granted but that he hadn't been able to do in several years.

As I left his room, I felt real satisfaction. I had given hope to the hopeless. I had opened his tunnel to the light of day. He could live in the present. He was truly reborn. Then my euphoria was broken by a loud, deep voice behind me.

"Dr. Nagel?"

I turned to see six doctors approaching, the head surgeon in front with residents and interns ranged neatly behind him.

"Yes?" I answered.

"We noticed that you have put Mr. Smith back on pain medication," the head surgeon said.

"Yes, I have," I replied, struggling to keep my voice from trembling.

"Are you aware that you are addicting this gentleman to medication?" he replied, bringing "medication" to a crescendo.

Surprisingly, my fear was replaced by an anger that I had never felt before. I had always been the one to back down from confrontation in the past. But now I had no urge to run. I stood my ground, longing to hurl these doctors into the vortex they had put Mr. Smith into.

"I am not sure what you are talking about," I said.

"Percocet, sir," he replied firmly. "Doctor, you are condemning this man to a life of drugs."

I was incensed. I remembered every karate movie I had ever seen. The minute you lose your composure your opponent has beaten you. I somehow found a way to regain mine.

"Doctor," I said, "I clearly remember seeing this man unable to move before I started the medication. It is my job to get people back on their feet and back into life. It seems that my treatment is accomplishing that. Perhaps our goals are conflicting. However, since I am now his primary physician, I will continue to prescribe until I see that the medicine is doing him harm."

The surgeon stood speechless. "I will talk to your attending about this," he replied with the same whine children use to shout, "I'm going to tell your mother on you!"

I took care of Mr. Smith for the next three months. The surgeons never returned, and my attending physician (who supervised me) never said anything. Mr. Smith gradually improved and left the hospital. I don't know what happened to him after that. I have always wondered. Short-term successes do not always lead to long-term ones. On that day, though, I learned to think for myself. I learned to look into my patient's eyes. I learned to stand up for what I thought was right, no matter what the sages said. I learned to trust my instincts, and I learned to trust the patient. Patients truly are the experts. They know what they are feeling and struggle to communicate their feelings to us.

Perhaps it is we doctors who are disabled. Although we parade around in our white coats with our "sheepskins" stuck on our walls, we really are ignorant. We cannot feel what our patients are feeling. We struggle to take the pegs they give us and stuff them into the holes that represent our theories. Sometimes the peg fits, sometimes it doesn't. If it doesn't, perhaps it makes more sense to reshape the hole than it does to keep trying vainly to stuff the patient's story into our preconceived notions.

We have all seen poor men who walk the street in search of an opportunity. Hope. Holding a sign: "Will work for food." Person after person walks by, staring at anything, everything except that sign.

Mr. Smith also held a sign. He held it up to his doctors, but they walked by, staring at anything and everything except that sign. Mr. Smith went from doctor to doctor—"doctor shopping," as it's called, and considered a certain sign of psychological distress. Maybe it was a sign of common sense—a sign that he was looking for someone to give him a chance.

A Doctor's Education in Pain

> I have always held firmly to the thought that each one of us can
> do a little to bring some portion of misery to an end.
> Albert Schweitzer, *Out of My Life and Thought*

I grew up going to Catholic schools, where the nuns taught me to clothe
the naked, feed the hungry, heal the sick, give hope to the hopeless . . . to
love others as ourselves.

"Where are the naked? Where are the hungry? Where are the hopeless?
Where are the sick?" I recall asking.

My teachers answered: "They are all around us. Whatsoever you do to
the least of these, that you do unto Jesus."

I longed to do what I was taught. I longed to use the gifts I had been
given and be the best I could be. In school, I wasn't the smartest, or the
most athletic, or the most artistic. But I was the Outstanding Senior Boy.
I remember being happy when I was told that this was because of how I
treated others.

When it was time to find a career, I wanted to find one in which I could
do what the nuns had admonished. After much reflection, I chose rehabilitation medicine, the home of the poorest of the poor of the medical world.

My education was hard. Much of it did not occur in the classroom. One
summer, I asked to work with the dying in a cancer hospital. There I learned
to laugh with, to touch, and to hold those in pain. When I did so, I noticed
that their pain and their loneliness left, if only for a moment. In the short
time I was there, I said hello, and good-bye, to many new friends. When
they left, I wondered what place they went to.

Dolores, who was stricken with breast cancer, became one of my best
friends. One day, she lay gasping for breath. She knew her end was near.
She looked up at me and said: "My whole life I wished for big breasts. All
of a sudden, I had one. At first, I was proud. Then the ulcer appeared [when
her breast cancer erupted through her skin], and I realized why my breast
was so big. I wonder why God did that to me."

I remember smiling at her, as a façade for the tears I struggled to hold
back. The next day, she was gone. The surgeon feared by most residents
took me aside and said, "The ability to help people die is a gift. Nurture
that gift." The rest of that summer, he made sure I was assigned to all the

terminal patients. I relished this role. I did not realize my big test was to come soon.

Two days before my third year of medical school was to start, my mother woke me suddenly.

"Get up, David," she cried. "Your father needs you in Kenny's room."

My brother Kenny had been a diabetic since he was four years old. Despite his disease, he was full of life. He was about to start college the next day. Wondering what my father needed, I ran to Kenny's room and found his lifeless body and my father engaged in a futile attempt to perform CPR. There was no response. Kenny was cold. My father slowly accepted the hell that fate had bestowed. He walked out of the room and to the kitchen where my mother sat, waiting. Then I heard the screams, screams that echo in my head to this day.

Many people attended the funeral. Person after person shared kind reflections of Kenny with the family. It is so unfortunate that we need death to make us realize the treasures we possess. Two days later, I was back in medical school. I was in a daze. "Life goes on," my father said.

Two months later, the head of the internal medicine department called the young students together. He told us that Ed, a friend and fellow third-year student, had been found dead in his car. He had committed suicide.

I saw death everywhere. I needed to get away. I drove to the snowy mountains, where I pitched my tent, lit a fire, and drank hot bourbon and cider to my heart's content. Two weeks after Ed's death, I returned to school and threw myself into my work. My heart was not in it. Still, the attending physicians were amazed by my diligence. One said that I was one of the best medical students he had ever had. But when we got our grades, I had a B-. When I asked for an explanation, the course director showed me my teachers' comments. All but one had given me Honors, the highest grade.

"I don't understand," I said angrily.

"Did you really need that week off?" he asked.

Lesson learned. Do your best. Accept your limitations. Take care of yourself. Let the chips fall where they may. You cannot always control others' judgments of you.

In my fourth year of medical school I met a new friend. A beautiful smile. A pretty face. A wonderful relationship. We did everything together. Fourth year over, she went to Boston, I to Hanover. Despite the distance, we still did everything together. She called every day. Soon I had placed a ring on her finger. We needed to make plans; Christmas was approaching. Her calls came less frequently. Suddenly there were none. I had an ICU rotation, 130 hours per week. Where was she? What was she doing? I tried calling, but there was no answer. What was going on? On my day off, I drove to Boston and walked into her apartment. There I found the answer, in her bed and in her arms.

A knife had been thrust into my heart. Life goes on. Does it? I longed to go back to the mountains to get a rest.

"Sorry, we are short-staffed. We need you here."

My life became a blur. I couldn't go to Boston; I couldn't go home. It all became too much and culminated in a trip to the emergency room. I was given two months off, put under a psychiatrist's care, and given medications. But they didn't work any better than hot bourbon and cider. I couldn't go back and couldn't go forward. I was stuck. Suddenly I understood despair, because I felt it. My scientific mind began to analyze it. I saw myself in an abyss, a crevasse. Slowly, with the help of many, I climbed out into the bright sunshine.

Back at my internship, Rosie, one of the nurses, looked at me: "Glad to have you back. We missed you!"

As the surgeon had done, she found the hopeless patients and gave them to me. One was Ray. Ray's face was disfigured by cancer, his lungs by smoking, and his hip by too much use. His only wish was to fish. His face and his lungs didn't stop him from fishing, but his hip did. His life was over, or so he thought. I looked into Ray's face as if into a mirror. I saw despair. We talked and hit it off. A smile came to Ray's face for the first time in months.

Two months later, I was called to see a patient who didn't seem to be responding to anything.

"Why do they want me?" I wondered. "I'm only an intern!"

I ran to the fifth floor, and when I arrived, I saw Ray.

"He's in a coma," they said. "We don't know why. His niece thought you might be able to help. All his blood tests are normal. His head CT was fine. We are clueless."

I walked slowly to Ray's bed, grabbed his hand, and looked into his eyes. I saw a spark. I felt a bond. I knew where Ray was. I had just been there. Stuck. Can't go back. Can't go forward.

"How ya feelin,' Ray?" I asked.

"Like shit," Ray answered, clearly and deliberately.

Lazarus had arisen. Ray wasn't comatose. He didn't want to die. He just didn't know how to live. He said his hip was killing him and he was worthless. The doctors said his heart wasn't good enough for a hip operation. I told Ray I had some ideas. Only two months before I had crawled out of the same abyss that Ray was in. I thought I could help him get out.

I started Ray on an antidepressant and got him an orthopedic and cardiology consult. They agreed to operate if Ray could get his energy back. Slowly Ray improved. Soon the surgery was scheduled. Ray was ready. He saw the fishing boat getting closer and closer.

A few weeks after his surgery, I was called again to the fifth floor. Ray was back in. I went to his room. Ray didn't move. This time I didn't see life in those eyes. I knew Ray was gone. You can call it starvation or coma or whatever. All I knew was that the spark was gone.

The resident said that his blood tests were all screwed up. Ray wasn't eating. I looked at Ray's meds.

"Where is the antidepressant!" I shouted.

"The cardiologists stopped it because his QT interval had widened," came the reply.

Tears of anger came to my eyes. "That medicine gave him his life back!"

Too late. Ray was dead . . . but he had his new hip.

Ray was gone, but I got the message. You cannot fully understand what a person is feeling unless you have been there. To give hope to the hopeless, you need to have been hopeless. To help someone climb a mountain, you must have climbed it yourself. Armed with those lessons, I realized for the first time that I truly could give hope to the hopeless. Were my experiences gifts from God? I think so.

My mom had an infectious smile. Everyone said so. It was fortunate, because the smile hid her deformed joints. Every major joint in her body had been operated on. She had taken every poison the doctors had given her to try to stem her disease, rheumatoid arthritis. She was diagnosed in her twenties. By her seventies, she suffered as much from all the treatments as from the disease. Every small chore was an event. Dressing, walking, bathing—never mind driving.

Her smile distracted me from thinking about her disability. I grew up thinking she was like everybody else. When I became a doctor, I realized she wasn't. She was better than everyone else. She smiled through her pain in a way nobody else could. She tried to do everything on her own and cried alone, hiding the tears from others as if she didn't want them to feel what she was feeling. Most doctors treated her well. Some didn't. To them she wasn't a whole person, but just the hip in room fifty-five. She overwhelmed them. They didn't have time for all the problems she presented them with.

One year, her pain changed. The antiinflammatories didn't work. The pain burned down her leg. Her doctor thought it was her arthritis and tried medicine after medicine, every one but the right one. The pain wasn't from arthritis. Her steroid-soaked spine had collapsed, compressing a nerve. She lived with that pain for a year and a half. Nerve pain and nociceptive pain (caused by injury to tissues) are not the same. They respond to different treatments. Lesson learned. Thanks, Mom.

"Listen to the patient! She might be trying to tell you something!" Dr. Robert Joynt had taught me. As she described her symptoms, my mom was telling her doctors the answer to the medical riddle the whole time. All they had to do was stop, listen, and think. Sometimes, the truth is right in front of our eyes. But if we are blinded by our preconceived notions, we can't see it. Fortunately, one person was able to listen to my mother, figure out her problem, and get her the treatment she needed—a surgery that at least eased her burning pain.

As I grew older, her smile no longer distracted me. When I was with her, I started to feel her pain. How could anyone live with this? Could I? I longed to flee. School and job were ways to get away. She couldn't flee. Whether she wanted to or not, she educated me about pain. I watched how she responded to each treatment and what helped each type of pain she experienced. I realized that the textbooks told me nothing of this.

I longed to understand pain. Perhaps I couldn't help my mom, but I could help others. I dove into books and studied the sages. I studied my patients and looked into their eyes. There I saw my mother. "If this were my mother, how would I want to treat her?" I asked myself.

My mother taught me an entirely different perspective on pain and life that my medical textbooks rarely talked about. I read the writings of others who had ventured into the forest. They wrote about pain in a manner totally different from the textbooks. They came to understand that pain was not mere cause and effect. They realized that the pain system is much more complicated, and that each person's experience of pain is unique, and so must be the treatments. These were the giants of pain: Livingston, Melzack, Wall, Foley, Portenoy, and many others. I realized I was not alone.

How I Became a Pain Management Specialist

My area of expertise is pain management. More specifically, I am an "interventional pain management specialist." That means I treat pain problems by placing long needles in my patient's bodies. Usually I inject some substance into the painful body part. Sometimes the needles provide electrical stimulation. At other times they intentionally damage, or denervate, nerves associated with pain. For some odd reason, physicians have come to believe that spending fifteen minutes placing a needle is an intervention, while sitting down with an individual for several hours over the course of several visits; listening to his symptoms, thoughts, and concerns; and then developing a concise treatment plan that addresses all his needs, is not. This latter approach is referred to as comprehensive pain management. While placing needles accurately in painful structures might seem to be technically more difficult, in reality it is not. Moreover, it takes less time, creates less stress for the practitioner, and pays much better. Because of the financial windfall, corporate medicine encourages interventional pain management.

Comprehensive pain management is what I used to do until both legal and economic pressures, to be described later, forced me to stop. It takes more time, is much more stressful, and pays poorly. Corporate medicine shuns such practitioners, and making a living in this form of practice is challenging, at best. For reasons of pure economic survival, it is becoming a dying specialty—yet it is much more important for the patient's well-being than interventional pain management.

Pain management was not my initial passion, but it is where my path through life led me. I did know I wanted to be a doctor and, as I mentioned, spent some time working in a cancer hospital. Interestingly, even there I didn't notice my patients' physical pain. I was drawn to their mental pain. They suffered alone with disfigurements brought on by their disease and its treatment. Some died. Some lived with new disabilities to which they struggled to adapt. Most were discharged after treatment with little thought for the rehabilitation and adaptations they would need. When I inquired as to the reason for this neglect, I was told there was no need to rehab someone who would die soon. However, as treatments improved, many of these patients were no longer dying from their cancer. It did leave permanent physical and psychological damage, though, and they needed help. I longed to be the person who helped with their transition.

I was quite conscious that I would be going into a field where cure was not the goal, but rather helping people adjust to a new life. I realized there would be no quick fixes and little glory. That suited my personality. I am simultaneously obsessive and patient. I don't like being the center of attention. If I see that something needs to be done, I do it. I thrive on common sense. Those are traits that serve the rehabilitation specialist well. That was the career for me!

I entered medical school with that goal in mind. All the electives I chose had to do with rehabilitation. I chose a medical school, the University of Rochester, that valued and taught doctor-patient communication, a topic I had already written two papers on. I had many wonderful instructors, although to this day, the instructors I remember most were my patients. I was entering a field where little was written and common sense reigned supreme. Treatment was by trial and error, and my patients showed me the way by allowing me to observe their successes and failures. The instructors who taught best were the ones with their own disabilities. I observed how they adapted to life's big and little challenges and how they found their way around the barriers life provided. They truly lived the adage: if life gives you lemons, make lemonade!

Still, I was blind to pain. It was not taught and barely mentioned. The "gate control theory of pain" was referred to in passing, but that was it. In the 1960s, Ronald Melzack and Patrick D. Wall had collected all the knowledge that existed on the phenomenon of pain and used it to develop a neurophysiological model of pain processing. They called it the gate control theory because they theorized that at every level of the nervous system, "gates" exist in the form of neural mechanisms that control the sensory input and the motor response to pain (that is, the pain signals the brain and spinal cord receive and the signals each sends out to the muscles in response). As happens to many theories, the gate control theory was later shown to have limitations. Still, it served as the first model to guide experimentation on pain and contributed greatly to our understanding.

While this model was acknowledged in our training, we never really were taught why it was important. There were no lectures on the neurophysiology of pain or on its treatment. If such an enlightened institution neglected this area, how was it handled at other institutions? This question never occurred to me. We were taught by implication that the only pain of significance was caused by an injury to tissue, and that by treating that tissue, one would relieve the pain. That meant surgeries and drugs. If a patient did not get better, it was because of flaws in her "unconscious," and the only hope was psychotherapy. This concept was never taught formally, but it clearly determined all behavior toward patients.

After medical school, I went on to a year of internal medicine at Dartmouth, which is where I confronted my first back patient. We were given a "back pain algorithm" for treating these patients, which had been published in an authoritative textbook. All got antiinflammatory medications and two weeks of bed rest. They were not supposed to get up for any reason, even to go to the bathroom. If they did not follow this rule, they were chastised. If they did, but still didn't get better, they were sent to the surgeon. Once that happened, the internal medicine residents never saw them again, so we never learned of their treatment outcomes. We assumed the surgeons had a fix for these problems because that is what they led us to believe. In fact, they never did fix them. I don't mean to criticize surgeons—they were mired in the same cause-and-effect theory of pain as the rest of us, so they were no more or less at fault than anyone else.

I brought that level of knowledge with me to my physical medicine residency (physical medicine is the same as rehabilitation medicine and is also called physiatry) at the va hospital. Most of our education was devoted to learning how to work with people with all sorts of disabilities. It was at this point that I started to notice that pain was frequently a part of these disabilities, and sometimes the primary part. My eyes were opening, and I started to see chronic pain not as a purely psychological disorder, but as something more. And then I met Mr. Smith, who challenged the little I had been taught about pain.

And I must repeat, it was very little. At the va, we were given the opportunity to treat pain patients, but not really taught how. Residents taught residents; the blind led the blind. Fortunately for me, one of my fellow residents had done a fellowship in pain management, and another had been a physical therapist. He and a third resident had an interest in treating musculoskeletal pain and had spent a lot of independent time learning about pain. I learned from them and from their example, and this education included much that I didn't want to know. I learned about the often-violent differences of opinion regarding pain treatments, the inability of the people holding those opinions to communicate with others who disagreed with them, and their need to spread their delusions to others. I learned that the more impressive the degree people possessed, the more effective they were in spreading their ignorance, forever dooming their disciples. I began to look at pain as the elephant being examined by the blind men. I yearned to learn as much as I could from as many people as possible. In the beginning, though, I refused to believe that we had no cure for chronic pain. I saw chronic pain as similar to acute pain, and believed that with the right combination of medicine, surgery, and therapy, we could cure it. I surveyed the sages—the foremost academic experts in the field of pain—to find the answer.

The first thing I discovered was that what I had been taught in my internal medicine residency was all wrong. Bed rest was bad. I concluded that activity, not passivity, was the best treatment and that injected medicines were better than oral. I developed a strange faith in surgery, perhaps because surgeons possessed the most powerful credentials. Given what happened to Mr. Smith, that faith is surprising, but I assumed Mr. Smith had been subject to the wrong type of surgery, so the cure must be another type of surgery.

Somewhere along the road, I gave up my dream of becoming a cancer rehabilitation specialist. Most of the best jobs in physiatry were in musculoskeletal medicine, so I spent innumerable hours during the last year of my residency learning about this. I read books, went to meetings, and moonlighted at a friend's clinic and at a pain clinic. I thought I was ready.

I found my first job in New Hampshire as an occupational medicine specialist. Only once did I go to a job site, so I'm not sure what the occupational part of the specialty was! For the most part, I treated patients with back pain, neck pain, or back and neck pain. From the very beginning, for reasons not clear to me, I was viewed as an expert. Like most people, I enjoy having my ego massaged, so I gladly accepted this new title. Over the next few years, I learned much from the school of hard knocks. For example: people only consider you an expert when you see things their way. One day, I confronted an insurance company about the way they were treating (or mis-treating) one of my patients. They didn't like what I had to say. Suddenly, they no longer viewed me as an expert. I came to understand that in the business world, consultants are only viewed as experts when their opinions satisfy the needs of the referral source's bottom line.

I submitted my patients to all the treatments I had learned from the sages. Many got better, despite my ministrations. Some, no matter what I did, "refused" to get better. According to the medical establishment, these people must have a "screw loose." Over the years, though, I saw patterns emerge. I began to think it odd that an awful lot of people had the same loose screw. Perhaps there was a lot more to chronic pain than structural cause and effect: structure injured, repair it, and all will be fine. That was clearly not true for these patients, and I was determined to find what was missing. Though I now realized that the sages I had chosen didn't have an answer for me, I still naïvely believed there was a cure for this scourge.

I sought guidance. If the sages couldn't provide it, perhaps someone else could. I met some other pain management specialists and asked where I could learn more. I joined several pain societies and read their journals. I shared my observations with others. I went to meetings. I examined every treatment, conventional and unconventional. I came to believe that there is a place for all at the table of pain treatment and sought to learn from all. Each piece helped me understand the puzzle better. I learned the neurophysiology of pain, what we understand and what we don't; that chronic pain and acute pain are not the same; and that chronic pain is not simple cause and effect, but rather an entire complex restructuring of how the nervous system interprets pain that is unique in each individual sufferer (chapter 2 explains this in more detail). There are patterns, but there are dozens of them. I learned that in order for treatment to be effective, we need to understand these patterns better and become more specific in our therapies. All I had been taught was wrong. And I came to acknowledge that there is no cure. This meant that pain needed to be managed, much like any other disability. The question was, how?

I studied Chinese medicine. Descriptions of acupuncture used to treat pain date back to 5000 BC. My impression is that acupuncture originated as purely an instinctive treatment used to "dig out the pain." Many of my patients feel that if I could just "dig out their knots" they would be fine. Perhaps surgery for pain is just an extension of that primal instinct. The contribution of the Chinese to pain management, though, is not acupuncture. Many other cultures shared this treatment. The real contribution of the Chinese was that they studied their patients, *listened* to them, and *accepted* their symptoms. They observed pain patterns shared by groups of people and attempted to create a model to explain these findings. Ironically, all breakthroughs in medicine begin with this bold, surprisingly courageous step of listening to patients and believing them. The Chinese described pain syndromes such as fibromyalgia thousands of years ago. They understood pain referral, meaning that pain will radiate from its source in predictable ways depending on its nerve supply. They created novel pain treatments we still use today. They didn't understand how the nervous system works; but with the patient as their guide, not their bane, they came to believe in a system of meridians, or channels through which energy flows through the body, and they developed treatments directed at them. By trial and error, they found treatments that worked. I was quite disconcerted to find that they knew and understood more about pain two thousand years ago than we know now.

I studied Silas Weir Mitchell, who investigated the pain created by nerve injury in dozens of patients during the Civil War. He recorded his results and began to develop theories of pain based on them. He listened to his patients and accepted what they said. Weir Mitchell observed that the pain of nerve injury is different from somatic pain (pain from injury to structures other than nerves) in that it requires much higher doses of opioids.

I studied William K. Livingston, MD, who is credited with starting the first university-based pain management program in the world at the University of Oregon in 1947. He saw patients of all types, examined them, and strove to understand them. In 1943 he published *Pain Mechanisms,* a book that challenged contemporary thoughts about pain. In another book, *Pain and Suffering,* he described his thoughts about the mechanisms of chronic pain, including the importance of spinal modulation of pain (the notion that spinal mechanisms alter the sensation of pain), sensitization (the idea that nerve cells associated with pain sensation may become more sensitive to stimulation), and neural plasticity (the central nervous system's ability to adapt and change in response to a stimulus from its environment). These concepts are widely understood in the pain community, but remain foreign to most health-care providers in the general medical world, even though Livingston did his pioneering work in the 1930s, 1940s, and 1950s, and Weir Mitchell did his work shortly after the American Civil War.

I studied Melzack and Wall's gate control theory of pain, and later modifications to it. I also studied Melzack's subsequent work, in which he encouraged physicians to take pain seriously. He outlined the carnage of untreated pain and offered guidance in using opioids to treat it. He published a paper in *Scientific American* in 1985, outlining his observations for general health-care practitioners, yet it apparently remains unknown.

I felt my eyes had been opened, and it bothered me greatly that I never had been exposed to these thoughts during my medical education. I was also very disappointed that I was learning not about recent breakthroughs, but rather about ideas that were decades, centuries, and millennia old. It distressed me to realize that the problem in pain management is not what we don't know, but that we naïvely think we know more than we really do. We place blind faith in individuals who tout the values of their treatments, often at considerable profit to themselves and at great expense to the affected patient and society as well.

My research, as well as my experience as a practitioner, has convinced me that the scourge of chronic pain is not merely a physiologic derangement but a societal one. It is evidence not only of the misplaced transmissions of some angry neurons within the pain patient's body, but also of the way people interact with each other. There is no mere pharmaceutical creation that can solve this problem. The solution must address all levels of society, and all levels must be willing to participate actively and honestly—willing to acknowledge what they know, what they don't know, and what they can contribute.

Another of my transforming moments occurred in September 1983. I was a "clinical clerk" (a polite name for a very naïve third-year medical student) on the wards at a local geriatric facility. We were assigned to one patient per week, and our job was to get to know that person and his or her medical problems very well. Viola was my first patient. Her superficial problem was that she had lupus and suffered not just from her disease, but also from the effects of the steroids used to treat it. Her bones had thinned, and as a result had fractured several times. She could no longer function on her own and had been sentenced to a nursing home for the remainder of her life.

But Viola had a deeper problem. She had been sentenced once before, when she was young. A sentence implies a crime. Hers was that she was Jewish. Her judges were the Nazis. Her sentence was Auschwitz. She survived, but she was never released from her mental prison. The memories haunted her forever.

One day, I saw Viola on the ward.

"Hi, Viola, how are you?" I asked dutifully.

"Why do people ask that question when they don't really care about the response?" she said.

I felt naked. She had looked through the cover of my soul. She was right. I was in a hurry, and I really didn't care how she was feeling. She was the depressed old lady in bed three. Everyone knew it. I wasn't going to change her depression. I wasn't going to give her a new life. I wasn't going to erase the haunting memories of her past. It wasn't convenient to care. I was late for a meeting.

Twenty-eight years later, I think of Viola every day when I ask how someone is doing. I try hard to hear the response. There is no greater gift one person can give another than listening.

Two other transforming moments occurred merely because I heeded the lesson I learned from Viola. The first was an encounter with a homeless man on a street in Seattle who held a sign reading "Will work for food." At first I assumed he was a worthless bum. After spending time with him, I found he was an interesting, inspiring man who had been through more trials than any human had a right to suffer. Rather than ask for a handout, he was asking for a chance to find meaning in his life. The second moment was meeting Mr. Smith. I began to see a similarity between the cycle of poverty and the cycle of pain. Both are destructive, downward spirals brought on by many factors. Both destroy a person's self-esteem. Both require action and energy to reverse. The first step in ending both is to stop the spiral. The second step is to reverse it. I sought a way to accomplish this, at least in the area of pain management. As time passed, though, I came to realize that the problem was broader than I had ever imagined.

TWO

What Is Pain?

Its Neurophysiology and Psychology:
Chasing Two Moving Targets

I never believed anyone's pain until it happened to me.
Quote from too many patients

In medical school, I was taught that pain was a simple cause-and-effect problem. It began with an injury to a body structure. This resulted in a neural (nerve) signal to the spinal cord, and then on to the brain. Once it arrived there, the person would feel a sensation of pain, the severity of which was directly proportional to the tissue injury. Over time, the structure would heal itself, or a physician would intervene to assist in that process. Once healed, the pain would go away and the person would be fine. Structures don't always heal perfectly, so the person might be left with some limitation, but pain shouldn't be a part of it. If the person's pain persisted and became chronic, that was due to one of two reasons. The first was that the problem was overwhelming in nature, such as rheumatoid arthritis or cancer. The second was a character flaw in the patient.

For the most part, these teachings were implicit, though they were based on the published work of Sigmund Freud, my mentor George Engel, and many others who believed that "persistent pain associated with emotional distress in the absence of organic findings is primarily due to psychiatric illness."[1] They also were based on a dramatic overconfidence in our ability to diagnose and understand pain. For all practical purposes, we were saying that if we couldn't see it and we couldn't treat it, it didn't exist, except in the flawed psyche of the patient. This head-in-the-sand paradigm has dominated education about chronic pain and its diagnosis and treatment and continues to do so, with unfortunate consequences for those who suffer.

Nothing is ever so simple. It has been recognized since the 1930s that this cause-and-effect model is flawed, and that chronic pain is rarely due to a character flaw. Yet this model still guides how the concept of pain is taught to health-care providers and the public as a whole, and how they relate to those who suffer from chronic pain. It amounts to a slap in the face to those who suffer, a challenge to their integrity that unnecessarily burdens their ability to adapt to and manage their pain.

To help those who suffer from chronic pain, then, it is critical to understand what pain is. To begin, a few definitions are in order. Definitions rarely capture the whole of a complex phenomenon like pain, but they are an important starting point.

The International Association for the Study of Pain has defined *pain* as: "an unpleasant sensory and emotional experience associated with actual or potential tissue damage, or described in terms of such damage."

We differentiate *acute pain* and *chronic pain* arbitrarily by how long they last. Acute pain is usually defined as pain that lasts less than three months, and chronic pain as pain that lasts more than three months.

Acute pain is also referred to as *nociceptive pain.* Nociceptive pain serves an important purpose. It alerts us to a problem within our body. We then take steps to protect that body part, which enables it to heal. Once healing has occurred and the signal is no longer needed, the pain goes away.

Chronic pain does not serve a useful purpose. Once healing has occurred, the pain persists. It is not serving as a signal, and it unnecessarily restricts the sufferer. It is considered a disease process in itself and is referred to as *pathological pain.* There are two types of chronic pain, which are not mutually exclusive: *inflammatory* and *neuropathic.* Inflammatory pain results from damage to nonneural tissue, and neuropathic pain results from damage to neural tissue.

We must make one more very important distinction: between *pain* and *suffering.* Pain is the body's physical (nociceptive or biological) response to tissue injury. Suffering is the person's psychosocial response to the injury. Pain can have very different meanings depending on the situation. For example, a boo-boo on my pinkie may not be a big deal to me; however, to a violinist, it may be career threatening and emotionally devastating. An injury to my back at home will provoke some stress. It will provoke much more stress if it happens at work, where people are counting on me to get things done, where my boss has little patience for wimps, and where a worker's compensation claims adjustor sitting in an office hundreds of miles away questions the validity of my complaints.

How much a person suffers, then, depends not just on what happens to him, but also on the setting in which it occurs. This creates dramatic ramifications determining how he responds to the challenge of pain medically, psychologically, functionally, and socially. In managing pain, it is critical to understand the distinction between pain and suffering.

The Neurophysiology of Pain

Understanding our reaction to pain also requires awareness of our current understanding of pain itself. Be aware that what follows is grossly simplified and also that there is a lot we don't know. Sometime in the mid-2000s, I sat in a lecture hall and listened to a prominent neurophysiologist promise his audience that we were on the verge of understanding pain, or more precisely, chronic pain. I sat in awe. Over the next few years I anxiously awaited the fulfillment of his revelation. Alas, I waited in vain. A few years later, I attended another lecture by that same individual, ready to be enlightened as to the new knowledge. He did not let me down gently but began his talk by saying:

"We don't understand chronic pain, and we're not sure what we don't understand."

His intellectual honesty was refreshing. So taking his statement as a given, let me lay out what we do understand. The accompanying diagram outlines the body's pain system.

Pain, like all other sensory phenomena, starts with a stimulus to a nerve ending. What makes pain unique is that the nerve endings involved are "silent nociceptors"—that is, they are usually quiet. It takes a lot to excite them. This makes sense, since we don't want to feel pain all the time. If a stimulus is of sufficient intensity, two things happen. First, a signal is sent from the nerve ending to the dorsal horn of the spinal cord, a region of the cord that contains sensory nerve cells. Second, a soup of inflammatory

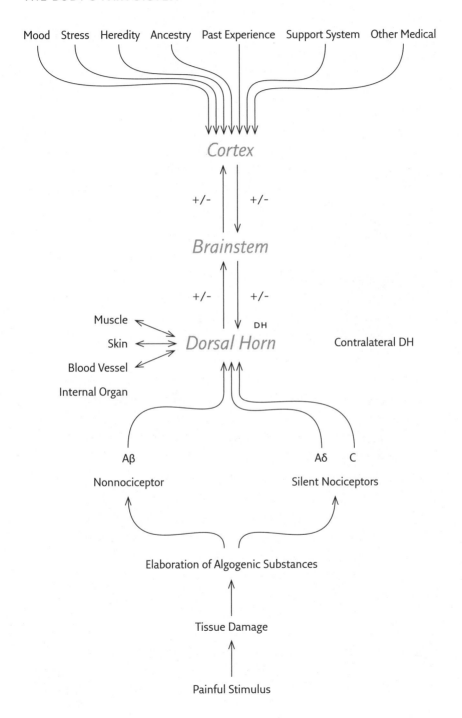

substances develops around the nerve ending, making it more sensitive. This is referred to as *peripheral sensitization.* This process lowers the firing threshold of the peripheral nerve (a peripheral nerve is one that is outside the brain and spinal cord), making it much less silent.

The dorsal horn is the relay area of the spinal cord. All peripheral sensory information converges here. It is not used to handling a lot of pain information from any one area of the body. If it starts hearing a lot from a no-longer-silent area, one of three things can happen. It can ignore the signal, it can relay it to the higher neurological centers and maintain it, or it can amplify the signal. If the dorsal horn maintains or amplifies the signal, that is referred to as *central sensitization* (*central* refers to the brain and spinal cord). The result is a *centrally maintained pain state* (CMPS).

At this point four things may occur:

> First, a descending or efferent signal (meaning it travels away from the brain or spinal cord out to the periphery of the body) is sent to the area where the pain originated, leading the nerve endings to dump more pain-inducing (algogenic) substances into the inflammatory soup. This aggravates the peripherally sensitized neuron, creating a vicious cycle.

> Second, efferent signals are sent to structures that share the nerve supply of the injured structure, sensitizing them as well. These structures include skin, muscle, blood vessel, bone, and internal organs—all of which become more sensitive and dysfunctional. That is how a "simple" herniated disc leads to muscle spasm, swelling in the arms or legs, skin hypersensitivity, and bowel and bladder problems.

> Third, dorsal horn sensitivity may spread up and down the spinal cord to adjacent levels. This is referred to as *enlargement of receptive fields.* It may also spread to the opposite side of the body, which is called *mirror imaging.*

> Fourth, the dorsal horn will send signals to the various centers of the brain, which repeat this whole process.

The critical element is what happens at the dorsal horn. If sensitization occurs, a cascade of adverse effects can occur. Fortunately, sensitization usually does not occur, and the pain goes away . . . sort of. Unfortunately, the dorsal horn does store a memory of the experience, and the next time an injury occurs in that area, the pain response occurs more quickly. With each successive injury over time, the likelihood of a CMPS increases.

But why does a CMPS occur at all? The reality is that we don't know. We understand what has happened neurophysiologically once it happens, but we can't predict if it will, and we don't really know why sensitization occurs in any individual case. Some people with a catastrophic injury have minimal if any pain, while others with a seemingly trivial injury develop substantial pain. To make matters more complicated, one individual can undergo the same trauma in two different situations and experience minimal pain in one, but disabling pain in the other. For example, if the back injury I referred to above happens in a supportive environment where the individual has time to heal with little stress beyond the injury, then she is likely to do better than if it occurs in a stressful environment that makes high demands on her.

We do know that the dorsal horn relays all sorts of information. Some sensory information ascends from the periphery of the body. Some information descends from the brain. Some comes from adjacent levels of the spinal cord. This information can be either excitatory or inhibitory. The sum total of the pluses and minuses determines whether a CMPS develops and to what degree. Numerous factors play a role, such as past pain experience, stress level, mood, supportiveness of the environment, and so on. Culture and heredity are also important. For example, I once had a patient with a somewhat trivial Achilles tendon injury. He didn't have a lot of pain, but he was emotionally distraught about the injury because in his Middle Eastern culture, the cutting of the Achilles tendon was thought to be a punishment from God.

What is critical to understand is that we can use these factors to minimize or even prevent the development of chronic pain. Thus we must take all of them into account in developing a prescription to manage the pain.

There are several points to be made based on this discussion:

Pain has both a structural and a neurological aspect. Structural injury may incite the pain, but a neurological adaptation or maladaptation maintains or amplifies it. Treatments that attend only to the structural element are bound to fail in chronic pain.

The neural response is not static. It changes constantly. This is referred to as *plasticity*. Chronic pain is a moving target, further complicating successful management.

Each person's pain is unique. Each person brings different intrinsic and extrinsic factors to the pain experience. Each person processes the sensory experience of pain differently, with very different outcomes. Each patient must therefore be treated individually. There is no single recipe that will help everyone, and the search for a "magic bullet" is futile.

For these reasons, *we cannot understand another person's pain based on our own experiences.*

While chronic pain may be pathological, it is physiologically *real*. It is not a character flaw or a purely psychological problem. Psychological dysfunction in those who suffer is most often the result of chronic pain, not the reverse.[2] A patient who had had chronic back pain for three years came to see me. I gave her an injection that relieved the pain for about three weeks. In that period of time, her family noted that she readily became the person she had been before her injury. If you remove the pain, the psychological distress usually goes away.

Despite all the ads in the media from doctors and nondoctors alike suggesting otherwise, there is no cure for chronic pain. We can only manage it. More important: we must not unnecessarily aggravate it.

The evolution of chronic pain in an individual is based on both internal and external factors. All who come into contact with a pain patient play a significant role in the outcome, for better or for worse—not just the doctor and the patient.

The Experience of Chronic Pain

Every year I receive multiple mailings from various medical groups asking me to send money for one medical cause or another. There is no question that the ones that show a deformed child attract my attention the most. I find it interesting that despite my profession, I never receive any mailings requesting money for a cause related to chronic pain. I had never really thought much about that until I wrote these words. I wonder why? Perhaps it is because we don't really think of someone who suffers from unremitting pain as worthy of our attention. We don't believe that pain is really a problem. We think the sufferer should just suck it up and get on with her life. It's also difficult to believe in someone for whom there is no poster child. Pain patients look just like you and me. Frequently there is no test to explain their pain.

Too often we believe that pain worthy of our attention only accompanies a life- threatening illness. Over the years, I have heard many people, colleagues and lay people alike, say to a pain patient: "It's not like you have cancer." Do cancer patients have a monopoly on severe pain? In medicine, we make an arbitrary distinction between malignant and nonmalignant pain. Why? It seems to me that by doing this physicians are, in effect, making a value judgment that pain of malignant origin is more legitimate and more worthy of our attention. While cancer pain may be easily explainable, I do not believe we should be any less supportive of those who suffer from nonmalignant pain. While cancer pain can be horrible, so is nonmalignant chronic pain.

Imagine that you sign up for a 5K race. You run as hard as you can, sensing the finish line approaching. But when you arrive, there is no finish line. There is only a race official who tells you that there was a mistake, and the race is really 10K. You are discouraged, but you decide to continue on. You slow your pace since you spent much of your energy in the first 5K. However, you know you can last a little longer. You soon approach the 10K mark, where you find the same race official telling you there's been another mistake, you are not at the finish line, and you must keep going. This cycle keeps repeating. Eventually, the race official tells you he has no idea how long the race really is, but you have no choice but to continue.

Now, imagine there are no longer any rest stops, bathrooms, water, or food. There are no crowds to cheer you on. They all left and went home after the first 5K. But you can't stop. What would you do?

The race is the pain. The finish line is the cure or death. The rest stops are the diagnostic tests, diagnoses, and treatments. The race official is the doctor. The cheering crowds are the people who provide treatment and support. In the cancer pain race, there is usually a definitive diagnosis and a well-defined finish line. Treatments are liberally provided. The runner is well cared for. The families, friends, and caregivers support the "runner." The race is still grueling, but at least it is usually well managed.

In the race of nonmalignant pain, there is no clear finish line. There is no cure and no endpoint. Diagnoses are frequently lacking. The rest stops are unpredictable and often undersupplied. The patients are undermedicated. The crowds are gone.

Which is worse?

Imagine what it is like to lose your ability to do everything you value—an experience exacerbated by an unremitting pain that pervades your entire existence. Imagine such a life, in which not only do you receive no sympathy or empathy, but few people even believe in your predicament, and most people blame you for having it. Is it surprising that depression, anxiety, and suicide are prevalent among chronic pain sufferers?

Too often, those around the patient unnecessarily aggravate or even create these secondary psychological disabilities. By questioning their symptoms, we challenge patients' sense of self, their integrity. We make them doubt themselves. They begin to question their own sanity. "Is the pain really all in my head?" they ask themselves.

One of the greatest losses pain sufferers experience is a loss of control over their destinies. Their lives too often become a rudderless voyage controlled by others, one they feel powerless or incompetent to take control of—a perception created by other people's judgments.

I recall a time when I did something previously unthinkable for me. I let my son drive us to Buffalo and back. I am a terrible passenger. I need to be in control. To be honest, my son did a great job. Still, for me the round-trip was sixteen hours of hell. My stress level was off the charts. It took me several days to recover.

Imagine if I had to live that way every day. Perhaps I could get used to letting him drive. It's more likely that I would go nuts. We are all quite aware of the effect stress has on our various bodily functions. I would most likely die an early death due to some cardiac event.

We are well aware of the effect of stress on our immune, cardiac, pulmonary, renal, and gastrointestinal functions. But as the previous discussion indicates, stress and other psychological conditions play a central role in pain and healing. Loss of control and challenges to integrity create stress and depression that feed into the pain system negatively through descending input from the brain to the dorsal horn. This is the physiological mechanism by which stress and depression can aggravate chronic pain or, worse, create a chronic problem that might not otherwise exist.

GRIEVING AND CHRONIC PAIN

> The most beautiful people we have known are those
> who have known defeat, known suffering, known struggle,
> known loss, and have found their way out of those depths.
> Elisabeth Kübler-Ross, *Death: The Final Stage of Growth*

We devote much energy to understanding pain, which as noted prior is a moving target because of neuroplasticity. There is another moving target affecting people with chronic pain and its associated disability that is just as important to understand and address, but is frequently ignored: grieving.

Grieving is a mental and spiritual process we go through when adapting to a significant loss. It is important to recognize that it is not a pathological process. It allows us to heal, and therefore it is important for us to experience it. Too often, we treat it as a disease state that needs to be alleviated. Perhaps we feel this way because grieving entails suffering, and we assume that suffering is a bad thing. However, as Dr. Kübler-Ross's statement implies, we grow by going through this process. Medicating it only serves to deny the sufferer this opportunity. It is critical, then, that those who care for people who have experienced a loss understand what grieving is and how best to manage it. As the next chapter explains, chronic pain creates many simultaneous losses for the sufferer, and grieving is an innate part of the process of adaptation. Since the rest of the book frequently examines how grieving affects the experience of the chronic pain sufferer, here I give a general overview of the process.

In *On Death and Dying,* published in 1969 and based on her work with the dying, Kübler-Ross not only defined the process of grieving, she also changed how people looked at it. While she described the process that the dying and their families go through, her work is clearly applicable to our response to other, non–life threatening losses.

She described a series of five stages that the bereaved go through: denial and isolation, anger, bargaining, depression, and acceptance. It is beyond the scope of this discussion to describe these in detail, but I want to point out two important lessons of her book. First, grieving is not a linear process.

As Dr. Kübler-Ross says, "The five stages . . . are a part of the framework that makes up our learning to live without the one we lost. They are tools to help us frame and identify what we may be feeling. But they are not stops on some linear timeline in grief." Indeed, moving in a straight path from one stage to another would be unusual. I see this all the time in my patients. On one visit a patient may be in denial. On the next he may be angry, then back in denial, then depressed, and so on. Sometimes people experience more than one stage at the same time. I find it most challenging when an early stage reappears after the patient has seemingly accepted her situation. Cycling back and forth this way is also normal, and the caregiver must understand this as well. Caring for patients who experience loss becomes much less frustrating when the caregiver understands that grieving, like pain, is a moving target.

I think the stages that challenge the caregiver the most are anger and depression. Dr. Kübler-Ross says: "It is important to feel the anger without judging it, without attempting to find meaning in it. It may take many forms: anger at the health-care system, at life, at your loved one for leaving. Life is unfair. Death is unfair. Anger is a natural reaction to the unfairness of loss." The caregiver needs to understand what the anger means. Above all, she needs to understand that the anger is directed at the loss, not the caregiver. To me it is almost sinful to take advantage of this anger, but that is what personal injury attorneys do, by encouraging lawsuits that delay adaptation, and this harms more than helps.

Depression is normal. Yet being around this emotion is a struggle for caregivers. I think we want to rid the sufferer of it in order to treat ourselves, more than him. It is easy for me to write a prescription for a drug that has as much potential to harm as to help, then walk away. But that is a form of abandonment. Sometimes the most important intervention is to just be there for the person, to lend an ear, a hand, and a hug. I firmly believe that being there is much more therapeutic, but it requires great energy. As Dr. Kübler-Ross said: "I say to people who care for people who are dying, if you really love that person and want to help them, be with them when their end comes close. Sit with them—you don't even have to talk. You don't have to do anything but really be there with them."

The second lesson involves understanding the duration of the grieving process. Kübler-Ross envisioned that for family members of someone who has died, this should take a year. Grieving lasting longer than that is considered pathological. While that may be true in the case of death and dying, I do not find it to be true for adaptation to chronic pain or other disabilities. I am reminded of a friend who became quadriplegic at thirteen. Her injury occurred in the early 1970s, and at that time, community support was lacking. In her case, family support was lacking as well. After her acute care, she was placed in a nursing home, where she lived for the next thirteen years. She cycled through all the stages of grieving throughout this period, but never came to any state of acceptance until she turned twenty-six. She is not sure how it happened, but one day she realized she did not have to live like that. She had choices and could take control of her life, which she proceeded to do. She got her GED, college degree, and then her master's. Eventually, with the help of many, she became a social worker who worked with people adapting to spinal cord injury and lived independently. She told me she had observed that her grieving experience was typical, that acceptance does not come in a year. It takes a long time.

In my experience, the same is true of chronic pain. The time frame can be quite variable. For some, a few months suffice. For others, it takes years, and this is more typical. Some never come to acceptance. Many factors play a role in determining this time frame, such as severity of pain, age at onset, type of pain, and level of functional impairment. The most important factor, though, is the response of the people around the person. If the environment is nurturing and supportive, the patient adapts better. If the environment is hostile or enabling, she does not.

The natural process of grieving should be supported and not denied. Grieving can become pathological, though. The challenge is realizing when this is the case. Usually an individual is stuck in a specific stage or is experiencing a particular stage too intensely. In such a case, intervention is needed. For example, a patient of mine was so angry about his injury and the treatment he was receiving from his doctors and his insurer that he threatened them with bodily harm. That behavior had to be confronted. It is not easy to confront someone so belligerent. However, by summoning more than a bit of courage, I was able to talk to him and deflect his emotions in a more productive direction (although I could not have done that if I had not already earned his trust). I find that a useful litmus test for differentiating between physiological and pathological grief is the patient's level of function. One can grieve, yet still be working toward maximizing function despite limitations. When this work is not occurring, there is a problem.

POSTTRAUMATIC STRESS DISORDER AND THE PAIN PATIENT

Posttraumatic stress disorder (PTSD) is an underappreciated accompaniment of chronic pain, and it plays a role in many ways. Posttraumatic stress is a severe anxiety disorder that develops after exposure to any event that results in psychological trauma. Such an event may involve the threat of death to oneself or to someone else, or a threat to one's own or someone else's physical, psychological, or sexual integrity, overwhelming one's ability to cope. Diagnostic symptoms include reexperiencing the original trauma through flashbacks or nightmares, avoidance of any stimuli associated with the trauma, and increased arousal such as difficulty falling or staying asleep, anger, and hypervigilance.[3] This response is an exaggeration of the "fight versus flight" response and involves multiple areas of the neural and endocrine systems. In effect, it backs the pain patient into a corner, and as I have explained, it has the potential to amplify and perpetuate the response to pain.

PTSD in pain patients is often ignored. Yet failure to acknowledge and treat it can have negative effects on outcome. I have observed four different types of PTSD in the setting of chronic pain.

First, PTSD can precede the pain disorder, as for the many chronic pain patients who have a history of physical, verbal, or sexual abuse. While cause and effect are not fully understood, it is likely that these patients have a different neuroendocrinological response to perceived threats, such as pain, than other people, a response that increases the risk of developing a chronic pain state. Note that not all patients with PTSD will develop chronic pain when so exposed, but their risk is higher. Note too that not all pain patients have a history of PTSD.

Second, pain patients can experience posttraumatic stress related to the event that brought on their pain. For example, individuals who have been involved in motor vehicle trauma may develop flashbacks and exaggerated psychological reactions to a car they see approaching quickly in the rearview mirror. For this reason, they may develop avoidant behaviors, in extreme cases avoiding motor vehicles altogether. Individuals injured at work may fear returning to work and avoid the workplace. While some would characterize this behavior as malingering, it is the result of a very real anxiety disorder that needs to be respected and treated as a separate entity if rehabilitation is to be successful.

Third, PTSD occurs in those whose trauma is the result of abuse by insurance companies, the courts, attorneys, or the workplace. Sad to say, I see this regularly. The trauma is usually caused by these actors' unwillingness to accept the patient's complaints as real and the constant sense of belittlement that ensues, assaulting the patient's self-esteem. Many patients tell me that if they had known how badly they would be treated by the workers' compensation system, they never would have filed a claim. All they need to trigger a full-blown PTSD attack is the mention of a labor board hearing. Some of my patients have developed panic attacks just from hearing the name of the claims adjustor or attorney who handled (or mishandled) their case. One patient of mine had moved to the United States from Australia. She was a very active woman who had been injured in an automobile accident. Her only goal was to get back to full function and have her medical bills paid, and she did everything in her power to make this happen. Yet she was so abused by a system which belittled her that it took her years to get over the totally unnecessary assault on her self-esteem.

Fourth, the trauma may be inflicted by the medical system. Jane, whom I described in the prologue, is a prime example. Her back surgeries with their terrible outcome constituted such a devastating experience that when she developed a threat to her spinal cord from a re-herniation, she refused to go to the hospital for three weeks out of pure fear. When I later admitted her to the hospital for pain control, she went into uncontrollable shaking fits. On top of this, she suffered such abuse from the workers' comp system that she became homebound and paralyzed, afraid that anything she did was being watched by her rehabilitation nurse or a hired private investigator. After another patient of mine got hurt, no physician would acknowledge her problem as real; both her doctors and the insurance company's representatives clearly communicated this judgment to her. To this day she must be premedicated just to go to a doctor's appointment. Even with premedication the mere thought of seeing any health care provider causes her great suffering. When it later became apparent that her problem was real, she received no apologies.

These third and fourth types bother me the most, because they are fully preventable and are caused by the sometimes conscious actions of those who should be helping the sufferer.

In managing the pain patient, it is critical that PTSD be acknowledged, for doing so can have a huge effect on healing, both physically and psychologically, as well as a huge effect on return to function. Although providers may find it convenient to refer to this condition as malingering, it is a very real psychological disorder. While we can do little to change the past, we must still acknowledge the wounds of the past and certainly avoid creating new, secondary wounds inflicted by our treatment.

Belief Is Therapeutic

It is also critical to understand the consequences of not believing the patient. Belief is healing, even though it may be challenging. I once bumped into Jill, an old patient who had challenged me greatly several years before. Her problem was refractory to care, and her pain persisted. She had one of those old New England stone faces that showed little emotion. Every time she came in to see me, that look made me believe she thought I was failing her. I could not have been more wrong. After she left my care, she took control of her life and found a meaningful job. At our chance meeting, her typical stone face was replaced by a smiling, gracious one. She gave me a huge hug that left me speechless. Reluctantly, I asked how she was doing. I expected to hear that she had found some pain guru who had solved all her problems. Instead, she thanked me and told me I was the only one who had helped her. I struggled to take that in. For years I believed I had failed her. So I asked what exactly I had done for her. She said that from the beginning I had believed in her, and that never changed throughout our time together. Maybe you can't bill for it, but it is powerful.

Each of our lives is a book, and the world a library, full of wonderful stories. Some books have pristine covers adorned with gold and leather. Others have worn, tattered covers. We tend to judge by the cover, which is easier than taking the time, energy, and courage to appreciate what lies within. But judging others on their appearance alone does them a great disservice. The greatest harm we can do to others is to rob them of their dignity, their self-esteem, their ability to believe in themselves. Yet when we judge superficially, that is exactly what we do. Initially the accused may be able to ignore the world's judgment. However, when they hear it again and again, they start to believe it. They begin to act as if they don't deserve respect, and their behavior changes accordingly.

As I have said, trying to eliminate chronic pain is futile. A better goal would be to acknowledge the needs of those who suffer and to minimize their suffering to the extent we can. That requires listening to these bereaved people and acknowledging their concerns. We must also take care to "do no harm." A misplaced word or action, conscious or not, can easily make the problem worse.

Do you believe in miracles? Taking time to believe can be miraculous.

THREE

You *Do* Have to Suffer...
Just Not as Much as We Make You

We cannot solve all the problems in the world, but never bring
in the worst problem of all, and that is to destroy love.

Mother Teresa, *Love: The Words and Inspiration of Mother Teresa*

The mystery of pain is a puzzle that has tormented humanity more than any other puzzle in medicine. It has baffled the medical world for centuries. Each generation mocks the one before, thinking it is closer to solving the riddle. But pain has many forms, and we are still far from understanding its varying nature. We don't understand the many neural pathways that convey pain information, we don't know how to describe each person's pain, and we don't have any way of predicting who will respond to what treatment. And since we see this lack of knowledge as a sign of weakness, doctors concoct theories rather than acknowledge their limitations. Then they pretend that their theories explain everything and that they are experts. The less we know, the more experts there are. In reality, like the blind men touching only part of the elephant and basing their conclusions on just that one part, each expert only understands a small piece of the whole. But in my opinion, the person who is willing to ask, "What do we know, and what don't we know?" is the true expert, for you can only seek answers if you are willing to admit to yourself that you don't know them.

Sir William Osler, MD, said: "The greater the ignorance, the greater the dogmatism." In few areas of medicine is this statement truer than in pain management. Experts abound, often convinced that their point of view is the correct one and all others are wrong. I struggle to understand why people tend to think that their answer is the only answer. The problem is that this intellectual stubbornness puts patients in a virtual crossfire between experts. Their heated disagreements impair our ability to systematize goals and outcomes. Worse, these controversies create an implicit, artificial hierarchy by which we judge the pain patient, often to his detriment. Four factors determine a patient's place on this patient ladder:

First, the patient's problem must be understandable. No matter how devastating the illness may be, if a patient follows the "rules"—meaning that her problem is easily explained by current theories—her stock rises and she occupies an upper rung of the ladder. Patients whose problem is poorly understood defy these rules, and their stock plummets. They challenge the contemporary paradigms. When confronted with a paradigm crisis, it is easiest to ignore the "aberration." So these patients are relegated to a lower rung.

Second, the patient's problem must be treatable. Patients can go a long way toward satisfying the egos of their caregivers by responding to treatment—even if what has really happened is that the patient got better *despite* the treatment. "He had what the doctors called 'bilious fever.' But in spite of the fact that the doctors treated him, bled him, and gave him drugs, he recovered" (Leo Tolstoy, *War and Peace*). The patient whose problem does not get better despite all attempts at treatment challenges the integrity of the caregiver. In such circumstances, the caregiver may protect her integrity by denigrating the patient: "Must be all in his head."

Third, the patient's problem must be simple. Patients whose problem fits neatly into a fifteen-minute spot are cherished. Those who don't fit into the schedule are feared. Time is energy. Time is money. Such patients cost energy and money. Keep it simple and avoid them.

Fourth, the patient's problem must be billable. Patients are prized as long as they present a pot of gold. Once the pot runs dry, the care often does too.

Patients whose problem we don't understand, who do not get better despite our best efforts, whose concerns occupy too much of our time at great cost, sink to the bottom of the medical ladder, a status that is readily communicated to them. We believe such patients amplify their symptoms and deserve their lot in life. Because those symptoms defy our attempts to explain them, we assume the patients must be making them up. We send them away.

In a very real sense, those who suffer from chronic pain are the lepers of the current medical world. Just as the lepers of old were exiled to the outskirts of the community, physicians today shun the pain patient. In the past, when leprosy was not understood, sufferers were abhorred because of their disfigurement. It was assumed that the affliction was a punishment from God for some apparent misdeed, and the sufferer was "unclean." There was no need to provide treatment, since only God could commute the patient's sentence. Leprosy is a simple problem compared to the challenge that chronic pain presents.

We shun chronic pain patients as though they were lepers. We don't invoke the "will of God" but rather resort to the modern explanation that their problem is all in their head. Having committed a crime against our theory, they are sometimes treated almost like criminals, as if they are deliberately fabricating their ailments. As a society, we deny these patients not only medical care but jobs as well. Like the two people who passed the victim by in the story of the Good Samaritan, we leave pain patients on the side of the road, hoping someone else will come along and minister to them, ignoring our responsibility for their plight.

But it's not a crime to be in pain. All the patient wants is to be free of pain and regain his or her lost sense of self. One physician noted that my patients act like victims. I responded that, in fact, they are victims. They did not ask for pain; they did not ask to be disabled. They did not ask to be dependent. They *are* victims. The question then is: do they have to act like victims? Life is a gift with opportunity around every corner. Just as at a yard sale, one person's junk is another's treasure. One can find riches in any situation in life, if one is willing to look. What stops a patient from looking?

In questioning a patient's behavior and forcing him to prove himself, we question his integrity, backing him into a corner. Forcing people to prove themselves, rather than accepting them as they present themselves, makes them angry and depressed and condemns them to stay in the present, rather than work toward a better future. Those are natural reactions to being backed into a corner. Unfortunately, as we saw in chapter 2, anger and depression add to pain. Rather than help these people, we have further victimized them. Who is at fault, the victim or the ones who create the victim? As two physicians wrote in 1977, "quacks" do make "crocks"—that is, bad doctors make bad patients.[1]

Doctors also victimize patients by offering treatment after treatment hoping to one day hit the jackpot. But what if there is no jackpot? What if the only solution is to accept the way things are? When do we stop? There is in fact no agreement about how to identify the point at which all reasonable treatments have been exhausted, and the goal of treatment should shift to adaptation.

For the most part, I don't believe doctors victimize patients on purpose. It is easier to try one more treatment than to admit that we have nothing else to offer. There is an endless array of treatments for pain, all with varying potential risks and benefits. At what point does the risk-benefit ratio become so high that we say "enough?" I don't know. I don't believe anyone does. That said, there are some unscrupulous physicians who do victimize on purpose, for their own financial gain. I will discuss them further later in this book.

Physicians behave as they do for a number of reasons. We have an irrational belief in our ability to understand the human body. We have so many wonderful diagnostic tools, and we think they can explain all conditions. We also have an irrational belief in the power of our treatments. We believe we have the cure for everything. We also fear the patient with a condition we can't explain or treat. We fear admitting to this patient that we don't understand his problem and don't have a solution.

We fear taking responsibility. There are few things harder than telling someone he will have to suffer forever. We fear the patient's reaction. There are few things harder than being in the presence of someone in pain. Rather than take responsibility, we run and hide; and we find many creative ways to do this. Blaming the victim is one way. Another is to "turf" responsibility by transferring care to someone else who we hope is more skilled (rather like dumping a baby on someone else's doorstep), hoping never to see the patient again. That is why patients go from provider to provider, conveniently allowing us to comfort ourselves by affixing yet another label to them: doctor shopper. Eventually, when nobody has assumed responsibility, the frustrated patient, in a last stand, assumes responsibility for his own care with no guidance and too often winds up at the mercy of those willing to take advantage of him.

Another reason is laziness. Most health-care providers are busy. We like simple problems that fit nicely into the routine, even if most such problems would get better without us. In fact, we like those problems more because they make us look better. "Challenging" problems require more energy. We must admit that we don't understand them, then "think outside the box," questioning our preconceived notions, in order to solve them. It takes energy to guide a patient through the maze of specialists, treatments, and diagnostic tests; to hold the patient's hand, be there when times are bad, and help her grieve. Yet that refusal to abandon patients, to accept their experience of what they are feeling, is exactly what they need. Unfortunately, that is more than many of us are willing to do, and we fear patients who ask it of us. So we shift the problem to someone else, who may be no more willing to assume responsibility than we are.

Chronic illness causes wounds to all levels of the self. While we may bear no responsibility for having caused these wounds, we don't want the responsibility of caring for them either. If we can somehow reason that the wound was self-inflicted, we can free ourselves from responsibility, allaying our sense of guilt. Some of this process is unconscious, a defense mechanism. We cannot believe that someone could suffer so much, and therefore, it must be her own fault. When I see a victim of any kind, including those who suffer from pain, it is only with great psychological effort that I do not join in the chorus of those heaping abuse.

Beyond this, I think we are protecting ourselves from a sense of our own vulnerability. To paraphrase John Bradford, "There but for the grace of God go I." It is hard to accept that we could someday be in the same shoes as the person with whom we are confronted. Blaming the victim mitigates our own fear of vulnerability. We tell ourselves that as long as we don't behave like a victim, we won't become one.

All these factors come together to make the management of chronic pain like a game of "hot potato" as each provider, frustrated and unable to manage the patient, transfers, or attempts to transfer, care to someone else. As the transfer occurs, labels are affixed to the patient. Communication between providers often begins with an apology, as if that will soften the blow. It goes on to assess whether the patient's problem is "real" or not. Once transfer is accepted, the responsibility is shifted, and the referring doctor often subtly closes the door on the patient. Each doctor extracts fees from the patient, perhaps helps him somewhat, and when the doctor runs out of options, he transfers responsibility to another provider. In the process the patient acquires more labels, many uncomplimentary, which add more reasons to fear the patient.

Physicians share an unspoken understanding that they are judged by the patients they see. Comprehensive pain management specialists, who have the courage to take responsibility for the pain patient, often wind up at the bottom of the medical hierarchy, valued only as the ones with the "asbestos gloves" who are willing to take the "hot potato" and protect everyone else from it. While surgeons and "interventionalists" (also called "procedural-ists"—physicians who primarily perform a physical intervention such as surgery, injecting painkilling drugs, or inserting a catheter to deliver drugs over time) extract large sums from patients that pad their status in the medical hierarchy, they often are unwilling to actually take responsibility for the pain patient. "I'm a surgeon, I operate, I don't prescribe . . ." Or, "I'm an interventionalist, I inject, I don't take care of the patient."

Yet the proceduralists are not willing to share the financial remuneration of their labor with those who do take responsibility. That would be bad business, and after all, medicine is a business. This added burden of responsibility without appropriate compensation for their efforts makes it even less desirable for other physicians to comprehensively manage these patients. No wonder the pain patient has trouble finding care. The system so created provides incentives to providers to take on only a part of the patient's problems, and no incentive for anyone to see the big picture—that is, to coordinate care.

The entire process frustrates patients and clearly communicates not only that their problem is not worthy of attention, but that they themselves are unworthy. This message obliterates their self-esteem, aggravating what is already an overwhelming problem.

Pain practitioners generally assume that the goal of pain management is to maximize the pain patient's physical, psychological, functional, and so-cial well-being despite his pain. They also assume that all those who come in contact with the patient share this goal—physicians, insurers, employers, lawyers, family members, and so on. Mostly, this is a myth. Perhaps I am cynical, but it seems to me that everyone—not only physicians—who comes in contact with those in pain first consciously or unconsciously assesses their own needs and then acts to maximize their own self-interest. If the patient happens to benefit, that is a pleasant side effect. Acting in one's self-interest is not necessarily destructive, but when one does this without any thought for the effects on others, the outcome is always destructive.

Each person's motives may be different, but they are shaped by similar considerations. One is how each views chronic pain, which will vary depending upon her level of education, openness to new ideas, and personal experiences. The second factor, not unrelated to the first, is how the patient in pain affects him or her, directly or indirectly.

Suppose I am a claims adjustor for an insurance company. I have no direct medical knowledge about pain through either personal experience or education, so I rely on someone who may or may not know much about pain, but is labeled an expert. I have no fund of knowledge to evaluate his advice, so I accept his judgment without question. I am told that my department must cut costs. My expert tells me that a particular chronic pain patient, whose claim is costing my department lots of money, has no "objective basis for his complaints." My motivation will be to deny care because my expert says this patient is milking the system, and I need to save money.

This very well paid expert shares my interest, which is to be more responsive to the needs of my employer than to those of the patient. We share a bias against the patient: the expert because he profits monetarily by rendering judgment against the patient (since experts who too often find in favor of the patient find themselves no longer being hired by the insurance company), and I because accepting the expert's opinion protects my bottom line and my job. So we take an action quite destructive to the patient. Would I feel differently if I had a similar pain disorder? What if the patient were my mother, or a close friend? In that case I might be more sympathetic to the plight of those in pain and more willing to help them navigate the same stormy waters that I had to navigate.

Or suppose I am a physician with a busy practice. The care of pain patients is time and labor intensive and fraught with controversy. The effort of caring for the chronic pain patient, when added to the needs of my other, more straightforward patients, may cause me great physical and psychological duress—in other words, burnout. Consequently, I may be more willing to listen to those who say the pain problem is merely psychological, beyond my level of expertise and better handled by a psychiatrist. Believing that, I may "turf" the problem to someone else, abandoning the patient.

In either scenario, as long as my line of reasoning benefits me, I will be inclined to ignore any information suggesting that another approach is more appropriate. Since opinions on the nature of chronic pain and its treatment vary so widely, everyone involved in the process is free to choose their own point of view. My premise is that each will choose the option that benefits his or her self-interest.

At some level, everyone who participates in managing a patient's pain must interact. Their points of view either clash or reinforce each other. In order to maximize their self-interest, each attempts to maximize his or her level of control. Some groups inherently have more power than others. For example, surgeons bring in more money to medical institutions, and as a result they have more clout in the decisions made by health-care organizations. Insurance companies control the flow of dollars to health-care providers, and thus they can control physician behavior with implied or actual threats to withhold payments. Managers of corporate medical practices control physicians' behavior by controlling salaries and job security. Some parties naturally align themselves with others to create a more powerful entity. For example, doctors may align themselves with insurance companies as experts to deny pain patients care, enriching themselves in the process. The battle rages. Though nobody really wins, some benefit more than others. Physicians benefit by providing expensive, fragmented care that maximizes their revenue and minimizes their responsibility. Insurance companies benefit by limiting care. Corporate medicine benefits by excluding care.

Eventually all parties reach an equilibrium, a status quo maintained by those with more power. Once this happens, changing it requires great effort, especially since making a change requires that all participants agree this is necessary. One participant may rock the boat, but is unlikely to have the power to tip it over. Many years ago, as described in chapter 1, I tried to create a system of coordinated care in my town for those who suffered from back pain. My plan required that competing entities work together to make the flow of patients through the system faster and more efficient. If the plan worked, the hospital would benefit through increased business, so they readily backed my proposal. The problem was that none of the individual physician or therapy groups saw any potential benefit. They feared losing patients to their competitors. They feared working with their competitors. In the end, the more powerful among these groups made sure the plan was defeated.

Among all these people, the one with the least power and the least control over the system of care that results is the pain patient. That is, the system is inherently biased against the patient, who is forced to go along with it. Sometimes the system works to the patient's advantage; sometimes it doesn't. The patient is thus very much like a poor man holding a cup on the street, begging for help.

If the system produces a maximally beneficial outcome for the pain patient, it is constructive. If instead it maximizes the benefits to the individual participants despite having a negative effect on the pain patient, it is destructive. In my observation, more often than not the system is destructive. Those who come into contact with chronic pain patients, physicians and nonphysicians alike, become frustrated by the patients' inability to get better. While the caregivers could accept their limitations and learn from them, most often they blame or ignore the victim, and the system fails the patient.

Is it possible to change this system to emphasize the patient's needs? The first step is to acknowledge the system's deficiencies. Then we can work to change the status quo. I believe that with more than a little altruism, that goal is achievable; although after twenty-eight years in the field I am skeptical, especially because of the "MBA-ization" of medicine, which means that the bottom line increasingly reigns supreme.

Around the beginning of the millennium, rather than admit defeat by the Goliath of pain standing before us, many in the pain community regrouped and offered a series of new strategies. In May 1998, the Federation of State Medical Boards (FSMB) recognized the rights of patients to receive opiate mediations for their pain and of prescribers to write prescriptions for these medications without undue regulatory pressure, and the FSMB published a set of guidelines for opiate prescribing. This policy was quickly accepted in various forms by all the states. In 1999, Congress, with the support of President Clinton, took this policy a step further and passed the Pain Relief Promotion Act. Its intent was to encourage practitioners to prescribe and administer controlled substances to relieve pain and discomfort. Practitioners were encouraged to treat pain aggressively. On October 31, 2000, as a result of the efforts of the Pain Care Coalition, Congress passed legislation providing for a "Decade of Pain Control and Research," to begin on January 1, 2001. Lawmakers recognized that pain management lacked a significant constituency at the federal level, and they hoped that this designation would bring a much-needed focus on pain to both the public and private sectors.[2]

So what exactly was the decade of pain control and research? The best way to answer this question is to say what it was not. It was not a unified attempt to better understand the phenomenon of pain. There was no specific agenda and no specific guiding force. In retrospect it is troubling to realize that this designation was largely window dressing with little substance, and that most people were unaware it ever happened.

What, if anything, did it accomplish? The answer requires exploring six major areas that those involved in the field of pain believe need to be addressed.

First, we need a better understanding of the neurobiology of pain. There is no question that we have come a long way in understanding how pain works in our bodies. That is a good thing.

Second, we need to use this understanding to develop novel and better treatments for pain. We have found many treatments that benefit laboratory mice, so I am sure they are quite happy. But there are no new treatments for pain in humans. What has changed is our use of two old remedies: opioids and cannabinoids. By the early 1980s, many in pain management realized that opioids were one of the few effective treatments for pain and recognized that it was inhuman to deny this treatment to people suffering with pain from terminal illness. By the mid-1980s, many in pain management suggested that opioids could be used to treat chronic pain from nonterminal illnesses.

After the release of the FSMB opioid policy, physicians' prescriptions of opioids skyrocketed, creating an epidemic of prescription drug abuse, misuse, and death from overdose. As a result, many individuals involved in medicine, public policy, and law enforcement began to question the use of these medications, and regulations were developed to curb this epidemic. Physicians, fearing the ramifications of prescribing—the loss of their license, arrest, and so on—became more reluctant to prescribe opioids. Although regulatory action against physicians was not common, the fear of a potential investigation and the adverse publicity it brings increasingly limited the availability of opioids for those who suffered.[3] In 2014 a law enforcement official, unaware that I was a pain specialist, told me, "Those pain doctors are the problem. They should be punished. Their patients don't know what pain really is." Such comments are chilling reminders of the risks physicians face in prescribing. The decade of pain control showed us that many people are helped by opioids and many are harmed. But we don't know how many fall into each category, and we don't know how to predict who will be helped or harmed. (Chapter 13 will discuss the use of opioids in more detail.)

Third, in order to better understand pain and develop new treatments, we need better research. Research costs money, and therefore better funding is needed. As of this writing (2015), funding for pain research is still lacking, and less than 1 percent of the NIH budget is spent on the symptom that most often brings a patient to the doctor.

Fourth, we need increased awareness of the problem of chronic pain among health-care professionals, legislators, and the general public—awareness that the problem exists and is worthy of being addressed. Many organizations in both the medical and the public sectors are involved in this endeavor. Still, it is not at all clear that any change has occurred in public perception. Few, if any, physicians or otherwise, knew that the decade for pain control even existed. I myself was unaware of it until 2005. In 2010, a number of pain specialists, including myself, were summoned to Washington to talk to our representatives about the Pain Care Policy Act (discussed following), which had recently been passed as part of the Patient Protection/Affordable Care Act (PP/ACA), even though the issue had little to do with health-care reform. Our goal was to make sure our representatives knew about this act, which had bipartisan support, so it would not be lost in the appropriations process. I talked with the health-care expert for each of my representatives. None had heard of the bill, and none knew anything about the issues facing the management of pain. A few were eager to learn, although they were more interested in what we thought about the PP/ACA.

Fifth, medical education is needed, yet at the end of the decade, there was no increase in the teaching of pain in medical schools. Most physicians still see chronic pain as a symptom, not a disease process.

Sixth, in order to help teach about pain and treat it, more health-care providers who specialize in pain management are needed. Unfortunately, there has been no increase in the number of trained pain specialists, and there still is a serious shortage. And since many pain specialists subspecialize in interventional pain management, there is an even more serious shortage of those who actually manage pain. An important reason for this problem is the bottom-line mentality I described above, resulting both in inadequate compensation for comprehensive pain management (as opposed to interventions) and in the medical-industrial complex's control over the provision of health-care services and the behavior of providers. Comprehensive management is left to undertrained primary care doctors, often with little support from specialists. The result of this continuing trend is to fragment care and to isolate those with chronic medical conditions such as pain.

The Pain Action Alliance to Implement a National Strategy (PAINS) is an organization whose goal is to bring together a consortium of leaders working in professional societies, patient advocacy organizations, policy groups, people with pain, payers, and the private sector in order to work together toward a common vision and mission. At the end of one meeting, I listened to one of the leaders lament how much energy had been expended, yet with very little accomplished. While she may have been correct, the reality is that much foundation work must be done before you can build anything, and you really don't see much until that work is accomplished. It is too early to say how the structure of pain management will be built in the United States, but the decade of pain control spawned some hopeful signs.

One is the National Pain Care Policy Act (H.R. 756), passed in 2009. It provided the following:

That the secretary of Health and Human Services, together with the Institute of Medicine of the National Academies, convene a conference on pain to develop a report that would increase the recognition of pain as a significant public health problem; evaluate the adequacy of the diagnosis, treatment, and management of chronic pain; identify barriers to appropriate pain care; and establish an agenda to reduce such barriers and significantly improve the state of pain care research, education, and clinical care in the United States.

That the director of the National Institutes of Health continue and expand, through the Pain Consortium, an aggressive program of basic and clinical research on the causes of and potential treatments for pain.

That the secretary can make awards of grants, cooperative agreements, and contracts to health professions schools, hospices, and other public and private entities to develop and implement programs to provide education and training to health-care professionals in pain care.

That the secretary establish and implement a national pain-care education outreach and awareness campaign to educate consumers, patients, their families, and other caregivers.

If carried out, this act will remedy many of the problems pain management faces today. It is not window dressing; it has substance. Good things are already happening. The Institute of Medicine report was completed in June 2011 and will serve as the basis for many of the next steps. The National Institutes of Health Pain Consortium was created. One of its actions was to designate twelve institutes as centers of excellence in pain education, charged with the task of developing, evaluating, and promoting pain management curriculum resources for students of many health disciplines. By 2015 the NIH had developed a draft National Pain Strategy intended to serve as the blueprint for meaningful socioeconomic change in pain management.

The future is hopeful, but for the time being not much has changed, and it is still a challenging time to be a pain practitioner. While the legislatures legislate, the courts adjudicate, and the magazines publicize, the pain practitioner remains before all as the emperor with no clothes. The Goliath of pain still mocks our attempts to destroy it. We mix and match our armamentarium in new and creative ways. We struggle to understand pain and all its nuances. We hope and pray for a better future. But for the time being, we remain relatively powerless.

Aside from highlighting our impotence, the decade of pain control and research may have had some beneficial effects. For the first time in history, a unified drive existed toward understanding the causes and treatments of what we know as pain. Next, and perhaps more important, it elevated the social status of the pain patient and the families and providers who have had the courage to stand by them. If the result of this decade is that the pain patient no longer has to sit on a medical street corner with a sign proclaiming, "Will work for pain relief," and instead can count on kind and compassionate care from all of society, then it will have accomplished something really spectacular—and we really will have given hope to the hopeless.

PART TWO

The Cast of Characters

All the world's a stage,
And all the men and women merely players;
They have their exits and their entrances, . . .

William Shakespeare, *As You Like It,* 2.7.139–41

It seems to me that we treat pain as a fantasy, a drama that plays itself out on a stage, one that we can laugh or cry about, but one that to many of us is not real. The curtain and the stage separate us from that painful reality, unless some cruel twist of fate intervenes, and we, like Alice in *Through the Looking-Glass,* are transported into that fantasy. Should that occur, then we become the lead character. We become the person in pain, the sufferer. While we lament our fate, we stare out into the audience and shout, "Help me! Please! God forgive me! I never believed anyone until it happened to me! Please, listen to me!"

One fact that has become apparent to me in my years of treating those in pain is that how we feel about chronic pain changes dramatically when we become the one suffering from it. The actions of many affect the person who suffers. They are the supporting cast, if you will. For each member of this cast, their role is merely an act, one they can escape from by removing their costume and heading off to the cast party or the golf course. As they retreat, they congratulate themselves on their performance. To the audience, the performance is over, and they can leave the theater and return to their daily lives. To the person in pain, the lead actor of this play, this was not a performance. There is no party. There is no costume to remove. Rather, this is reality. There is no escape. Initially, the crowds throng to the performance; but over time, they become bored with the "typecast" actor, and leave him or her alone, doomed to a vacant theater.

The drama of unremitting pain is a reality play. It is played out in the lives of millions of lead characters each day. The drama is a tragedy, one in which the lead character, the person in pain, does suffer alone. They long for recognition. They long for hope.

We are all characters in this play, whether we know it or not. Most of us, like my younger self, are totally unaware of our role. Others are aware, but long to get off the stage. Still others are involved, but they read from the wrong script, forever dooming the production. Finally, others put their whole heart and soul into the production and do their best to bring about a happy ending.

An inevitable end to any drama is the feared critique. Criticism alone may create great suffering! However, it may serve a great constructive purpose. Constructive criticism serves the purpose of informing us what we are doing right, what we are doing wrong, and what we can do better. It is my intent, at this time, to critique "the play" and its actors, of which I am one. The actors are not only individuals; in this analysis, many are groups such as regulatory agencies. They also include social entities such as opioids, opiates, and cannabinoids and the highly emotional public policies associated with each.

FOUR

The Patient

Making Lemonade When Stuck
with a Lemon

The Chinese have a very good proverb: the bird of sorrow has to fly;
but see that it does not nest in your mind.
Yes, suffering is unavoidable. So let us suffer cheerfully.
Mother Teresa, *Thirsting for God*

Even though the system gives pain patients the least amount of power, they are still very active players, and their actions play a great role in how they are viewed and treated, even though they are burdened with the albatross of the chronic pain stereotype.

In chapter 3, I described the four factors that define a patient's place on the "patient ladder." I also have identified three types of pain patients:

Type A patients have easily definable problems and respond appropriately to our treatments. After treatment (or spontaneously), they return to their normal level of function.

Type B patients have an overwhelming disability that severely compromises their function. However, their illness is easily definable. More specifically, there is an "objective test" that verifies their problem, such as a spinal cord injury. It is clear to everyone that there is no cure, and the treatment regimen and outcomes are easily definable and predictable.

Type C patients have a medical problem that, despite great effort and expense, defies all medical explanation and does not respond to appropriate, well-intended treatments. For the most part, the pain patients I am concerned with here are type C.

Type C patients are subcategorized as subtypes 1 and 2, primarily according to their degree of motivation to improve. Both types say they want to get better, but for whatever reason, the type C-2 patient is all talk and no action. Be aware that these patients are not making a conscious choice. Many of the motivating factors are unconscious, beyond the patient's clear understanding.

To further understand these different types of patients, we need to look at "secondary gain" and "secondary loss." These concepts predate Freud, who coined the terms; essentially they amount to "we reap what we sow." Every action brings about a consequence. A positive consequence is a secondary gain. A negative consequence is a secondary loss.

On the surface, the pain patient's balance sheet would seem to be skewed toward the negative. For most, that is true. The list of negative consequences of pain is long. Patients fear their pain. They fear the cause, they fear the consequences, and they fear the future. They don't understand their pain. Their efforts to accomplish sometimes trivial activities may result in a searing reminder of what hurts and what is limiting them. Those who are not in pain criticize their grimaces, their gestures, and their hobbling. These involuntary responses, which physicians call "pain behaviors," are their signal to the world of their distress. We criticize them for their braces and their collars, even though these devices shield at least part of the blow the pain delivers to their body and mind. As they seek to avoid their pain, they become more and more functionally withdrawn. Paradoxically, this behavior actually worsens their condition.

Those in pain fear their loss of control. They feel helpless. Previously independent, they are now doomed to rely on others, sometimes just for putting on a sock. They rely on others' generosity, which is often in short supply. They also must rely on people they don't know if they can trust: doctors, lawyers, and claims adjustors.

They lose their family role.

They lose their social role: their job.

They lose their financial independence.

They lose their avocational activities, what they liked to do for fun.

They often lose their family and friends.

They become reliant on fearsome drugs.

They lose their ability to sleep comfortably.

They lose their ability to engage in sex.

They lose their ability to play with their children and grandchildren.

They lose their community mobility when they cannot drive comfortably.

Patients grieve these losses and experience all the emotions grieving entails: fear, anger, depression, and denial. Denial allows them to persist in the belief that all will be better someday. However, clinging to that belief may cause them to avoid doing what they need to do to make things better now, if not physically, then functionally.

They face a daunting adaptation process. They grieve their old self and certainly do not welcome the new one. Adapt they must, but they are not sure they want to, especially since our medical culture has promised them a cure and tells them they do not have to suffer! To the extent that patients believe this, they see no reason to adapt and focus instead on finding the right treatment. Thus, the "doctor shopping" goes on. To the patients, the endpoint is clear: it is the point at which they have no pain. But supposing that endpoint is not realistic? Many patients are blue-collar workers who rely on their bodies for their jobs. When their bodies don't function, they have few options to provide for themselves. No wonder they become depressed, anxious, and even suicidal.

So why would anyone want to be like this? There are some reasons, which involve the secondary gains.

Many injured patients earn a disability income. This may constitute either a loss or a gain. For some patients, especially those who work seasonally, an injury at the end of the season is a bonus. For those who have little motivation to work, whatever income they lose because of their injury is more than offset by the freedom from work. In a similar way, an injury releases still other patients from the responsibilities of the world. Before their injury, they never had expectations placed on them and never learned how to set goals. Every responsibility in life was a burden to them. The sudden freedom from responsibility comes as a joy!

For those who desire to work but have limited options, the disability check actually may be a secondary loss. They want to work, but they rely on that check for survival, and the current disability system is set up so that a person who tries to work but fails risks losing everything. There is no guarantee they will get that disability check back. Many patients calculate that the cost of failure is higher than the potential benefits of trying, so they don't try. They can't afford to. So for them, the apparent secondary gain is actually a loss, a disincentive to seek what they want: work.

Some pain patients have never had any good relationships; they have never known love. Sometimes, the only thing they have known that even resembles love is pain. Those who were supposed to love them physically, mentally, sexually, or spiritually abused them. They see punishment as part of love and covet it. Then love comes to them from an unexpected source as people shower compassion on them. They learn to embellish their symptoms in order to receive more of this magic potion. Misguided sympathy enables them to stay disabled.

One consequence of pain functions simultaneously as both a gain and a loss: anger. When people suffer, they become angry at those whom they see as the cause of their pain and seek vengeance in any manner possible. In our society, that means a lawsuit. When they go to court, they are not necessarily looking for money. They want to punish. But most of the time, the supposedly guilty party had nothing to do with causing their misfortune.

Anger is a destructive force. Patients become so eager for retribution that they fail to concentrate on recovery. Whether consciously or unconsciously, they reason that if they improve, they will lose the grounds for their lawsuit, and at the same time the satisfaction of successful vengeance. In the end, they are the only ones who suffer. Any money they receive does little to help their pain, and they are left years behind in the recovery process. The ones who win are the patients' lawyers and health-care providers. Patients see the hoped-for court victory as a potential gain, but in reality it is a loss.

For each pain patient the scale tips one way or the other. If secondary loss predominates, I characterize them as type C-1. These patients, though overburdened by their pain, seek a better life; and there is hope that with a lot of physical and mental work, they can get better, at least functionally. Where there is a will, there can be a way, assuming that we, as a society, are willing to provide them the care and support they need without enabling their misbehaviors.

If secondary gain tips the scales, I characterize them as type C-2. There is not much hope for these people unless they can recognize the factors that motivate them and alter their behavior. These are the patients who drive their caregivers nuts. The providers try everything possible to help them, yet the patients return with a smile, proudly announcing that the treatment did not work.

Most patients will tell you they want to get better. In fact, I have never had a patient tell me otherwise. Even most type C-2 patients believe that they do, but most have limited insight into the unconscious motives that drive their behavior. For the astute practitioner, these patients will define themselves, but it takes time.

I must emphasize that for the majority of patients, secondary loss is a much bigger problem than secondary gain. In the literature on pain, though, one sees a predominance of attention paid to secondary gain. Why? Emphasis on secondary gain shifts the burden of responsibility onto the patient and off the doctor, the lawyer, the employer, the family, and the insurance company. It allows us to conclude that the problem is entirely the patient's fault, not ours, and certainly not the fault of our cause-and-effect medical model. In fact, the idea of secondary gain allows us to cling to that model. So we abandon the patient, exacerbating the downward spiral she experiences.

What can patients do to avoid the downward spiral? The basic steps are as follows:

First, recognize that they need to *take control and take responsibility* to the extent possible.

Learn to recognize passive and avoidant behaviors and to correct them.

Become physically, mentally, functionally, spiritually, and socially active in their own care.

Then, find a provider they trust. Together, patient and provider set up a series of goals designed to define the medical problem to the extent possible, treat it to the extent possible, and adapt to whatever change in lifestyle is imposed by the remaining disability.

It is necessary to grieve for a period. However, grieving is a way of looking back to the past. Patients also need to learn to look to the future, albeit an altered one, and take responsibility for creating it.

Patients also must learn to forgive. Forgiveness is the opposite of vengeance. They need to forgive themselves, those around them, and fate.

Whereas vengeance is destructive and holds them back, forgiveness is constructive and liberating. They cannot heal until they forgive.

They must learn to disregard the constant judgments they face. The lawyers, insurance companies, employers, and doctors will come and go, each rendering a judgment. However, none of them will ever live with the consequences of that judgment. Pain patients need feedback, but it must come from someone they trust, a person who can see the trees from outside the forest. It is crucial that pain patients find this person.

Finally, patients must have realistic expectations. Pain that has lasted for more than six months is less likely to be cured; however, people can learn to function despite pain, though it is important to proceed in baby steps. When a small goal is realized, one can look to the next goal. If someone's only goal is to be totally rid of the pain, he will never see any progress and will get discouraged. Discouragement feeds into the downward spiral of depression, which only aggravates the pain.

We all face barriers in life. Unending, persistent, chronic pain is a perpetual and unpleasant barrier that takes persistent, daily effort to overcome. In my career, I have found that the successful pain patients are not those whose condition is totally cured. Instead, they are the ones who, while always maintaining some reasonable degree of hope, take responsibility for their condition and their actions, and do what they can to move on.

Lot's wife looked back and was turned into a pillar of salt, a virtual monument to those stuck in the past. Those who adapt put the past behind them, where it belongs, and focus their attention on making a better future for themselves. With great effort and help from those around them, they make lemonade from the lemons they were stuck with.

FIVE

Family, Friends, and Community

*Of all the preposterous assumptions of humanity, nothing
exceeds most of the criticisms made on the habits of the poor
by the well-housed, well-warmed, and well-fed.*

Herman Melville, *Poor Man's Pudding and Rich Man's Crumbs*

Some time ago I was preparing a big meal, trying to show off my culinary skills for my sons and some of their friends. I zoomed about the kitchen, a man on a mission. The recipe called for doing several different steps simultaneously. Timing was critical. As I chopped some vegetables with a knife that was apparently sharper than I realized, struggling to keep up with the schedule, I became distracted by something cooking on the stove. I turned away from my chopping and neatly sliced off a piece of the tip of my index finger. Initially, I felt no pain, and the finger was not bleeding, so I assumed I had done no real damage.

Since I am an obsessive person, completing my mission was more important than attending to the wound, so I protected the finger with a paper towel and continued cooking. Soon the towel was saturated with blood. Nevertheless, I finished my tasks, just changing the paper towel as necessary. Only then did I attend to my finger.

I removed the paper towel and tried to assess the damage, though it was difficult because blood flowed every time I tried to dab the finger dry. I saw a large flap of skin, but did not think I would need stitches. Besides, a trip to the emergency room might adversely affect my gastronomical masterpiece. I thought it best to wash the wound and apply pressure until the bleeding stopped. As soon as the water hit the wound, I felt a searing pain, but I summoned the courage to continue. It took several hours, but eventually the bleeding stopped.

I bandaged the wound, but any attempt to put pressure on the tip of the finger caused pain. Worse, though, I really couldn't feel anything there. Buttoning a button or undoing a zipper became a challenge. I wondered if

I would be able to perform my job, since virtually every aspect of it required finely manipulating a needle with index finger and thumb.

At night, the wound throbbed, interfering with my sleep. Unable to pinch, unable to sleep, I became miserable. Short-term discomfort with a well-defined "finish line" is tolerable. Uncertainty is not. I began to worry that this insult would affect my long-term functionality and comfort.

The wound looked trivial, and I was sure that if I complained about my misery and disability I'd be dismissed as a whiner. Assuming my difficulty would be short-lived, I attended to my daily tasks as best I could. But as the days passed, I began to wonder what I would do if the feeling did not return to the tip of my finger. I worried that I had cut the cutaneous nerve and a phantom pain would develop (a pain experienced as being in a body part that has been lost). My cushion of security had been damaged, and I began to fear a future different from what I had expected and planned for.

The wound did heal, and now I am fine. Still, the experience gave me the sense of what it's like when your feeling of invulnerability is shattered, and your life is changed forever by pain and disability.

Think for a moment of a pain you have experienced that substantially affected your life, if only for a short time. How would you describe it and communicate your suffering to others? How did it affect your ability to function, to live your life the way you wanted to? To perform your job? To engage in the activities that define you, such as what you do for fun? How did others react to your plight, especially those who were counting on you? What if that pain had never gone away? How would those around you have reacted? How did you react when others complained to you about their problems, especially when their plight had an adverse effect on your own life?

Now think of someone you saw suffering, a person who had been healthy—especially someone whose suffering had an adverse effect on you. Perhaps it was someone at your job, whose inability to work increased your own responsibilities. How did you respond? How did you treat that person?

Saint Maria Faustina Kowalska is known as the "saint of divine mercy." Her message, thought to be born of divine inspiration, was one of mercy, not just of God toward His children, but also of His children toward each other. Elaborated in her diary, this message inspired the people of Poland during World War II. It also inspired her countryman, Pope John Paul II, known as the "great mercy pope," throughout his life.

Saint Faustina suffered physically and spiritually, and endured harsh treatment from her fellow nuns, who did not believe she was sick, but instead was malingering to avoid the rigors of religious life.[1] She wrote in her diary: "When I fell sick after my first vows and when, despite the kind and solicitous care of my Superiors and the efforts of the doctor, I felt neither better or worse, remarks began to reach my ears which inferred [sic] that I was making believe. With that, my suffering was doubled."[2] Saint Faustina died of tuberculosis at age thirty-three.

In my experience, we often think of people who suffer as "wimps" and assume that if we were in their shoes, we would respond much more courageously (although when we are the ones in pain, we respond just as they do, while somehow assuming that we are different—that our problem is worse than theirs and we are more courageous). Unfortunately, this attitude is counterproductive, if not harmful, for, as Saint Faustina stated, "Those who live with such a person should not add external sufferings; for indeed, when the soul's cup is full, the little drop we may add to it may be the one drop too much, and the cup of bitterness will overflow. And who will answer for such a soul? Let us beware of adding to the suffering of others."[3]

The behavior of those in chronic pain is often counterproductive as well. At some level of their psyche, they reason that if they can more effectively communicate how they suffer, others will listen. They therefore learn to exaggerate their pain behavior. The extent to which they do so depends on the circumstances.

Many people with chronic pain choose to hide their suffering because, despite their suffering, they may still believe that chronic pain is a personality disorder and not something real. As long as they remain silent, they can pretend it does not exist, or that it will get better on its own. Few people realized how much my mom suffered because her smile hid her pain so effectively. In fact, my mother-in-law knew her for four years before she became aware of my mom's illness. Other people hide their pain because they fear the response of those around them. The pain sufferer remembers how he responded to the suffering of others before he developed chronic pain himself; or he has seen how others berate, ignore, and abandon people with chronic pain, and he is afraid of being treated the same way.

This abandonment of people in pain occurs even in a medical setting, and especially when the health-care professionals have nothing to offer. The physician will assure the person that she is just fine. The assumption is that in the absence of "objective signs," she must be fine. The reality that she is not is irrelevant. In essence, the physician just walks away, perhaps handing her a "boo-boo bunny" in the form of a useless prescription as she leaves. I am amused by how difficult it is for health-care professionals to use the word "pain." Instead, they prefer "discomfort," a word that minimizes the effect of the person's suffering on the caregiver. But sugarcoating the word does little to alleviate that suffering or communicate any understanding of what she is experiencing.

I see this scenario played out every day. When I inject spines, I frequently inflict pain. When I feel and see the patient wince, I have a natural inclination to just ignore it and move on. But I have taught myself that I can cement our relationship merely by acknowledging that this hurts. No matter how far behind I am, no matter how much I may be struggling with the procedure, I always stop and ask, "How are you doing?" If the patient says he's fine, I insist, "No you're not. People don't jump like that for nothing." Acknowledgment is powerful. It allows the person an open door to communicate his pain, and treatment can only begin when one acknowledges the scope of the problem. Asking only perfunctorily how a person is doing closes the door and communicates to the person in pain that you do not understand, do not care, and do not believe.

Together, we find out if there is something we can do to make the procedure less painful. If there isn't, I honestly tell him that the procedure may hurt, but only for a while, and I will take all steps necessary to minimize his discomfort. My goal is to restore as much of the patient's sense of control as possible. Letting him know he is not alone helps tremendously. When we feel lost, this sense of loneliness only aggravates that feeling of being out of control.

There have been times when I was not so empathetic. But I have learned that when I ignore a patient's plight, perhaps because I am more focused on where I need to be at 5:00 PM than on being with her right now, all I do is create a greater problem. I create an agitated patient. If I choose to attend to the agitation that I helped create, I wind up spending more time with that patient than I would have otherwise. But if I ignore the agitation, I know I will spend even more time at 2:00 AM listening to her when the loneliness of nighttime intensifies her fears, or during other visits when I must undo the damage done, or when I hear from her attorneys several months later, or when I hear from other people what a rotten doctor I am.

When people in pain seek help and acknowledgment, the way caregivers respond has a dramatic impact on the quality of their lives. We make the assumption that they are "OK" only so we can avoid the responsibility of helping them. But denying their plight creates a bigger problem, not just for those in pain, but also for society as a whole, which is stuck with the burden of problems that could have been prevented if only someone had taken a moment to extend a compassionate hand.

I have noticed that many long-standing pain patients exhibit much more dramatic pain behaviors when in the presence of others to whom they wish to communicate their plight. When such communication is not needed, they don't exhibit these behaviors. The longer a pain patient's suffering goes unacknowledged, the more dramatic these behaviors become. The problem is that as the drama increases, the less likely the patient is to elicit the compassion she craves. Health-care professionals use such labels as "symptom amplification," "catastrophizing," and "somatization" to describe such behaviors. These labels merely serve to mask our own denial. When such pain behavior occurs, it becomes almost impossible to ignore. The response among would-be caregivers is often violent opposition. Some people, convinced the individual needs help, take on the role of the Good Samaritan. Others are convinced it is all in the person's head and she needs to suck it up. Arguments ensue, with each party convinced he is correct, fueled by preconceived notions and past experiences. Their unwillingness to bend only aggravates the problem. This is referred to as "staff splitting," in which, rubbing salt into the patient's wounds, the caregiver assumes that the patient is the cause of the pain. In adversarial situations, we too often seek a single cause and effect, ignoring the complexity of the situation and often ignoring our own potential role in creating it. We seek to blame someone else, who often turns out to be the one at the bottom of the hierarchy.

The problem the pain patient creates is also the result of the variance in individual responses to pain. Some people are stoic to an extreme. They will ignore pain and disability to their detriment, and often to the detriment of those around them. Others are incapacitated by minimal trauma.

Sometimes it is not the physical insult that is the problem, but rather the emotional meaning. The bumps and bruises of physical abuse may heal, but the emotional trauma never does. Perhaps this explains why those who have suffered emotional as well as physical trauma overwhelm the ranks of those in chronic pain.

The first step each of us must take, health-care provider or otherwise, is to acknowledge the problem. We must be willing to take a break from our own lives and attend to the needs of those in pain. We must accept their experience of what they are feeling and put our own judgments aside. Our questions must be open-ended to allow them to convey what they feel, even if this entails periods of silence. We must never answer the questions for them. Second, we must take our own pulse. Most destructive reactions begin with a desire to treat our own fears before attending to the needs of the suffering. Only by taking a deep breath and acknowledging our fears can we put them aside to focus on the one in need.

Let me illustrate. I love the desert. Once, traveling from New Hampshire to San Diego, I had a few extra days, so I flew to Phoenix in order to drive through the desert to San Diego. As I drove out of the Phoenix airport, I was greeted with an unseasonably cold and windy, yet sunny day. As I approached the mountains, the wind picked up. Signs cautioned truckers about the wind danger and urged them to drive slowly.

I became lost in the beauty of the day and the surrounding landscape, but my reverie was broken suddenly by a large suv towing a camper, which flew by me at what seemed an unsafe speed. Just after it passed, the driver lost control, and the camper began fishtailing. Soon the car was off the road and the camper overturned. Miraculously, the truck remained upright.

As I slowed down, I had a choice to make. Even though I had allowed myself plenty of time to get to San Diego, I was still on a schedule, and I was not in any mood to have my plans ruined by the stupidity of someone whose misfortune was clearly the result of their own poor choice. But I also thought of the stupid things I had done that created problems for myself and others. I thought of the kindness of others who had taken the time to assist me. In effect, I "took my own pulse" and, choosing to pay forward the kindnesses of others, stopped to help. Many other cars passed, rubbernecking but not stopping, perhaps assuming everything was ok. Only one other person stopped to help.

I got out of my car and rushed to the truck. Its occupants were an elderly couple. The woman had been driving. I was shocked that she had been going 80 mph in such poor conditions, but right now that was irrelevant. We all make mistakes. She had gotten out of the truck and was frantic. She needed kindness, consolation, and help.

I quickly ascertained that both members of the couple were physically fine, but mentally shaken. She was much more concerned about her cats, which were in the camper, and begged me to get them. After some effort I got the cats out, at the cost of a laceration on my palm. Soon, the police arrived. Everyone was safe, and after exchanging addresses and hugs, I was on my way. Several weeks later, I received a letter of thanks and some canned salmon from the woman, who said I was her "Good Samaritan" and had restored her faith in humanity.

In fact, my choice to help benefited me just as much, for it helped restore a sense of faith in myself. Had I kept going, my life would have been no better or worse. But I feel it has been infinitely enriched because I did take the time to check in with myself and stop.

I have a sign over my office desk that says: "What would Jesus do if he were here right now?" Whenever I want to run away from whatever faces me, I look at it and think. This gives me the courage to put my cares aside for fifteen or twenty minutes and attend to the needs of the person in the examining room. Each time I do this, I am rewarded with much more than money and prestige.

While acknowledging one's own feelings, it is also important to acknowledge the uniqueness of the sufferer. We all come into new experiences with preconceived notions shaped by past experiences. It is important to note that the situation and experiences of the person we seek to help may be quite different from ours. It is often difficult to avoid superimposing our own notions, but in order to be truly helpful, we must approach the other with an open mind.

I once had a patient with a standard whiplash event who complained of persistent neck and arm pain of a type consistent with a specific nerve pattern. However, her MRI was read as normal, and her caregivers chose to believe the MRI rather than the patient, even though we know that whiplash trauma may not show up on x-rays for years after an injury and that the pain from it may persist. They insisted nothing was wrong with her. They did not say so explicitly to her face, but in effect she was told that the problem was all in her head. The more her problems were dismissed, the worse her complaints became.

What was not apparent was that she had been viciously physically and verbally abused in the past. She had sought help for the emotional scars that resulted, but her requests fell on deaf ears, provoking a steady crescendo in her calls for help, which finally could not be ignored when the abuse became physical and the bruises and broken bones were obvious. While the physical wounds healed, the emotional ones did not. Now she was crying again for help, and her caregivers, with their irrational belief in the infallibility of the MRI, refused to listen. This only provoked her to cry louder.

As I came to know her better, I began to question the wisdom of those caregivers. Her pain fit a pattern well described in the literature, and I became convinced it was real. I explained that her pain was caused by a damaged cervical disc. I was amazed what a therapeutic effect this simple action had. Her pain behaviors lessened, as did her anxiety and her depression, even though I did nothing to cure her problem. Within two years, her MRI showed an abnormality in her neck right where the literature predicted it would be.

I am convinced that had her early caregivers acknowledged the reality of her problem rather than dismissing it, she would have suffered less and had a better outcome. At the same time, there was no cure; she would have to suffer. Most inspiring of all about her story is that her very physically able husband stood by her all this time, never questioning the legitimacy of her problems. His behavior inspired and humbled me.

It is also important to be versatile in offering solutions. While we tend to disdain those who maximize their problems, those who minimize them may create worse problems for everyone by not addressing their condition when a solution is possible. How often do we hear of people who ignore the obvious signs of a developing cancer and die needlessly because they did not seek treatment when it was possible? Ignoring the signs and living in denial only make the problem more difficult to manage later, not just for the sufferer, but also for everyone around him or her. So it is important that minimizers be confronted.

Maximizers also need to be confronted and taught that their behaviors are counterproductive, though in an encouraging way. Compassion does not always mean being kind and gentle. Changing a pattern of behavior often requires a stern reality check. But "tough love" is quite different from abandonment. It resembles the behavior of a coach who knows what an athlete needs to get ready for an event, who will accept nothing less than the athlete's best, and who will not allow the athlete to give up. The coach remains by the athlete's side, encouraging, sometimes quite forcefully. The challenge is to push, but only hard enough, since the limits of those in chronic pain are lower than other people's and need to be respected. We find out where those limits lie through a gradual approach.

Achieving a better level of function in the face of pain requires energy and commitment, which the patient must summon for him- or herself. Trying to do this for him only enables his destructive behaviors. Tough love is tough! It is much easier to do it for the person. But I have heard of many caregivers who did steadfastly push a person in chronic pain toward a goal. Great pain and suffering was involved, not just for the affected person but also for the caregiver, who could hardly bear to watch. Maybe days, weeks, months, even years later, the goal was met. Only then was the caregiver willing to admit that she cried herself to sleep wondering if pushing so hard was the right thing to do. This is why helping a person with chronic pain sometimes requires a lot of faith.

The Family: On the Front Line

> The Family is a haven in a heartless world.
>
> Christopher Lasch, *Haven in a Heartless World: The Family Besieged*

It is one thing to periodically visit a patient in chronic pain. It is quite another to live with one and witness her daily suffering. It is very painful to sit by and watch someone suffer, especially when you know there is little you can do to help. Often your presence alone is of great support. However, being present with this sense of impotence creates great anxiety in pain patients' family members. The urge to run away is strong. Yet love and support are the greatest gifts we can bestow on the afflicted. It is well known that the one factor that predicts a successful outcome for rehabilitation from any disabling illness is a strong, supportive family. That is also true in pain medicine. The family and the patient must truly be one and treated as such by the caregivers. Everyone involved in the patient's care needs to understand that it takes great courage to stay and care for the pain patient. Sometimes that courage will wax. Sometimes it will totally fade away.

How the family responds to the challenge of chronic pain is, once again, dependent on their understanding of pain and the nature of their self-interest. Most often, the family shares the same understanding or misunderstanding of pain as the patient. They learn about pain through what they read in magazines or on the Internet and through personal experience. Most people have little understanding of chronic pain. They know that most people who experience pain get better, and they fear pain that does not get better because they think it indicates either a deadly disease or a psychosomatic illness. That is what the experts tell them, and it takes great courage and intuition to believe otherwise. As long as the family maintains those beliefs, they will be of no help to themselves or to the pain patient. It is crucial that they become educated about the pain process and what the long-term ramifications may be. Still, even the most educated family members will tend to act in their own self-interest. Their response to the pain will lie somewhere within the extremes of abandonment and overindulgence. Neither is healthy. Helping them find the "happy medium" is critical if pain management is to be successful.

Chronic pain creates a dramatic change in the function of the family that poses a mental and spiritual challenge for each member. The family may lose income. Medical bills mount. The family can't do all the things they used to do. Others must take on the patient's previous duties. The family must adapt or dissolve. All members feel the stress of this challenge, and how they respond to it will determine whether they stay. If they stay, the nature of their response will determine whether they are a help or a hindrance to the patient. The greatest gift they truly can provide is love. However, pain stresses the bonds of that love.

Like the patient, each family member grieves the losses. Often they deal with these losses by denying the severity of the problem and its permanence. In the beginning, they may seek comfort in denial. Over time, they begin to realize that things will never be the same again, at least as long as they remain with the person in pain. They long for the old life. While the patient is stuck with the pain, the family members are not. All they have to do is abandon the patient and start all over. For many people this urge is irresistible. I have seen it happen often, with disastrous effects on those in pain. One patient woke up one morning and found a note from her spouse informing her that he could not take the pain and its effects on their lives anymore and was leaving her. The next time she saw him was in divorce court. Others do the opposite. They readily adopt a "soft-love" stance and cater to the patient's every whim. This enabling encourages the patient to lead a passive existence, which is quite contrary to the goals of successful pain management. The goal is activity and responsibility for one's life, not passivity and responsibility shifting.

Most families' behavior lies somewhere in between enabling and abandonment, but all experience the overwhelming stress. We can handle only so much stress before we break. Families vary in how close they are to this breaking point. Some require very little to put them over the edge; for example, a workers' compensation denial or hearing can be devastating.

To function properly, the family needs both education and support. It is also crucial that they be involved in the treatment process. The caregivers must correct misperceptions and teach the family about what the patient is experiencing. Family and patient should be educated about the nature of the patient's condition, what treatments are available, and what the long-term expectations may be. They need to know that the health-care provider and the entire "cast of characters" are sensitive to their needs. They need instruction on what the patient should and should not be doing, what help he or she may need, and what kind of help is appropriate. They need to be reassured that sometimes the patient needs "tough love"—no matter how tough it is to provide.

Many family members, especially enablers, feel guilty about attending to their own needs. That creates a separate sense of loss in caregivers. It is important that they acknowledge this sense of guilt, but equally important to get a respite now and then. That may mean time away, or an enjoyable family or personal activity. If you don't take care of yourself, you can't take care of someone else.

Family members need to develop a capacity for introspection. Living in the presence of unrelieved pain creates powerful emotions, which carry a hidden meaning. Failure to understand those emotions can make for bad choices. Introspection often requires a sounding board, someone who can objectively stand back and explain the situation to the family member. That is where counseling and support groups come in. The family must understand that it is not a sign of weakness to ask for help. The family is a system. When stress builds up within a system, it needs to be let out, just as steam is let off from a hot water heater. If it is not, it builds up and can destroy the family. A caring outsider can go a long way toward allowing a family to "blow off steam."

How the family functions as a unit, how much it loves, and how intact it remains will often determine both its own strength and the strength of each member in the face of adversity. We get by with a lot of help from our friends, and there should be no better friends—friends we can always count on—than our own family members. Knowing they will always be there for us is powerfully therapeutic. People around the family can help strengthen their bond, for even families in crisis can remain intact through great stress when showered with love and support from others. Pain management providers need to remember what huge burdens chronic pain and the resulting disability are for a family. A wrong word or impression can destroy this basic therapeutic unit. A moment taken to provide an encouraging word can lessen the stress and provide inspiration for a lifetime.

My mom suffered with chronic pain throughout her life. My dad, who had always enjoyed wonderful health, had every opportunity to run away. He never did. Quite the opposite—he was always there for her. His example, born out of love, stabilized our family and showed us how to live our lives not just for ourselves, but also for each other.

This is something every person involved in the care of the chronic pain patient needs to think about. Actions taken in our own self-interest have a domino effect, with ramifications far beyond our own gratification that are often negative. They unnecessarily stress the person who is suffering—who, as Saint Faustina wrote, often cannot handle even a little additional stress. If the stress breaks the sufferer, the family dissolves, and the pain patient is truly left alone. By contrast, a kind word, an acknowledgment of suffering, recognition of the challenges faced by the entire family, momentarily putting aside one's own needs and those of the bottom line for the needs of a suffering fellow human being boosts the family, and with it, the hopes and function of the patient.

Saint Faustina made a curious observation, which many of us would struggle with. She wrote: "In suffering we learn who is our true friend."[4]

Perhaps that is why those in pain are often so lonely: because those they thought of as friends and caregivers chose to walk away. Saint Faustina challenged all such caregivers with these words: "Help me, that my ears may be merciful, so that I may give heed to my neighbors' needs and not be indifferent to their pains and moanings."[5]

SIX

The Physician and the Pain Patient

Poorly Equipped for the Role?

The eternal providence has appointed me to watch over the life and
health of Thy creatures. May the love for my art actuate me at all
times; may neither avarice nor miserliness, nor thirst for glory or for
a great reputation engage my mind; for the enemies of truth and
philanthropy could easily deceive me and make me forget my lofty
aim of doing good to Thy children.

May I never see in the patient anything but a fellow creature in pain.

Grant me the strength, time, and opportunity to always correct
what I have acquired, always to extend its domain; for knowledge is
immense and the spirit of man can extend infinitely to enrich itself
daily with new requirements.

Today he can discover his errors of yesterday and tomorrow he can
obtain a new light on what he thinks himself sure of today. Oh, God,
Thou has appointed me to watch over the life and death of Thy creatures; here am I ready for my vocation and now I turn unto my calling.

The Oath of Maimonides

In the traditional medical model, the physician has primary responsibility for the care of the patient—including responsibility for easing suffering
and doing no further harm. Society recognizes the doctor as the expert on
the diagnosis and management of pain. More than 70 percent of all patients'
complaints to a doctor are for a symptom of pain. Since there are nearly three
hundred million people in the United States, and only four-thousand-plus
trained pain physicians, it is incumbent on *all* physicians to be knowledgeable in pain management. People assume that all physicians receive
adequate training in this subject, but this assumption is not valid. In fact,
a large number of U.S. medical schools do not teach pain at all, and an
equally large number devote fewer than five hours over four years to this

topic. Veterinary students receive more education about pain than medical students.[1] This fact alone creates a crisis in pain management.

Despite their limitations, most physicians are caring people who really desire not just to ease suffering and do no harm, but to go beyond that and *remove* suffering. For the chronic pain patient, this goal is not possible; and that sets up the first of several conflicts between doctor and patient, since the patient wants the pain to be removed. A second conflict arises when it becomes apparent that well-intentioned therapies based on the model of cause and effect may actually harm the patient. That is, when both physician and patient assume that pain is merely a signal that can be turned off—rather than a signal gone awry—the physician will pursue a series of treatments in a futile attempt to find a switch that shuts the pain off. The inability to achieve a cure frustrates the doctor and patient and unnecessarily prolongs rehabilitation and adaptation. The standard model ignores the fact that many factors contribute to the pain, and all must be addressed. We need a paradigm shift in our treatment model, which means that many bio-psycho-functional-social problems must be acknowledged and addressed.

A third conflict is that medicine has become a business, as this chapter explains in detail. A physician who seeks to be altruistic when treating a patient with a complicated problem does so at the peril of the bottom line. This is less of an issue for physicians who own their own practice, but those who are employed have less control. If the patient's problem fits nicely into a fifteen-minute spot and is well reimbursed, the conflict between altruism and the bottom line is minimized. But the pain patient rarely fits into this mold. All medical investigations begin with the history. In fact, 90 percent of the investigation comes from the history. But merely examining the body is insufficient. All factors—biological, psychological, functional, and social—play a role and must be examined. Such a broad examination does not lend itself well to the fifteen-minute office visit. Thoroughly investigating the pain patient takes time and costs money.

So how does the physician respond to these conflicts? *The first problem to tackle is understanding what pain is.* As we have seen, that is not easy. There are many opinions in the voluminous literature, but few facts and little consensus. What is more, there is virtually no support in the literature for any of the myriad treatments available. Thus there is no "party line" that the rank-and-file doctor and the public can rely on. This makes the physician's job daunting and confusing.

Like anyone else, physicians desire security. They look for a comfortable paradigm to guide them and choose the one that is most appealing. However, their choice is not always guided by rational thought. The most common way to choose a paradigm is to "follow the leader." We pick an expert we feel comfortable with and follow him or her, sometimes to our peril, or worse, our patient's.

I once watched a nature show in which the alpha male of a walrus community climbed to the top of a cliff and, for no apparent reason, jumped to his death. All the males blindly followed him. It was gruesome to witness the pile of writhing, fractured bodies at the bottom of the cliff. In the human world we are also likely to follow a leader blindly, assuming that this person is omnipotent and has all the answers. Often physicians choose to follow a professor from their medical school who guided them. Sometimes they choose an instructor or an author. Often such leaders have great charisma or power. They seem to have thought through all the problems and possess all the solutions.

Sometimes the expert is chosen merely out of convenience. The doctor, eager to be rid of a problem he does not understand, is more than willing to transfer care of the patient to someone who is willing to take the case, even if that person does not have the expertise. The rank-and-file doctor tells the patient: "You don't have to suffer. I have someone who can help you." He sends the patient off to follow the Yellow Brick Road to Oz, or the pain clinic, where she is subjected to innumerable invasive procedures and pharmacologic interventions with no predicable outcome. Sometimes the patient gets better, but that does not mean she is cured.

But supposing we discover that our professors are wrong? Do we continue to blindly accept what they profess? Or do we take the necessary, yet difficult, step of questioning our paradigm? In my experience the best teachers readily acknowledge their limitations and remain open to new thought. However, in the medical world this type of leader does not abound. Many people who are respected as leaders actually have no knowledge about pain; but oblivious to their limitations, they seem more than happy to lead others astray. Still, they may have great power, which guarantees many followers. Appearance counts too. They wear nice suits, drive big cars, occupy chairmanships, and make lots of money for themselves, their practices, and their hospitals. Often their success is not due to their work with patients, but rather, because of their skill at politicking. The skills that bring success in politics are not necessarily those that make a thoughtful, competent physician. To the extent that this type of "expert" drives the pain paradigm, the patient and the system suffer. Fortunately, there are many competent, humble people in the medical world who have much to share and do have the patient's needs at heart. The trick, for the rank-and-file doctor, is figuring out who they are.

As a substitute for a single expert or school of thought, physicians also may look to evidence-based medicine (EBM) for guidance. EBM is best described as "the conscientious, explicit, and judicious use of current best evidence in making decisions about the care of individual patients."[2] A thorough discussion of EBM is beyond the scope of this book, but awareness of its limitations is crucial for understanding how its use may adversely affect care for chronic pain patients. The definition quoted above implies that there is a body of medical evidence that can be used to produce a medical algorithm (an organized, stepwise plan of care) for each patient problem. It also implies that interpretation of the evidence base must be modified by the unique biological, functional, psychological, and social factors each patient presents. Not only is the initial assumption that there is a definitive evidence base for most medical problems false, but complex medical problems such as chronic pain involve the interaction of a multitude of factors, while EBM looks at the simple cause and effect of only a few variables at best. A 2007 assessment of 1,016 review articles from the most systematic evidence base in the world, the Cochrane Collection (which reviews many questions and interventions about various medical topics) found that only 44 percent of the interventions discussed in the review articles were likely to be beneficial, 7 percent were likely to be harmful, and 49 percent were inconclusive in that the evidence did not support either benefit or harm. The assessment recommended that 96 percent of the interventions needed further research.[3]

I conclude that there are four types of questions in the medical literature:

1. Those that have been answered beyond a reasonable doubt. Assessment of the Cochrane data suggests these are rare.

2. Those that have been addressed, but require further study, and for which there are no firm guidelines.

3. Those that lack guidelines because they have never been studied sufficiently.

4. Those that, because of their complexity, will never be studied satisfactorily.

The questions discussed here are types two, three, and four.

Despite the large holes in our knowledge base, insurers and academicians increasingly demand that physicians making clinical decisions refer to an evidence base that, especially in the case of chronic pain, is essentially nonexistent. Where does this leave the practitioner? Medicine remains an art, a mixture of study, experience, teamwork, and common sense. While EBM has some value, it is merely a tool that aids but does not supplant the art of medical practice. Failure to acknowledge the limitations of EBM can harm those who suffer from complex problems such as chronic pain.

Another problem that pervades the health-care community is overconfidence in our technology. What we can do medically for many ailments is amazing. However, in the world of chronic pain, little has changed. Five thousand years ago, there was opium, willow bark, and needles. In the twenty-first century, we are blessed with opium and its derivatives, willow bark and its derivatives, and all sorts of needles. Moreover, the degree of confidence we place in our technologies to diagnose and treat pain is not warranted. While MRIS, CT scans, PET scans, and EMGS are wonderful, they don't tell us if someone does or does not hurt. While we have wonderful surgeries for all sorts of problems, outcome rates for surgeries related to chronic pain have not really improved all that much. After decades of investing billions of dollars in all sorts of new and improved pain medications, we are back to morphine and ibuprofen.

We promise solutions we cannot deliver, which creates a crisis of honesty. Do we do this consciously, or are we just blind? I think there is a little of both going on. I once attended a surgical meeting where speaker after speaker presented the results of their surgical procedures, some very invasive and complicated. Each speaker touted a 90 percent success rate. I will never forget the last one. He ended his presentation with the line: "And, of course, we had a 90 percent success rate."

"Of course?" I thought.

He was talking about multilevel fusion spine surgery. Nobody has a 90 percent success rate with that procedure. Several years later, armed with much more experience and after having observed a more realistic 50 percent success rate for that same procedure, I asked a very well-known colleague how those surgeons came up with that 90 percent success rate.

He said, "They are either dumb, blind, or lying."

Early in my career, I read a study on cervical (neck spine) fusion that claimed a 90 percent success rate. I dissected the study and concluded that it was well done and its conclusions valid. Because of that study, I referred a number of patients for cervical fusion. At best, 50 percent got better. It was a classic case of following the walrus. I know my intentions were honest. Were those of the investigator who published that study? I am not sure.

Recall that Mr. Smith's surgeon assured him that he had a 99 percent chance of cure with the proposed surgery. I did not make that up. I have known several surgeons who promised such results. Where did that number come from? Certainly not reality.

After twenty-eight years, I have, of necessity, become skeptical and cynical. Just because it's in the literature doesn't make it accurate. I have developed the "Nagel 80 percent rule." If any pain researcher promises a better than 80 percent success rate with any treatment, I don't believe him or her. The problem is that it took many years of treating pain before I became that cynical. There are many out there, providers and patients, who continue to be misled by exaggerated claims.

Still another problem is created by what is known as the "law of parsimony." As students, physicians are taught to seek one cause for a problem, and one solution—a magic bullet. But that is clearly an inappropriate approach to disability in general and chronic pain in particular. The magic bullet does not exist, nor will it ever. Because chronic pain is a complex phenomenon, each patient requires a unique approach and a complex solution. Since "one size fits all" does not work, it is useless for a nonspecialist to research the success rates of an individual treatment. This reality further hampers communication between the pain specialist and the nonspecialist. Doctors like to know what approaches have a high cost-benefit ratio. They want a single number indicating what that ratio is. For the pain patient, that information is not available.

The reality is that treatments must be looked at not in isolation, but in combination with other treatments, and this is not easy to do. A "good" outcome for any single treatment may be only a 50 percent success rate, which would not be considered good in any other area of medicine but may be excellent in the world of pain. Perhaps a series of concurrent treatments could accomplish a better result. How does one study this and the relative effect of each individual therapy? These considerations further complicate the understanding of pain and its management, especially for the nonspecialist physician.

A related problem is that chronic pain patients are frustrating to treat and generate an unpleasant feeling of impotence in the physician, setting up a vicious cycle. The patient grows frustrated as each treatment fails and becomes more demanding, requiring more time and progressively more expensive and invasive investigations and treatments, which frequently do not resolve the problem. Mutual frustration creates friction between doctor and patient, which leads to them blaming each other. At this point, the relationship is poisoned, potentially to everyone's harm.

Making things still more difficult is the fact that pain and the psychological response to it are moving targets. Because of the nature of both plasticity and grieving, the pain system is constantly changing and adapting or maladapting. Timing in therapies may be critical. Some treatments may work well at some points in time, but not at others. The patient's pain system may adapt or become tolerant to a certain treatment, necessitating rotation to another. These changes further complicate the assessment and management of these patients. All these factors create fear in physicians, which adversely affects the entire process of treating pain.

Physicians fear feeling helpless. They are used to being in charge, and it is difficult to admit they may not be, that they may not have a solution for the patient's problem. In such a situation it would be best to acknowledge our limitations. If instead we pretend to have a solution, we wind up subjecting our patients to invasive, risky, and expensive procedures that may not have a reliable chance of success and may create even greater problems for the patient. In my experience, feigning knowledge is usually an unconscious behavior, which makes it even more dangerous, because we cannot act in a clear-minded and objective manner when we are unaware of our motives. We wind up misleading the patient and unnecessarily delaying adaptation.

Physicians fear their inability to measure pain objectively. Tests of the body structure correlate poorly with complaints of pain. How does one measure pain then? You have to talk to the patient and listen to him. How frightening. What do you do if you don't trust the patient, especially when the paradigm you rely on is not consistent with what the patient is telling you?

Physicians fear prescribing powerful drugs for chronic pain patients. The use of opiates and opioids has a clear endpoint in most patients with acute pain. With chronic pain patients, there are no endpoints, and after a certain point, these drugs may cause harm. Opioids do create addiction. They do create tolerance, and they do create dependency. They do create paradoxical hypersensitivity, meaning the more medication one takes, the worse the pain gets. The problem is that they also help. When does help turn to harm? The answer is rarely clear. Physicians fear harming a patient so much that they may err on the side of withholding drugs that may be simultaneously helpful and harmful. That creates a problem for the patient.

Physicians fear regulatory agencies. While regulatory agencies stress that punitive actions are rare, investigations are not. Investigations go on for months and years. They cost money and are stressful, especially to a physician whose only crime was to try to help a fellow human being in need. The fear is compounded by the knowledge that physicians have been tried in criminal court, and some have been convicted. While this outcome may be rare, the fact that it happens creates a legitimate fear in all physicians.

Physicians fear going to court for their patients and being the "big brother" standing up for them against the insurance companies, the employer, the courts, and the lawyers. Though most physicians who treat pain patients never see the inside of a criminal court, nearly all spend time in a civil court, defending either themselves or their patients. In this odd world, a physician may be sued for overtreating and undertreating pain in the same patient. To the physician the courtroom is a foreign world, where there is only black and white, no shades of gray. Lawyers want "black-and-white" answers, yet any such answer invariably distorts the truth. In addition, time in court is time out of the office, which costs money.

Physicians fear the burden of record keeping that managing a pain patient requires, which eats up both time and money.

Physicians fear the complexity of pain, which requires a considerable expenditure of time if the physician wishes to remain current in his or her thinking.

Added to all of these problems is the reality that health care has become a business. When this transition has been made, the ethics change, and that is a problem. The behavior of health-care providers changes, because with every decision doctors have to think of the effects of our treatments both on our patients and on our bottom line. This creates a conflict between the patient and the business. The way this conflict currently is being resolved poses a great threat to the quality of care we provide for patients in general, and pain patients in particular.

Physicians are basically selling out to businessmen, a process known as the *corporatization of medicine*. The primary factor driving it is the dramatic increase in the complexity of practicing medicine, due to factors including excess government regulation, tort risk and associated insurance costs, and technology requirements. Becoming a physician and establishing a private practice are increasingly costly and require assuming a large debt, one most individuals do not have the stomach or the ability to tolerate. Many practices operate in the red, something that seemed impossible only twenty or thirty years ago. Physicians are increasingly unable to function independently and, as a result, are selling out to hospitals or private health-care conglomerates. When I started out in medicine in 1989, over 80 percent of physicians were in private practice. Now fewer than 20 percent are.

As a result of these changes, the physician is no longer the captain of the medical ship. Physicians have become employees who must "produce" for their employers. I heard of one such employer who no longer refers to doctors as physicians, but as "providers," asserting that when doctors became employees, they gave up their right to be called doctors.

As corporatization proceeds, quality of care becomes less important than productivity and profitability. Physicians are expected to generate revenue. If they don't, they are gone. One of my friends is widely recognized as a warm, caring, and competent physician. He was noted for spending time with his patients. As a result, he tended to see more complicated patients. Needless to say, in the corporate world, he was not productive. When his clinic was bought out by a corporate entity, he was soon let go because he could not and would not restrict his patients to their allotted ten-minute time slot.

There are two ways to generate revenue. The first is to get really good at one thing. That means *specialization*. The second is to perform as many procedures as possible. I refer to this as *interventionalizing*. Specializing and interventionalizing pay; managing patients does not. Increasingly, each individual physician does more and more of less and less, taking care of only a small part of each patient's health. Consequently, fewer and fewer physicians see the big picture. This situation is referred to as *fragmentation of care* and is especially problematic for those with complex medical problems such as chronic pain. Doctors who manage care are becoming obsolete, so patients have a tough time finding someone to take responsibility for their overall care, someone who knows them from "cradle to grave." This shift toward specialization creates a plethora of cracks in the mosaic of the system, through which a patient may fall. The more complicated a patient's problem is, the more health-care providers become involved in his care, and the less likely any one assumes responsibility for managing the big picture.

Why are physicians succumbing to this model? The answer is survival. Physicians are more often being dictated to by larger and larger entities, public and private. If they don't follow the party line, they can easily find themselves out of a job, something which was unimaginable in the not-too-distant past. Still more concerning, this process is also being driven from within medicine. Greed is increasingly permeating this field. Clinical decisions are too often made based not on what is good for the patient, but rather, what is good for the provider's bottom line. The bottom line thus takes precedence over the stated goals of health care: the needs of the patient and doing no harm. I contend that the more attention we pay to the bottom line, the more harm we do, especially to those whose problems do not respect the bottom line.

These issues challenge not only the physician but also us, the larger society. The first step toward resolving any problem is recognition. The second is to develop creative solutions. These solutions must come from all spheres, but the medical world should lead.

Solutions: Changing the Trends of Medicine

It is imperative that there be incentives for the physician to treat the pain patient. At this time, for the rank-and-file health-care provider and the pain specialist alike, the disincentives present a major obstacle. Therefore, viable solutions to the problems of pain management must involve changes in the practice of both pain specialists and general physicians and in the practice and business of medicine as a whole. I acknowledge that the suggestions that follow may seem impossible to implement. Yet the carnage that our current system creates for pain patients in the courts, the marketplace, the workplace, and the home is frightening, so it is incumbent on all of us to take whatever steps are necessary not only to minimize pain, but also to minimize the secondary ramifications of poor pain management on those who suffer.

All solutions begin with honesty. Pain specialists must come to a consensus on what we know and don't know about pain diagnosis and its treatment. As Dirty Harry so wisely stated, "A man has to know his limitations." Pain physicians also must be honest about what we tell people outside our specialty, making sure that what we say is for the good of all, not just our own ego. As a united front, we must communicate realistic expectations of pain therapy honestly to rank-and-file health-care providers and to the world. We have to stop telling people that "they don't need to suffer," when they do. Remember, the goal is to ease suffering, not erase it, and the goal of pain management is to manage pain, not eliminate it.

Honest communication must begin in the medical schools. Since pain is such a large part of the typical physician's experience, medical students need to learn a great deal about it. It is a sad indictment of our system of medical education that so little attention is paid to this important symptom. Moreover, while acute pain is a symptom, chronic pain is a *disease process*, worthy of attention in itself. Medical educators always have assumed that pain is merely a symptom, and that ridding the patient of the underlying disease process will eliminate the pain. As we saw, that is not true for chronic pain. Yet medical school education too often emphasizes cure over management, which means that patients with long-standing, incurable illnesses that create long-term disability receive too little attention. The problems of type C pain patients are ignored in medical education. No wonder physicians fear them!

Education on pain as a disease entity should become a priority in medical schools. When I was a medical student in the early 1980s, much was known about pain, but not many people knew it. Now, much more is known, and lots of people know it and can teach it. It is imperative not to let this knowledge go to waste.

In managing pain, doctors must learn to examine the whole patient— biologically, psychologically, functionally, and socially—something Dr. George Engel emphasized more than sixty years ago when he developed the concept of the "biopsychosocial" model of medicine and began teaching it to medical students at the University of Rochester. Frequently, the genesis of the pain and its ramifications go beyond the biologic sphere, and if we don't examine the entire patient, we will miss something.

Doctors must use a different model to work with pain patients. There are three basic models of doctor-patient communication:

In the "passive model," the doctor does everything, and the patient accepts what is given. This model is usually applied in an emergency setting, or when the patient is not mentally able to comply with treatment.

In the most common model, "guidance-cooperation," the doctor makes a recommendation and the patient follows through.

In the "mutual participation" model, doctor and patient have a mutual exchange of ideas, generating hypotheses, setting goals, and measuring outcomes.

To truly empower the pain patient, the doctor must rely on the third model, which requires that she effectively communicate and work with the patient to set reasonable goals and measure progress toward them. In my experience, this is the model most patients prefer when addressing functional adaptation to any disability. The physician has some knowledge about the medical basis for pain. The patient knows what it is like to live with disability. Together, they can work out creative solutions to the problems the patient faces. Including the patient in the process gives a firm message that the doctor cares what the patient thinks. This is both powerful and empowering. This model also requires that the physician respect the patient and validate the patient's complaints. If there is no validation, there can really be no relationship. This does not mean that the physician should not redirect the patient when the patient goes astray. In any loving relationship, there is criticism, which may at times be harsh. But it should be constructive and oriented to the present, not the past.

Physicians need to understand that there is no objective test for pain that has a high rate of accuracy. So do patients, lawyers, and insurance companies. Diagnostic tests are useful only in a context, and it is important to create that context by developing an overall view of the patient, instead of seeing him merely as a test result. In my experience, the greatest harm to patients comes when physicians and society place excessive trust in a nondiagnostic test.

"I'm sorry, Mrs. Jones, your MRI was negative. There is no objective reason for your suffering . . ."

"I'm sorry, Mr. Jones, you have three Waddell signs. You are clearly embellishing your symptoms and in need of psychiatric help . . ." (Waddell signs are based on a set of physical tests said to indicate a nonorganic component to pain, meaning that the pain cannot be explained merely by a physical change. But one should never assume a psychological cause.)

"I'm sorry, Ms. Jones, your MMPI shows a 'conversion V' pattern. You need a therapist. There is nothing I can do for you . . ." (The MMPI is a personality test, and the conversion V personality type is associated with chronic pain. When this connection was first made, it was assumed that the cause of the patient's pain was largely psychological. We now know that the development of chronic pain usually precedes the development of this psychological abnormality, suggesting that pain causes distress, a fact that is hardly news to anyone.)

Possibly each of these Joneses actually does need psychiatric help. But more often the physician is misinterpreting the test, which harms and victimizes the patient.

Because of these limitations, physician and patient must have the courage to be creative together. They are venturing into the unknown, seeking information that is not in the textbook. Each patient's situation is unique and will require novel approaches. Through trial and error, the two must work together to find ways to help the patient adapt and minimize his or her suffering.

It is quite well understood in the world of "disability medicine" that no one individual has all the answers to solving complex problems. The physician and the patient must acknowledge their limitations and be willing to ask for help. They must work as a team with many others: family members, therapists, psychologists, counselors, other physicians, spiritual guides, pharmacists, vocational counselors, support groups, and so on. The house of pain treatment has many rooms, and all are valued. And it must be recognized that the patient is a very important inhabitant of that house. It is inevitable that conversation will go on in the patient's absence; however, the patient must be informed of those discussions at some point.

Despite its importance, working as a team is quite difficult in a bottom-line world. Communication requires time that is rarely reimbursed, except, perhaps, in pain clinic settings—and most pain treatment does not occur in that setting. Reimbursing time spent on communication may be helpful.

Scheduling time in the day to communicate is helpful. Working consistently with a specific group of team members, with whom a physician communicates regularly and comes to know and trust, is very helpful.

Doctors must remember that their primary responsibility is the patient—not the lawyer, the insurance company, the employer, and so on. It is inevitable that at times we will have to stand up to people in the interest of our patients, even if doing so may cost us financially or otherwise. That is now and always has been the role of the physician.

Physicians must be aware of the lure of power and the way it distorts reality. As I noted previously, pain physicians do not occupy positions of power in the medical hierarchy. But they should not be valued merely as people stupid enough to take the "gomers" off everyone else's hands. Their practice should be seen as challenging and physically and mentally stressful, requiring real courage to try to ease the suffering of people we really do not know how to help.

It is critical that health-care providers take control of medicine back from the businessperson. I acknowledge that the practice of medicine is not just a profession, but also a business, but I insist that the bottom line should never take precedence over the patient. As the business of medicine has grown more complex, out of a sense of helplessness physicians have abdicated this aspect of their practice to the businessperson. While I am not opposed to this, I am opposed to the increasing control the corporate interest has over the practice of medicine. Too often the business side of the practice dictates which patients can be seen, how much time can be spent with each, and how the visit is documented. Much worse, the business managers are increasingly dictating what interventions are provided and how they are allocated. More and more, caring physicians who challenge this status quo find themselves without a job.

To me, this is not acceptable. I admit that I have little interest in the business aspect of my practice. I am busy, and I don't have time for such *unnecessary* complexity. For the time being, I acknowledge the complexity exists, and I am willing to defer to the expertise of the corporate officer. However, I am not willing—nor should any physician be willing—to concede power to the business managers. Instead I propose that the business managers have a seat at the table to assist doctors in making business decisions. In that respect, they are invaluable. But the final decisions in the practice of medicine always should rest with the physician, no matter how big the organization. Most important, the business managers should never be in a position where they direct the physician's behavior. For example, in my practice I give each patient as much time as he or she needs. I don't watch the clock. If I get behind, I get behind. My patients learn that if they ever need the time, they will get it. That is the only way you can address complex problems. I would suffocate in a system that mandated I see a patient every ten minutes, and I would be ineffective if I were only allowed to address one problem per visit. Yet the business managers judge the physician's performance by these criteria.

Physicians need to work together with patients, government agencies, and insurers to close the ever-widening cracks in our health-care system that specialization creates. America has a top-heavy, inverted pyramid of medicine in which physicians who manage medical problems are increasingly being replaced by specialists who proceduralize care. While this fragmentation may not be a problem for simple medical issues, it is a huge problem for complicated medical situations such as chronic pain that require the input of several health-care professionals. The system fails patients with such problems because no person accepts overall responsibility for their care.

For example, every day I see postoperative patients who have not done well after their surgery. They are referred to me for an injection that, everyone hopes, will save the day. My injections rarely work immediately. Sometimes it can take six to eight weeks to know whether they will help. In the meantime, the patient is suffering and seeks some short-term relief—specifically, pain medicine. Inevitably, the patient asks me for a prescription. I explain that it is the role of their referring physician to oversee their medical management, which includes medication prescription. The next question is: who is that physician? The surgeon says it is the primary care doctor. The primary care doctor says it is the surgeon. At some point, while waiting to see if the injections will provide a long-term benefit, both become frustrated, abdicate responsibility, and point the patient toward some as yet unidentified "pain doctor," who typically has a several-monthlong waiting list. In the meantime, the patient suffers needlessly.

This is not even as bad as things can get. Too often patients fall through the cracks and get totally lost. I believe that we can close these cracks by empowering those who manage problems, both simple and complex.

I would argue for a three-tier medical system.

The first tier consists of primary care physicians. Their role is to manage a patient's overall health care, preferably for decades as their recent medical ancestors did. Practice longevity allows the physician to actually get to know the patient.

The second tier consists of practitioners who assist primary care physicians by managing complex medical problems beyond the primary care physicians' expertise. This tier would include psychiatrists, who manage complex mental health problems; physiatrists, who manage complex physical disabilities; and pain management doctors.

The third tier is occupied by the specialists, who treat a single problem within the overall care of the patient. The care they provide should be directed by the first two tiers, preferably all communicating with each other and with the patient.

Stressing the value of the primary care doctor is not new. Adding a second tier, to the best of my knowledge, is unique. This tiered system would right the inverted pyramid of medicine, decrease the cracks between providers by maximizing communication, increase the efficiency of care, and improve its quality. What is more important, this system would decrease the overall cost of care, for both simple and complicated problems.

For such a model to work, we first must recognize the value of the second-tier practitioners, who manage complex problems and incentivize physicians to go into those fields, which does not happen now. Currently, there is every incentive for physicians not to go into these fields, and the number who do so is not sufficient to manage the need. Equally important, we need to increase the incentives for physicians to stay in those fields.

I strongly believe that the vast majority of medical problems can be successfully managed by a primary care doctor, and that the point of entry for all medical problems should be with a primary care doctor. Only in this manner is someone truly overseeing all care. This was the premise of managed care. It failed because both specialists and patients refused to accept this model. Specialists lost money. Patients didn't trust their primary care doctors to be fully knowledgeable. At the same time, insurers put too heavy a burden on primary care doctors by penalizing them if they referred patients to specialists too often. The system was not fair or appropriate. However, I do believe that such a system, with some adjustments, can work.

The first step is to provide incentives to those who manage care, whether first or second tier, starting in medical school. One reason young physicians go into specialty care is that the cost of medical school is high and they need to recoup costs. They simply cannot afford to go into primary care. I suggest we create a system parallel to the National Health Service Corps, in which doctors who make a commitment to go into primary care or second-tier fields will have a portion of their education costs covered. Once these physicians leave medical school, they should receive subsidies to help them set up offices. It is unnecessarily expensive to set up and run an office, even for specialists, without resorting to selling out to a corporate entity.

I would take this a step further by looking at what creates these costs: excessive reliance on technology (e.g., electronic health records or EHR; see the discussion that follows), malpractice insurance, defensive medicine (unnecessary diagnostic tests and treatment performed to prevent or address a potential lawsuit rather than to treat a current, legitimate patient need), regulatory red tape, and so on. For example, is it cost-effective to require EHR? Is it cost-effective to require computer hardware and software upgrades on a regular basis? Are those who create regulations looking at how their decisions affect the day-to-day functioning of the practice? Solutions to problems do not always require mandatory regulations.

While I do believe that specialists should be paid at a higher rate, I also believe there should be cost shifting from specialists to first- and second-tier doctors. Subsidies and incentives are an indirect way of doing this. Another way is to revise fee structures. I propose equal pay for equal work. Why should a spine surgeon be able to charge more for a five-minute evaluation for a nonsurgical problem than a primary care doctor can charge for a one-hour comprehensive assessment? A more reasonable fee structure would reward the surgeon less for that five-minute visit, and a first- or second-tier doctor more for spending time with the patient. In this case, I argue, there should be no difference in fee per minute spent with the patient.

I would also empower primary care physicians by including education on pain and its treatment and on the management of complex disability in their training during both medical school and residency. Armed with such knowledge, they may be less dependent on second-tier doctors to manage complex patients.

To effectively close the cracks in the system over the long term, it is mandatory to incentivize both first- and second-tier physicians to stay in practice and patients to stay with the same doctor, ideally for a lifetime. My mom had the same rheumatologist for thirty-five years. The strength of that relationship played a great role in her ability to live a long life despite such a debilitating illness. It is a serious problem that physicians are retiring younger and changing jobs too frequently. Gone is the day of the doctor who chose a place to practice, hung out his shingle, and stayed there until he was old and gray. As a result, patients are forced to change doctors way too frequently, which magnifies the cracks in the system and undermines continuity of care.

All these changes will empower primary care doctors, increase their job satisfaction, and encourage them to stay in practice for a long time, especially when strengthened by portable insurance allowing patients to keep the same provider through insurance change.

My final piece of advice is that in order to survive the challenges of treating the complex pain patient, the doctor needs to know herself. This work is stressful! It generates the standard stress-related reactions: anger, anxiety, sadness, inadequacy, fatigue, and so forth. Introspection is critical. It is important to ventilate, to let off steam. Support groups and counseling are helpful. Working in a team setting is also helpful, since responsibility can be spread out.

The Computer: Help or Hindrance?

> The covetous man is never satisfied with money, and the lover
> of wealth reaps no fruit from it; so this too is vanity. Where there
> are great riches, there are also many to devour them. Of what use
> are they to the owner except to feast his eyes upon? Sleep is sweet
> to the laboring man, whether he eats little or much, but the rich
> man's abundance allows him no sleep.
>
> Ecclesiastes 5:9–11

In my second year of medical school, we were assigned to debate whether the computer should have a role in medicine. I took the negative side, arguing that I saw two adverse effects of computerization. First, in relying on the computer, we risked losing the innate skills we bring to medicine, specifically our ability to touch, to listen, and to feel, things the computer is incapable of. I argued that the computer would dehumanize medicine. Second, I argued that we would risk worshipping the computer, believing it to be infallible and losing confidence in our own ability to think and solve problems. In the process, for the sake of the computer, we would give up our common sense. These consequences have come to pass, and with devastating effects on the pain patient. What is more, the computer actually has decreased our efficiency in providing medical care.

In the old days of medicine, even if the doctor spoke in unintelligible words, at least he faced the patient. He touched her, and he listened to her. Now, the doctor faces the altar of the computer, which is against the wall, so his back is to the patient. In an absolutely absurd example, a patient of mine told me that during an office visit, after he described a symptom, his doctor insisted he needed to use a different word or words. When the patient asked why, the doctor replied that the computer template did not have a box to check for that symptom! This story illustrates a pervasive, troubling problem the computer has created. Rather than attending to the patient's needs, we put greater emphasis on those of the computer.

It bears repeating that the most important part of any evaluation is the patient's history in her own words. If you facilitate the patient in an open-ended manner, she will tell you what you need to know. What you hear will guide your inquiry. I supplement my questions by having patients fill out a "pain drawing." This drawing, which costs less than a penny, gives me more information than a $2000 MRI scan. In fact, when I do a spinal injection, what I do is based solely on that diagram, and the MRI serves only to validate the drawing and tell me if a condition, such as a tumor, exists that may give me a reason not to inject. What the patient tells me helps me create a pretest likelihood of what the potential results of the test may mean. The value of any test, no matter how sophisticated, is only as good as this pretest likelihood. The computer does not talk to the patient. The doctor does.

The most important tool of medicine, then, is the doctor-patient relationship. The basis of this relationship is empathy, which is developed by listening, touching, and feeling. One cannot enlist the patient's trust by facing a wall. Yet our irrational faith in the computer is replacing this critical element in medicine. For example, a patient comes in and tells us he has pain in his back that radiates down the right leg. The MRI shows a disc protrusion on the left side, the opposite side. Who is right, patient or computer? We have known for decades that many patients with severe back pain have normal MRIS and that many with no pain have severe abnormalities on the MRI. In other words, the sensitivity and specificity of the MRI (terms that indicate its reliability) are shockingly low. Yet we believe the test because it is objective, instead of listening to the patient!

The computer was introduced to make medicine more efficient, but I would argue that we see fewer patients and we see them less efficiently than we used to. We spend much of our visit with the patient serving the needs of the computer, too often at the patient's expense. Forms must be filled out, information entered into the system, bills generated. Much of this is done in the name of "defensive" medicine, "risk management," and the needs of the bottom line. Still, time spent on it takes away from time spent actually listening to, touching, and helping the patient. Often I hear patients complain that their physician was so busy pecking away at the computer that she failed to listen to them and did not examine them. They question how the physician could ever make any rational recommendations without doing so. The physician may justify such actions by stating that disease patterns are consistent and can be obtained from the history and decoded by the computer. But all pain patients are unique, and the computer does not decode those unique features. That is only done with time, listening, patience, compassion, and experience.

Meanwhile, the computer has not lowered cost. Cost has increased, and not just because of the need to create medical and legal records or the increasing use of technology for diagnostic and therapeutic purposes. Computer systems are expensive. They become obsolete quickly and need to be upgraded. Training is required, and experienced people must be hired. The physician is at the mercy of such people, and their needs come to dominate the practice. They need office space and tools. When the computer goes down, as it inevitably does, everything in the office stops until the IT person solves the problem. At such times, I must vacate my office. Yet these systems are required by Medicare and Medicaid. When I was young and my dad's medical practice was in its infancy, his office was run by my mother, armed with her manual typewriter and a box of 3"-by-5" index cards. She didn't even need an electrical outlet. Now offices are run by legions of business people and computer geeks whose motivations are not clearly related to good patient care.

This infatuation with technology has another adverse effect. We are infatuated not only with the computer but also with the treatments it has made possible. The physician seeking the magic bullet for his patient turns to sophisticated interventions such as radio-frequency lesioning, spinal cord stimulation, intradiscal therapies, robotic surgery, and others, which the computer has made possible. Patients also seek these interventions, having learned about them from alluring websites created by the medical-industrial complex. Outcome studies, when objectively done, frequently show that these interventions are not as helpful as promised, and many harm a substantial number of patients. The creators of these technologies are also the ones who successfully created and promoted the myth of the computer. They reap the profits, but the patients do not see any benefits.

People who are loved and cared for, who are treated honestly and with respect and are valued, have better outcomes. They return to society and contribute. This is the type of treatment that saves money and is better for pain patients and everyone else.

SOLUTIONS: BEYOND THE COMPUTER

My prescription for overcoming our infatuation with the computer is to return to the basics. The first step is to objectively acknowledge both the value of the computer and the problems it creates.

Next, health-care providers need to take patient care back from the computer "geeks" (and the businessmen and the lawyers). We need to rekindle the basic qualities of good medicine, specifically, the desire to listen, to touch, to provide compassion. My mentor George Engel pointed out over sixty years ago the importance of acknowledging these qualities and also of teaching them to students as we would any other skill. We need to make the computer an ally in this aim, rather than an enemy of it.

Medical education is like a Play-Doh Fun Factory. You put in a blob of Play-Doh, and out comes something with a different shape. The medical student is the blob. She brings very special qualities to medicine, and it should be the role of the education process to enhance these qualities, not destroy them. But by ignoring these qualities and shaping students to conform to a computerized world, I fear we are squeezing out humility, empathy, and common sense. Students are impressionable. They imitate those who control their fate. It is critical that we, the older generation, serve as role models stressing the importance of these qualities.

There are ways to reconcile the needs of the computer and of the patient, and I offer the following suggestions, which apply not only to pain but to other complicated problems such as depression and anxiety that are beyond a computer's ability to ascertain.

The visit must always begin with a touch. A warm handshake communicates to the patient that his or her needs are valued. The patient is then seated, and a history taken in the patient's own words, not the computer's, reinforcing the statement that the doctor acknowledges the importance of what the patient says and feels. The touch inherent in an examination conveys curiosity and compassion, a desire to reach into the patient's world in order to help. Pecking away at a computer conveys quite the opposite.

Certainly the computer is a part of this interaction; however, it should be kept in the background. All demographic information should be entered before the patient walks into the room so that time spent on the computer is not taken from the patient's fifteen minutes. The computer should be placed so that there is eye contact between patient and physician, or at least the physician should apologize for turning his back. I strongly recommend that physicians not use templates when evaluating pain patients. A template can be a time-saving device for simple problems, but for complicated problems it risks forcing the patient's square peg of a problem into the round hole of the template designer's preconceived notions. Complicated problems often require thinking outside the box, and the template forces you into a box. Verbal inquiry, supplemented by patient-generated pain diagrams, pain scales, and patient questionnaires, all brought together by a well-thought-out and individualized dictated note, are more helpful and productive.

I was taught to directly communicate to my patients my entire thought process, including diagnostic and therapeutic possibilities as well as risks, and to put these thoughts in writing. When I included another physician in the process, the expectation was that I would pick up the phone and call her, or at least send her a detailed note describing what I knew about the patient, what my care plan was, and what I hoped she could do to help.

That sounds simple. However, in the world of teleconferencing, EHR, and ten-minute patient visits, it is not so simple. We don't have enough time in our days to communicate with our patients or our colleagues. Instead, we seem to think our computer-generated notes will serve the purpose. Yet that is not what the EHR is designed to do. The EHR is essentially a bottom-line-driven implement used to satisfy Medicare billing requirements so we can obtain the maximum revenue from the time we spend with our patients. It produces a very confusing document, with little, if any, space for a free-flowing narrative describing why the patient is being evaluated or why he is being referred. Yet this document is the tool physicians use to communicate with each other. Too often, it communicates very little about what really matters, the problem being assessed.

Physicians need to relearn how to communicate with each other, with our patients, and with society as a whole. There is no question that poor communication results in excessive and inefficient treatment, especially for patients with complicated problems requiring multidisciplinary care. The result is an exacerbation of the conflict between patient care and the bottom line.

Instead, we need to redirect the computer geeks to generate a document that serves our medical purposes, not our bottom-line goals. We need to relearn how to pick up the phone, even if that means communicating with a competitor. We need to inform the policy gurus that their attempts to control information and Medicare fraud are having an adverse effect on how we physicians communicate, much to the detriment of efficiency and cost-effectiveness.

Finally, we need to do what the 1960s generation learned to do: question authority. Today, the authority is the computer. Our inquiry will create questions, and the computer can help us answer these. However, we must be aware of its limitations and those of the tests we order. We need to assess the outcomes of our tests in light of the pretest likelihoods we generate from our patient interaction. If there is a match, that is great. If there isn't, we need to have the courage to trust our own instincts. When there is a mismatch, in my experience more often than not the doctor's instinct is correct, not the computer.

I don't suggest retracing our steps back to my father's office in the 1950s, which would not be possible anyway. I do espouse stripping away the computer's aura of omniscience and evaluating objectively its costs and benefits. We need to ask where computerization makes sense and where it doesn't. We need to strip away laws and regulations that impose computerization. Instead we must rely on the wisdom of older physicians and cultivate that wisdom in the young.

Computerization can be useful only when it rests on a base of compassion, empathy, understanding, listening, and touching—in other words, a base of love, which implores us to acknowledge our limits and, above all, put the needs of our patient above our own. The computer functions best when it is put in the service of the fundamentals of human existence that attract physicians to medicine in the first place.

THE PITFALLS OF E-MAIL

The computer has also affected communication between physician and patient through e-mail. E-mail is attractive because it is short and simple. We can communicate with patients directly, in straightforward language. However, most medical communication is not so simple, and e-mail does not lend itself well to complicated communication. Consider the following hypothetical exchange:

> "Patient X, the MRI of your brain showed a 'lesion' in your thalamus that may explain why you have severe burning pain on the right side of your body. Have a nice day."
> Huh?
> "What's a thalamus?!"
> "What's a lesion?!"
> "What do I do about it?!"
> "Will it kill me?!"

Some communication can be conveyed merely by words. Medical communication between patient and doctor cannot. The meaning of a simple phrase can be altered dramatically with a shift in body language or a difference in tone of voice. This is why I strongly oppose assessing a patient by only reviewing a chart. I am amazed by how often I misinterpret the intentions someone tries to convey in an e-mail. Medical information should never be transferred by e-mail, especially not test results. This principle is particularly critical in the world of pain.

My rule is to allow e-mail communication only for something simple such as an appointment time, and only when the patient has stated she wishes to receive communication in this manner. I never share test results or any other clinical matters by e-mail.

We live in an exciting time. We can help pain patients more than ever before in history. As always, a doctor can do no wrong if he or she is willing to put the needs of the patient above all else. In doing so, we should be guided by the words of Rabbi Moshe Ben Maimon quoted previously, as well as these of Hippocrates:

I will prescribe regimens for the good of my patients according to my ability and my judgment and never do harm to anyone . . .

In every house where I come, I will enter only for the good of my patients, keeping myself far from all intentional ill-doing and all seduction especially from the pleasures of love with women or with men, be they free or slaves.

All that may come to my knowledge in the exercise of my profession or in daily commerce with men, ought not to be spread abroad, I will keep secret and will never reveal.[4]

SEVEN

Regulatory Agencies and Pain Management

Overregulation Breeds Underregulation

When critics sit in judgment it is hard to tell
where justice leaves off and vengeance begins.
Chuck Jones, American animator

At some point in 1998 I had one of those "I can't believe they are doing this to us" type conversations with a friend of mine. We were talking about medical board oversight of opiate prescribing practices in her state. She told me that her state considered prescribing an opiate for more than three months to a particular patient inappropriate practice and a sufficient cause to initiate a medical board investigation. Needless to say, this threat created a significant barrier to what was then increasingly viewed as compassionate and appropriate care of a patient in pain, especially someone nearing the end of life. When she asked what my state's policy was, I was embarrassed to admit I did not know.

I immediately consulted New Hampshire's rules. Since the state motto is "Live Free or Die," I was not that surprised to find that we had no such rules. I then reviewed other states' policies and was somewhat surprised to find that most had no formal rules governing opiate prescription.

At first I was relieved by this discovery. But the more I thought about the issue, the more I began to get a chill thinking about what would happen to my pain practice if a reactionary force took over and created a set of constrictive rules. That would devastate my ability to practice pain management. I concluded that we needed rules that would protect a physician's right to prescribe opioids for people in pain. I hoped that these rules would lower the barriers to such care.

My mother told me more than once to watch what I wished for, because it might come true. Still, I wished, and beyond that decided to take aggressive action. I e-mailed a friend who was influential in the New Hampshire Medical Society, a private organization that advocates for both physicians and patients, about my concern. I don't know what I was expecting would happen, but several months later, long after I had forgotten about sending the e-mail, I got a call from the director of the Medical Society, asking me to serve on the newly created State Pain Management Task Force. Our first charge would be to create a set of rules such as I had envisioned and present them to the state for consideration. He said my e-mail had been the impetus for creating the task force. I was quite proud that I had initiated the effort and also pleased and proud that our Medical Society agreed something needed to be done.

As it turned out, my mother was prophetic. Our state attorney general had a similar concern about the absence of such rules. But he wanted to curb prescription drug diversion, not improve access to medication for those in pain. Such a conflict rears its head again and again in this saga. He therefore created a set of rules that substantially raised the barriers to compassionate care. To his credit, though, the attorney general readily admitted his ignorance of the extent of the conflict and basically deferred to the task force to set the policy.

In this country the public policy pendulum historically has swung between the goals of controlling prescription abuse on the one hand and providing pain patients with the medication they need on the other. The assumption has been that conflict is inevitable, and that any policy developed must either risk diversion to satisfy the needs of those in pain or create barriers to compassionate care to prevent abuse. Where people stand on this issue depends on their assessment of the relative importance of each of these risks. Such determinations often are made myopically according to what each person sees. Pain management professionals seek ready availability, and drug enforcement officials seek limited availability. Our task force sought a middle ground.

We were not alone. At about the same time, the Federation of State Medical Boards had commissioned a "blue chip" panel of pain policy experts with the same charge. We began meeting just as they completed their guidelines. With some modifications, we accepted their guidelines and submitted them to the Medical Society, our sponsoring organization, which approved them. We were very fortunate that the Attorney General, when informed of our efforts, voluntarily withdrew his proposal and supported ours. Our next step was to "sell" our rules to the New Hampshire state medical board, the governmental body that enforces state rules regarding the practice of medicine and advises the legislative branch on policies relating to medical issues. Several task force members and a few members of the Medical Society at large journeyed to the state capital for this purpose. After our rather passionate presentation, one Medical Board member commented that he didn't see what the big deal was. He pointed out that they never had interfered with any physician's right to prescribe. The very next day, the headlines of the most prominent newspaper in New Hampshire announced the punishment of two physicians *by our Medical Board* for their opiate prescribing practices. One of the two clearly needed to be limited. The other case was not so clear. Still, the point was made in black and white to all physicians in our state in a rather chilling manner: compassionate management of pain may bring career- threatening repercussions.

These Medical Board actions foreshadowed what was to come, not just in our state, but throughout the country. The rules we had developed, which the state adopted with the hope of lowering barriers to compassionate care of pain, soon became a rope to hang the unwary physician, something that we had hoped to prevent, but which now happened more often, not less.

Regulatory Bodies

With respect to chronic pain, the most important regulatory bodies are state medical boards, the Drug Enforcement Agency (DEA), and the Food and Drug Administration (FDA).

STATE MEDICAL BOARDS

Oversight of the practice of medicine is a power reserved to the states. The executive branch of each state appoints a state medical board to serve this purpose. This arrangement acknowledges the reality that practice patterns vary from region to region, and each state should be free to determine what is appropriate for that particular locale. One advantage is that individual physicians have greater input into what is considered appropriate medical practice, especially in smaller states. A disadvantage can be that those who serve on these boards often have little knowledge about chronic pain, and their actions may be influenced by their preconceived notions. Reimburse-ment for such positions is limited, and service may, in effect, be volun-tary. Many qualified individuals can afford neither the time nor the cost of serving. This limits the pool of potential board members. This problem is much greater in smaller states, where a few people must regulate practice patterns for a broad array of specialties. They rely on consultants who are often heavily biased, tainting the quality of the information they provide.

Medical boards do not make medical rules; they enforce them. The rules themselves are made by the legislature, though often with input from the medical board and other sources (as exemplified by our experience in New Hampshire). The legislature is substantially less medically sophisticated than the board, and therefore even more reliant on experts to help it make the laws that set these rules. While anyone can have input into the cre-ation of public policy at the legislative level either directly or through a representative, usually only those with the most to gain or lose show up and offer advice. Moreover, such advice can be bought and sold, a practice that substantially skews the information the legislature uses as it seeks to understand the big picture.

Another advantage of a local board is improved access to the system, not just for physicians, but also for those in pain. Medical boards also hear patient complaints. As pain patients become increasingly empowered, their complaints of undertreatment are sensitizing the boards to the problem of untreated pain.

DRUG ENFORCEMENT AGENCY (DEA)

The DEA is a branch of the Justice Department, whose role is to enforce the controlled substance laws and regulations of the United States.[1] Centraliz-ing this function gives the DEA a broad ability to fight what is a truly global problem: the illegal manufacture, sale, and use of controlled substances. However, this same centralization distances and insulates the agency from those it serves, generating a certain myopia: the agency clearly sees the problems of drug misuse, but has a much fuzzier view of the potential benefits of drug use.

FOOD AND DRUG ADMINISTRATION (FDA)

The FDA is a branch of the Department of Health and Human Services, whose job is to enforce the federal Food, Drug, and Cosmetics Act and related public health laws. It monitors the manufacture, sale, and consumption of $1 trillion worth of consumer products each year, including food, cosmetics, medical devices, medicines, and radiation-emitting devices,[2] in order to keep consumers safe from those who would take advantage of them. While its mission is huge, its budget is limited and its labor force is relatively small. In addition, it must rely on studies generated by outside sources—often by the same industry it is trying to regulate—to make its decisions. Therefore, it must rely on the honesty of manufacturers seeking its approval. The FDA cannot possibly regulate all the products claiming medical benefits, and as the next chapter will explain, many fly under the radar, enabling their manufacturers to take advantage of unprotected and naïve pain patients.[3]

With regard to controlled substances such as opioids, the FDA is charged with "evaluating certain medical and scientific factors and making recommendations to the Attorney General as to whether the substance under review should be managed as a controlled substance, or removed from control, and the appropriate level of control."[4] The drug is designated as a controlled substance if it has a potential for abuse. The FDA also considers whether the drug has an accepted medical use and the likelihood of its use causing psychological or physical dependence.

Overregulation Breeds Underregulation

We do need regulation, but in my opinion we are overregulated. We seek a perfect system with an answer for every problem. In the real world, such a search is futile. There will always be exceptions to any rule, and not every contingency can be covered. Our response to each aberration is a new regulation, which creates multiple loopholes that we attempt to close with yet more regulations. The result is an ever-growing body of law that is increasingly costly to enforce, impossible to understand, and intimidating to live under. This is the antithesis of the Constitution, which was designed to be flexible in response to circumstances, and of the historic notion of "common law," which relied on the standard of what a reasonable person would choose to do in a given circumstance.

Inherent in overregulation is its opposite, underregulation. Because we do not have a rule for every possible contingency, and because we are not free to judge by common sense but must judge based only on existing law with little room for interpretation, we are inevitably underregulated. Because there are too many rules, too few who understand what needs to be enforced, and too few to do the enforcing, it is easy to flout the rules and take advantage of the system.

These problems are exacerbated by our inclination to simplify complex problems by seeing them through the filters of our preconceived notions. In a complex, black-and-white, artificial legal world, where all problems are either right or wrong, and right and wrong are not always clearly defined, it becomes nearly impossible to see the shades of gray in the big picture that more aptly represent the real world. Thus we are liable to misjudge and punish where no punishment is warranted. When a law enforcement official is educated about only the dangers of controlled substances and not their benefits, a pain patient reliant on pain medication becomes a drug addict, and the doctor who prescribes the medication a drug dealer. At times in our nation's history, both actions were considered illegal and were subject to criminal prosecution. It is of major concern that in trying to curb a growing prescription-abuse crisis, we seem to be heading back in that direction.

EIGHT

The Business of Health Care

Whose Bottom Line Are We Treating?

In these times of development, everybody is in a hurry and
everybody's in a rush, and on the way there are people falling down,
who are not able to compete. These are the ones we want to love
and serve and take care of.

Mother Teresa, *Love: The Words and Inspirations of Mother Teresa*

Increasingly, the health-care world is succumbing to the business paradigm, whose primary goal is to satisfy investors by maximizing profits. Customer (that is, patient) satisfaction only counts in terms of its effect on the bottom line. This reality conflicts with the health-care providers' mission of helping people in need. The interests of business management and stockholders are thus pitted against those of the patient. Such a system is potentially quite destructive to the pain patient.

When the bottom-line mentality rules, the end justifies the means, within the limits imposed by governmental regulation and common sense. As medicine becomes big business, medical ethics are stretched. Does medicine serve the bottom line or the patient? A balance must be struck so the needs of the patient are respected. In the time-consuming world of pain management in particular, where the patients' demands are so great and our ability to meet them so limited, the bottom line is winning, and that is a huge problem. As chapter 6 explained, health-care providers increasingly see what we provide as a "product" and our patients as "clients" or "customers" who are part of a "market." This shift is critical, because when we think in these terms, it is easier to justify our bottom-line behavior.

The business model of health care extends to the sale and marketing of products, both medical and nonmedical, that are used to treat chronic pain. The Internet has promoted the spread of this model by supplying a vast market for the sale of snake oil. The business model has also had a profound influence on academia, creating what I consider a crisis of dishonesty surrounding the research from which new products and treatments are developed.

Businesses market their products not merely to satisfy a perceived demand, but rather to *create* a demand. To that end they employ marketing people who deliberately distort the product. We are used to beer and whiskey ads showing a male consumer surrounded by beautiful women, implying that the product makes him sexually attractive. Such marketing preys on the consumer's unconscious needs or insecurities. It takes a strong person to resist these advertising lures. The same type of marketing is directed at the pain patient, and pain patients are rarely strong. They are desperate, and often willing to use any product that looks good. Thus pain product manufacturers create ads showing highly functional people doing all sorts of things the pain patient longs to do. Next, they add a testimonial from someone pictured in the ad, preferably someone famous. But the real killer is the "expert" endorsement: "Dr. So-and-So, with three hundred years in the field, developed this product in his own basement, and now wants to share it with you because he cares so much about you . . ."

Another creative technique is to get pain patients or their providers to *sell* the product in a pyramid-type system. It's no surprise that patients can be suckers. But the highly educated health-care provider is often as big a sucker as anyone else, and can easily be led to believe that the product is more useful than it really is. Just give her a free pen and a nice lunch. Provider and patient also are lured by the promise that they can make a handsome profit if they only work hard and create a big enough network. In the end, the patients don't benefit because the product is rarely if ever useful, while the seller finds her integrity shattered when her customers discover that the product doesn't work. Meanwhile, the manufacturer laughs all the way to the bank. Over my career I have been shocked to observe that a therapy, drug, or supplement always works best the first year it is "on the market." I know I am not the only one who has noticed this. I believe it is a mass placebo effect. The power of persuasion can be amazing.

Clearly, the pain patient needs protection. In the medical world, various government regulatory agencies provide abundant protection, though it is still not sufficient. In the nonmedical world, where many pain-relief products are marketed directly or indirectly, there is very little consumer protection. There is some civil protection through fraud claims, but this seems not to be very effective. Many companies are quite skilled at using "fine print" to protect themselves. They also realize that most businesses do not survive more than a few years. The key is to make a quick killing, disappear at the first hint of any problems, and then reappear with a new product.

Because legitimate companies are forced to compete with illegitimate ones, they too sink to deceit. In cities around the country, health-care providers are increasingly competing publicly. In the beginning, the competition is friendly; perhaps the parties put ads in the yellow pages. Everyone is busy, and everyone is happy. Soon, though, someone gets greedy and expands his marketing to grab a bigger slice of the pie. Advertising then pops up on city buses and billboards.

"Are you in pain? Come to our *laser* clinic where we can give you your life back . . . 'I wish I had met Dr. XYZ years ago. If it were not for him, I would be in a wheelchair by now.'"" The ad fails to tell you there is no clear indication for lasers in the management of spine pain, or that it is rare for patients with this problem to end up in a wheelchair, but it sure sounds good, and in my experience, it does get patients in their doors.

Soon, in order to survive, the other, previously more ethical providers are forced to sink to this low level, one with apparently no bottom.

Nonmedical Products: A Cure for Every Symptom?

While medical products come under the scrutiny of the Food and Drug Administration, nonmedical products, for the most part, do not. Nonmedical products cover a broad range and include nutritional supplements, herbal products, pills of all sorts, magnets, electrical stimulators, various topical salves and balms, bedding, and so on. I also include in this category people who provide services, such as faith healers, herbalists, and personal trainers. While these people may have some form of accreditation, it is not recognized by any responsible board or governmental agency, and they can set up shop with little or no training.

Although there may be some scientific basis for these products, and some pseudoscientific study may be cited as proof of efficacy, the products are rarely if ever systematically studied. In fact, it is to the potential detriment of a product to seek scientific justification. Studies are very expensive; and few, if any, of these products would ever meet any reasonable level of scrutiny. A wonderful example is the magnet industry. In the 1990s, "healing" magnets invaded our country. The manufacturers made incredible claims about efficacy, not only about magnets in general, but about their products in particular. They claimed that their bracelets, pads, and mattresses could not only cure pain, but also provide other health benefits such as improved sleep and increased energy. Yet they were unable, or unwilling, to provide any scientific evidence. They charged exorbitant rates and found many patients willing to try the products. Many of my patients not only bought these products, but also sold them. I like to refer to them as "closet products" because as soon as the patient finds they don't work, they end up in the closet, never to be used again.

Since these products are not submitted to any systematic quality evaluation, it is not clear what is in them. The consumer must trust the integrity of the producer, and quality control is often lacking. For example, several years ago, an independent analysis of Easter Herbal products demonstrated high levels of arsenic. Some supplements are actually spiked with harmful substances.[1] In one interesting advertising twist, a fish oil supplement manufacturer provides a testimonial from a pharmacist who recommends the supplement because the manufacturer submitted the product to some sort of independent evaluation of its contents. But they don't tell you there is little evidence that fish oil supplements provide any useful health benefit.

Nonmedical products, by law, are not allowed to make medical claims. In other words, while they may claim to ease a symptom, they cannot claim to be useful for an illness. This is because these products do not meet scientific scrutiny. Manufacturers carefully toe the line, promising results for symptoms, but never mentioning diseases by name. They also find ways to get around this restriction. For example, in a typical pyramid scheme, the manufacturer may make no claims for the product, but the independent contractors who sell it certainly do. I have heard these individuals, who are usually untrained and unsophisticated, proclaim the virtues of these products for every disease and symptom known to humankind. The contractor is liable for these false claims, but the manufacturer is not.

Nonmedical product manufacturers love to hone in on contemporary buzzwords. For example, many people are frustrated by the medical establishment's inability to heal every ill, as well as by the side effects of its treatments. They don't want established medicine to be in the driver's seat; they want to take control. Thus they seek another medical paradigm and look back in history for any paradigm that may make some sense. The wisdom of extinct cultures acquires value, and treatments that, say, "rebalance" our energy become the rage. Frustrated with the chemicals we put in our body, we seek an "all-natural" approach. We ignore the fact that many of these traditional paradigms arose from a need to explain phenomena these cultures had no way of understanding.

In fact, sometimes these cultures never fully embraced the treatment or concept being touted. A good example is acupuncture. In ancient China, some scientists and philosophers who could read and write and thus share their thoughts with future generations embraced acupuncture and the concept of qi, or vital energy. Their notion of a magical aura, or flow of qi, is in fact a normal manifestation of our neurophysiology, something Chinese scientists had accepted by the 1930s. In drawing their maps of the channels, or meridians, through which energy flows, the ancients, unencumbered by preconceived notions, observed patterns of symptoms that we are only now coming to understand as pain and symptom referral patterns. There is much to be learned from their observations, but our application of their treatments is somewhat myopic. While acupuncture may have a physiological effect, Chinese treatment was much more holistic (anticipating our creation of holistic medicine by two thousand years). In addition to needling, each treatment included herbs and stressed the importance of personal responsibility, exercise, proper nutrition, and stress reduction. This leaves it open as to which part of the prescription was responsible for a beneficial outcome. Most likely the outcome was the sum of all these interventions working together. It remains unclear what qi actually is, if it exists at all. Yet it remains an enticing concept to susceptible people. In addition, it provides a useful explanation for the failure of any treatment. The practitioner can blame the patient's "stagnant qi" or the will of God.

The search for natural therapies raises the question of what exactly is "natural." As I noted, nonmedical product manufacturers associate their products with the prevailing trends in our culture. Thus, they label products as "all natural" or "nonnarcotic" and claim they will tonify your liver or regulate your qi, whatever that means. Is it natural to pour all sorts of herbs, homeopathic remedies, and vitamins into our bodies, very few of which have any scientific basis or have undergone any reasonable quality control, merely because an unaccredited herbalist at the natural food store recommended them? Why do we assume these people are any more trustworthy than the big drug manufacturers? I once had a patient refuse an ibuprofen prescription. He informed me that he "doesn't do drugs," meaning medical drugs. The man smoked a pack of cigarettes every day, drank a six-pack of beer a week, occasionally smoked a joint, and took every vitamin and herbal supplement on the shelves, but he didn't do "drugs."

Often the appropriate management for many of our troubles in life, including pain, is a change in behavior. We need to simplify our lives, eat properly, exercise regularly, and stop smoking. But making such changes requires energy and effort. It's much easier to take a pill. So nonmedical pill makers hawk an "all-natural" pill loaded with Ginseng, Ginkgo, various miscellaneous herbs, *and caffeine,* promising it will give you more energy, focus your attention, and improve your brain power. There are few data to support any physiological effects of the herbs, which we think of as natural, but there is definitely a physiological effect of caffeine, which is not "natural" and is an addictive stimulant. Clearly the manufacturer has no confidence in the natural ingredients.

Another of our buzzwords is "outcome." We like to assess outcomes, and that is a good thing. But useful outcome assessment requires honesty and, ideally, a disinterested party. It is the rare nonmedical product manufacturer that submits its product to unbiased analysis. It is much easier to say, "Ninety percent of sufferers of this symptom get better with our treatment (operators are standing by to take your order . . .)." In fact, 90 percent of all symptoms we experience will go away without any treatment. The successful healer is the one who is lucky enough to be around and take credit for the spontaneous resolution of a symptom.

But in pain management, patients don't spontaneously improve. My own goal in treatment is not a cure, and I have had to get used to that. Once a friend of mine came to see me for an acute problem; she had sprained her wrist. I told her to ice it, put it in some range of motion, and take some ibuprofen. She returned to see me a week later, and I asked her how she was doing. She told me she was fine. I asked her again, and she repeated the same answer. Finally, I got specific and asked her how her wrist was. She said fine. After a long pause, she said, "You're not used to this, are you?"

I wasn't. I had actually cured someone. I was euphoric. I was so happy that I didn't charge her for the visit. I didn't care that she would have gotten better anyway. Neither do the nonmedical manufacturers who are more than happy to take your money.

After twenty-eight years in the field, seeing so many patients victimized by people offering false hopes, it is hard not to be cynical. Some products do have some value. There is a value to a nice bed. However, there is no particular type of bed that has cornered the market in relieving back or neck pain; and to claim that one has, even with the endorsement of a distinguished chiropractor who is getting paid a large amount of money, is ridiculous.

That brings up still another marketing buzzword. We don't just seek relief of symptoms. We want a cure and are willing to try products that promise a cure, even if doing so is illegal. Many product manufacturers openly taunt the authority of an overwhelmed FDA by making such claims. This is quite a significant issue. We are concerned with the astronomical cost of health care, yet according to the Federal Trade Commission: "People spend billions of dollars a year on health-related products and treatments that not only are unproven and often useless, but also sometimes are dangerous."[2]

I am not actually opposed to the nonmedical market. Some useful products have come from it. For example, electrical stimulation, in various forms, has been used to treat pain for over two millennia. The first recorded use was in 15 AD, when it was observed that accidental contact with a torpedo fish relieved gout pain.[3] Subsequently, electrical stimulation, although largely unproven, was used in various forms to treat pain. After the development of the gate control theory in the 1960s, it was thought that electrical stimulation could be used to close the gate on pain in the dorsal horn of the spinal cord. This hypothesis led to systematic testing and the development of various treatments such as transcutaneous nerve stimulation, spinal cord stimulation, and others that have had a great impact on pain management. Though I criticized the use of magnets for pain, the reality is that they may have some benefit. Placing a conductor, such as a nerve, in a magnetic field creates an electrical current. In theory, a magnet can do this relatively painlessly, unlike direct electrical stimulation, making it an intriguing potential treatment method. However, creating useful products requires scientific development, a step bypassed by many manufacturers. When such development has been done, positive treatment outcomes have created illuminating studies that have improved our knowledge of how our bodies work and how we can relieve symptoms. Treatments such as chiropractic care and acupuncture have become mainstream because they are effective and have been submitted to reasonable scientific assessment. Their practitioners have created a useful scientific literature and submitted themselves to an acceptable accreditation process.

Proper care begins with honesty. Honesty may involve some cost to the bottom line, but a society that prides itself on being ethical must have the courage to be honest.

REGULATION OF NONMEDICAL PRODUCTS

The FDA's role in regulating nonmedical products is limited, allowing charlatans to make medical claims whether there is evidence to support them or not.

For dietary supplements, including herbal agents and vitamins, homeopathic preparations, ointments, salves, and so on, oversight is provided in only three circumstances. First, if the manufacturer claims that the product affects the structure or function of the body in some way, the FDA must be notified within thirty days after the product has been marketed. The product is then required to carry a disclaimer saying that it has not been reviewed by the FDA and is not intended to diagnose, treat, cure, or prevent any disease. The claim itself is not investigated, approved, or disapproved. Therefore, the manufacturer can claim almost anything it wants, and so can the person who sells it at the local health food store, without fear of reprisal by the FDA.

Second, if a dietary supplement includes a new ingredient not marketed before 1994, the manufacturer must notify the FDA seventy-five days before marketing the product.

The FDA does monitor adverse effects of dietary supplements and may get involved if problems arise. For example, many adverse effects occurred in people consuming "energy drinks" (a polite way of saying stimulants) that contained ephedrine. The FDA reviewed this problem, stepped in, and banned ephedrine in nutritional supplements.

Devices such as magnets are not reviewed at all by the FDA as long as they do not make "structure-function" claims and as long as they emit no radiation. To date, no reliable studies have attributed any health benefit to these products, yet they still bring in considerable revenue for their manufacturers, which are under virtually no pressure to seek FDA approval.

While the FDA has little clout with nonmedical products, the criminal justice system may get involved if it can be proved that the manufacturer made fraudulent claims. For example, the manufacturer of an electrical simulation device promised that it would give the user washboard abs with virtually no effort. The claim was proved fraudulent and the product was taken off the market, but not until the manufacturer had made a con-siderable profit. But proving fraud is not easy, and many companies have mastered the art of disappearing when trouble arises, taking their profits with them, and then resurfacing later, either with a new wonder drug or a different use for the old one.

Private consumer protection agencies such as the Better Business Bureau do keep track of consumer complaints and maintain a database that can be shared with a potential user of these devices. Therefore, before spending money on any good or service, the consumer does have a way of checking for red flags.

While many of these products confer no benefit, most don't do harm either, at least physiologically. All have some placebo effect, and users may actually get results if they believe in the product enough. The problem is that desperate people spend money they cannot afford to at least "give the product a chance." Indeed, the nonmedical product industry consumes about two-thirds of the health-care dollar. Insurance companies do not cover these costs. These products do harm pain patients by tantalizing them with an unreasonable hope and delaying the rehabilitation that needs to happen.

I consider the nonmedical market a major problem, whose scope is well beyond the capability of the FDA, and it is unlikely that governmental oversight can or will increase. I do not have an answer for this problem other than preaching vigilance to my patients when they ask about specific products. The buyer does still need to beware.

Medical Products: Tools of the Trade

A partial list of medical products includes pharmaceuticals, surgical equip-ment, needles, syringes, x-ray equipment, durable medical equipment (that which is prescribed for home use), laboratory testing equipment, and so on. When used optimally, they can be very helpful, but when used improperly they can be very harmful. Thus their use is regulated, and only properly trained and accredited health-care providers are allowed to prescribe them.

The regulatory process is generally very thorough, and as a result, ex-tremely expensive because of all the hoops a manufacturer must jump through in order to bring a product to market. For every successful product, there are several failures. Someone must pay the cost, and to the extent possible, the manufacturer will try to pass it on to the consumer—that is, the patient, the health-care provider, and the insurance company. That reality explains part of the tremendous increase in medical costs. As our fund of knowledge explodes along with our ability to explore and treat the body through invasive and noninvasive therapies, the sophistication and cost of our interventions also increases. This cost of bringing a product to market is a huge barrier. That may be one reason why there has not been any major new innovation in the field of pain management in six thousand years. We do have some new adjunctive medications; but for the most part, we just have new ways of delivering the old modalities.

Once decisions are made, and medical products and services are made available, they are marketed, and clinicians "in the trenches" must decide whether to use a product and how to use it. Clinicians rely on established experts in their fields to help them make their decisions. They rely on personal experience and study. And increasingly, they rely on educated consumers (patients) who have studied the subject in great detail on the Internet. They also rely on representatives of the product manufacturers.

The marketing of these products used to be quite subtle. "Drug reps" would show up at a doctor's office with a few trinkets (pens, pads) for the doctor and his or her staff, and some medication samples to give to patients. The sales pitch was always bolstered by a free lunch for the staff. Softened by such an obvious display of generosity, the physician would be at the mercy of the salesperson's pitch, usually embellished by biased reports of the product's virtues.

Marketing is now much more aggressive. After a manufacturer has spent a huge amount of investors' money to create the product, it has every incentive to see a return on the dollar, and creative—and sometimes subtly deceitful—advertising that highlights the good and hides the bad aspects of the product is a proven way to ensure this. Manufacturers market directly to consumers by advertising in the media and by soliciting reporters to write human interest stories about their products. In this way they create a demand much as manufacturers of nonmedical products do. The intensity of the marketing pitch has a huge impact on what gets used.

We assume the physician is a savvy, well-educated gatekeeper who has the wisdom to see through the fluff and objectively assess the relative merits of the product. That most certainly is a false assumption. A doctor is as big a sucker for a sales pitch as anyone. The pitch is multifaceted and begins with a visit from a usually well-dressed, articulate sales rep, who starts her presentation by stating the benefits of the therapy, minimizing the side effects, and emphasizing the product's benefits relative to its competitors. After providing impressive scientific studies that she leaves for the doctor to review, she usually concludes by complimenting the doctor's intelligence and offering gifts such as pens, pads, dinners, tickets to events, and trips. While accepting such gifts is now considered unethical, it still happens. For example, if the rep shows up with a plate of pastries, are you going to let it go to waste?

I have discovered that there are three stages in the learning process:

Blind acceptance of everything we are told by those whom we believe to be experts

Hopeless cynicism, which occurs after we find out that these experts really don't know everything, and we realize we don't know whom to believe in for guidance

Equilibrium, when we realize that nobody knows everything, that we need to critically evaluate all information we are given, and that sometimes we must fly by the seat of our pants

Often we physicians blindly accept what sales reps say because the studies they provide look great. Closer analysis of these studies often reveals many flaws that may cast doubt on the therapy's true benefits. However, that analysis requires time and attention, something we are too often willing to entrust to our experts, so we wind up blindly following their recommendations.

When I was a young doctor, I pretty much accepted anything an academician recommended, even if he was paid by the company that made the product. I did not see it as my place to question authority. I prescribed all sorts of pills and therapies that were sold to me without ever critically analyzing them. Over time, however, I saw many treatment failures and became cynical. Now I don't do anything without thinking it through thoroughly. For example, I have concluded that epidural cortisone injections (ESI, injected inside the spinal canal) are a cost-effective treatment for back pain when done at the appropriate time in the treatment process. I also have concluded that radio-frequency ablation (RFA) of sensory nerves (deliberately damaging a sensory nerve with radiofrequency energy to impair its ability to transfer pain information) is not cost-effective. Therefore, I do

ESI and I don't do RFA. I fully accept that others do not agree with me, and I respect their opinions; but after much time and thoughtful consideration, I have chosen my own preferences.

Overall, regulatory scrutiny of medical products is a good thing that is lacking in the nonmedical world. It takes some of the burden off health-care providers to make decisions about the merits of various products. It serves an educational role for health-care providers, insurance companies, and the public. It does create larger barriers to new products, with significant ramifications for health-care costs and availability of therapies. To some extent, it limits the creativity of false marketing; but false claims still exist, and the buyer still needs to beware.

REGULATION OF MEDICAL PRODUCTS

Despite its overall benefit, FDA regulation of medical products—both pharmaceuticals and medical devices—is full of loopholes. The approval process varies depending on the product. All medical devices that pose a serious risk (for example, prosthetic heart valves) must be approved before they can be sold and used. A moderate-to-low-risk device (class I or II) can be approved more easily if it is similar to a device already in use that is approved. The manufacturer of such a product must submit what is known as a 510(k) request to the FDA ninety days before it plans to market the product. No clinical trials of safety and efficacy are required if the FDA concludes the product is similar to one already in use.[4] All pharmaceutical agents must be approved before being marketed and are monitored throughout development and production[5] (see chapter 13 for specific details about the regulation of opiates and opioids). It takes twelve years or more for a typical pharmaceutical to be approved, and at least that long for a medical device.[6]

As consumers, we feel comforted to know that a product has FDA approval. However, this means only that the FDA has determined that the product's potential benefits outweigh its risks.[7] This approach acknowledges the reality that nothing in the world is risk free. It is up to the physician to inform the patient of what those benefits and risks are, and this constitutes informed consent. In the end, it is up to the patient to decide whether to submit to the treatment.

Consumers also assume that the FDA has left no stone unturned when it decides to approve a product. That is rarely true. Although manufacturers are required to report adverse consequences that arise after the product has been approved and is in use, which the FDA can subsequently use to re-review the product, the FDA does not initiate studies of product safety before approval; it lacks the funds to do so. The manufacturer must conduct these studies and provide them for the FDA to review.[8] This creates an obvious conflict of interest. Manufacturers have a great incentive to present biased studies with flawed designs in order to show benefit while minimizing risk. Manufacturers also have the incentive to withhold information about risks, especially when the bottom line is at stake. As I explain in the section on academia below, consciously or unconsciously, most studies are infected with bias. It is quite clear that this bias affects the FDA's decisions.

Decisions made in the regulatory process often depend more on who is making them than on objective evidence. More specifically, who has power and influence is often more important than the relative merits of the procedure. Furthermore, which data are included for discussion is subject to the judgment of the person making the decision. If the evaluator has an inherent bias for or against a new technology, she may look only at the data that support her bias. Evaluators frequently do not have the knowledge base to make decisions regarding a new technology and must rely on a cadre of experts. Which experts they choose naturally affects their decision.

While FDA approval is not always needed for medical devices of moderate to low risk, manufacturers of these devices frequently seek it because insurance companies are often reluctant to pay for interventions that are not FDA approved. In most cases, the cost of getting FDA approval is more than made up for by subsequent sales. The 510(k) request streamlines the approval process, dramatically lowering the cost to the manufacturer. However, the consumer may be harmed, since there is no requirement for clinical trials of the new product; and in some instances, these products resemble products that were found to be harmful after being approved.[9]

Moreover, once a product is FDA approved, a physician can use it to treat any other problem if, in his or her judgment, the potential benefit of the intervention outweighs any risk. For example, pedicle screws were developed to hold supportive rods to the spine in order to improve outcomes in scoliosis surgery, and the FDA approved them for this purpose. Spine surgeons soon used them "off label" to treat other spinal conditions such as disc-related pain. To date, there is no convincing data to suggest that the benefit of this use outweighs the risks (a fact that plaintiffs' lawyers took advantage of when suing surgeons for bad outcomes), but the surgeons who used the product for these other conditions rode the coattails of the scoliosis indication to get away with doing so without approval—and it was from this use that the big profits came. However, the lawsuits over bad outcomes threatened the use of the pedicle screw for any purpose, prompting the manufacturer to get a separate FDA approval for disc surgery—which it was able to get in record time.

Conversely, at the same time the FDA would not approve IDET (intradiscal electrothermal therapy), a novel device for the treatment of spinal disc pain, an entity for which there was no clear surgical indication. This treatment heated a sensitized nerve above a certain point and "denervated it," with the hope of alleviating the pain. However, IDET was a novel technique that did not resemble an already approved product, and it was not approved. Second, IDET addressed pain "neurophysiologically" rather than with surgery. In my opinion surgeons were threatened by an alternative that challenged not just their source of income, but also their view of pain and its treatment. Surgeons have more clout than nonsurgeons, and my impression was that they used this clout to prevent FDA approval for IDET. Third, the creators of IDET, fueled by unusually positive initial outcome data, marketed the product heavily; and too many physicians began using it for all sorts of conditions. I was told I could substantially increase my income, not just from the IDET, but also from the discogram I would have to do first. When other outcome studies failed to support the initial data, insurers soured on the procedure, and soon it was impossible to get insurance approval. IDET has seen its time in the sun, and it is unlikely that it will ever be FDA approved, which, in my view, represents a problem with the system.

Many products enjoy the profits of off-label use, even though manufacturers are not supposed to market them for such use. Usually they don't need to; the physicians do it for them. Until the cost-benefit ratio turns against such a practice, it continues. Assuming the physician uses sound, unbiased judgment and carefully monitors outcomes, off-label use can indeed be beneficial. Unrecognized uses are discovered for many products; and if the product has already proven to be relatively safe by FDA standards, it is burdensome to require a new approval. However, physicians do not always use sound and rational judgment. Fibromyalgia is a painful disorder with few effective treatments. Duloxetine and pregabalin are FDA approved to treat it, but are probably no more effective than cyclobenzaprine and amitriptyline, which aren't. The latter two drugs have been used off-label for fibromyalgia for years, and they are well established. There was no sound financial reason for the manufacturer to seek FDA approval. The former two drugs were new, and the manufacturer's campaign for a wider market share justified the expense of getting FDA approval, which they widely tout in their ads. I have observed that physicians are more likely to prescribe one of these newer, more expensive drugs even though their safety and efficacy are no better.

Given its limited budget and the immensity of its task, the FDA may not be able to do a better job than it is doing.[10] In an ideal world, the FDA staff and budget would be larger, the approval process less costly and time consuming, information used to make decisions less biased, and individuals and specialties that can influence the process less motivated by self-interest. The reality is that the system does the best it can given its constraints.

The Internet: The Misinformation Superhighway

> Beware lest ye harm any soul, or make any heart to sorrow;
> lest ye wound any man with your words, be he known to you
> or a stranger, be he friend or foe.
> 'Abdu'l-Bahá, exemplar of the Bahá'í faith

The Internet has become the conduit through which the producers of health-care products, medical and nonmedical alike, sell their products to both health-care providers and the general public. As a fertile garden will grow not only beautiful flowers but also weeds, so history has proved that the garden of virtue also provides fertile soil for the invasion of human vice. The Internet has proved to be such a garden. Perhaps that is why in the story of Eden, God admonished humans to stay away from the Tree of All Knowledge. He fully understood their inability to handle such knowledge responsibly.

The Internet has multiplied the ability of makers of medical and nonmedical products to gull the public and take advantage of desperate pain patients. Those who perpetrate their greed on the vulnerable claim that they are only exercising their First Amendment right to free speech in order to make a living. They assert that controlling the Internet would cause them undue hardship—a claim that reminds me of the scene in the movie *Dirty Harry* where a character who has viciously murdered several people is dragged off to jail, crying out: "I have my rights . . . I have my rights." Harry Callahan, our vigilante hero, restrains himself with great effort from punching the man's face in.

It would be nice to think that the promoters of these products are just greedy, shady businessmen. But unfortunately doctors who have forgotten their Hippocratic Oath also take advantage of this marketing opportunity. Physicians who place the needs of their bottom lines above the needs and welfare of their patients find the Internet fertile ground for increasing their income. A physician group unashamedly tricks desperate patients into coming into their one-of-a-kind clinic offering "cutting-edge" technology guaranteed to eradicate the pain. "Ninety percent chance of cure!" they promise: one assessment, thousands of dollars of invasive procedures, most not covered by insurance and with virtually no scientific support, and no follow-up.

Seduced by the promises, patients submit to the procedures offered and anxiously await the promised cure, which rarely comes. I have seen patients waste tens of thousands of dollars on such hype. One of my patients spent $75,000 on this type of scam. To the misery of their pain is added a deepening debt owed to those they trusted. As they lament their fate, the man in the white coat sips his profits away at the country club or wherever such types spend their "hard-earned" dollars, apparently burdened by no sense of guilt or shame.

In my opinion, the solution to the misinformation of the Internet begins with personal responsibility and ends with some degree of governmental control. Thus I suggest that potential businesses that use the web should be responsible to some authority. We have long since abandoned the "let the buyer beware" ethos. The problem with the Internet is that although private and public watchdogs exist to advocate for consumers and protect our welfare, they only function when problems arise and there is need for investigation. Unfortunately, it is all too easy for a perpetrator to open up shop, milk the profits, disappear when the posse arrives, and then reappear on another site and under another name when the coast is clear.

In order to open a business and make claims for either a nonmedical or a medical product, one should be required to go through an approval process that includes peer review via professional journals. While this process is not perfect, it is infinitely better than what is happening now on the Internet. Any business that promotes any product, medical or nonmedical, should be liable to such review. At this time, as long as they cause no physical harm, such businesses flourish with impunity. Many of these products do cause harm, but the regulatory process is so limited that they can exist for months or years before they come to justice.

In the absence of governmental control, the only solution is personal responsibility. It is our responsibility to question. Providers of health-care services must constantly monitor the outcomes of their treatments, and this monitoring must ignore the bottom line. We must have the courage to question our interventions when they don't seem to be working. We must be willing to take the time to solicit feedback from those to whom we offer our treatments.

I once attended a meeting where one researcher told us he was unable to get funding for a double-blind, controlled trial of a particular procedure he was interested in. He told us the reason was that the manufacturer was making a lot of money on the procedure, and he was afraid that systematic study would demonstrate that the procedure did not work.

If you question the efficacy of what you are doing, maybe you shouldn't do it, and you certainly should not sell it.

Academia and the Business of Health Care

> As to diseases, make a habit of two things—to help, or at least,
> to do no harm.
>
> Hippocrates, *Epidemics*, 1.2

In my years practicing medicine, I have realized that all physicians are researchers and educators. We all observe the world, make hypotheses about what we see, test those hypotheses, measure the outcomes, and share our knowledge with others. I have learned as much, if not more, from doctors in small-town settings as from those in large universities. I have come to appreciate that everyone has something to offer. There is much to be said for the school of hard knocks, from which those in the Ivory Tower are too often insulated. Still, physicians in the teaching institutions serve an important purpose.

What differentiates a "teaching" physician from the clinician is that the clinician's educational process is very informal. There is no laboratory outside of the exam room and the hospital, and there is no classroom.

The student is usually the patient or the family. On the other hand, the teaching physician is engaged not just in education, but also in research. His endeavor is confined to a specific field, and the questions generated are pursued through basic and clinical research. It is then his responsibility to share those findings with students at the medical school and colleagues at various meetings. However, his responsibility goes beyond educating future doctors; he must constantly challenge the frontiers of medicine. He does take risks, but his position in a university gives him the relative freedom and time needed to take those risks.

Both of these aspects of medicine are of great value, and one cannot exist without the other. Clinicians are motivated by a need to help others and by the remuneration they receive for their efforts. Educators are motivated by a curiosity that drives them to ask and research questions and a desire to share that knowledge with others. The clinician with a broad practice relies on the observations of the academician, who presumably is more knowledgeable about the finite area she researches. How the academician chooses to share her knowledge has a profound impact on the care the clinician provides for patients.

The academician must have the sense of integrity that academic honesty requires plus a sense of a higher purpose that puts the needs of all above her own. She must be curious, willing to share, and above all honest about what she knows and what she doesn't. She must be courageous enough to acknowledge when she is on the wrong path and understand when it is time to turn back. We learn from failure, and it is actually more important to share our failures with others than our successes. For the courageous, this is easy. But for many, courage is in short supply, since the life of the academic is filled with incentives that may cause her to stray from these ideals. And when she does, her actions may have substantial adverse effects on clinicians and their patients.

It is easy to chastise dishonesty. However, I have come to understand how hard it is to be honest. The real problem, I think, is that the system actually is set up to punish honesty. In clinical medicine, we are rewarded financially and with a warm thank-you. The better we do, the more money we make and the more thanks we receive. But in the complex "publish or perish" world of academia, things are not so simple. Money is still a motivating force, but less directly. For a researcher to succeed, she first must raise money to fund her research. Then she must produce results.

Universities want to see results. Funders want to see results. And there is a huge bias toward seeing positive results, especially those that lead to a lucrative treatment or positive publicity for the university. I have observed that academicians who produce helpful interventions rise quickly up the educational hierarchy, both within their institution and throughout their field. Those who don't find it difficult to attract funds for their research. Too often they struggle to maintain a position. I have vivid memories of the thump I heard many years ago when such a researcher hit the ground after a fatal seven-story leap triggered by his failure to achieve "results," a failure that jeopardized his position at the university.

The problem is amplified in the commercial world where business directly hires researchers to "produce." In this world, productivity means big bucks, and those who produce are heavily rewarded. This creates an inherent bias toward "positive" results in the studies that researchers present to the outside world. Studies with negative results often are suppressed. This practice is unethical—a dangerous intellectual shortcut. When we reward only the successes and punish the failures, we create a distorted sum of knowledge.

The problem is that ideas, like all commodities, must be sold. Even though it may be better for all to admit "I don't know," that admission does not sell well. Those who buy value the positive, and those who sell value the accolades that go along with a positive result which may further the knowledge base. Whether it is real or an illusion doesn't matter. So researchers seek the positive result, in any way they can.

Thus there is a serious problem of bias in medical studies. In chapter 6 I described a surgical meeting where speakers claimed a 90 percent success rate. This was a prominent spine society that had historically focused on surgery, but was trying to expand the membership to include nonsurgeons. I was honored to be asked to join and excited to attend. Although I was shocked to hear surgeon after surgeon report "90 percent good to excellent" outcomes from some very aggressive operations, I believed what they said and sentenced dozens of patients to surgical slaughter out of a naïve belief that their statements were true. Reviewing the carnage, I found that the success rate was substantially lower than 90 percent, leaving me with two possible conclusions. One was that the surgeons to whom I referred patients were no good. The other was that the data were no good. It became quite apparent that the latter was true. Those data were used to justify a lot of ill-fated surgery, giving practitioners and patients a grossly inaccurate and overly optimistic estimate of the chances of success from these interventions.

The bulk of scientific research comes from academic physicians whose dictum is "publish or perish." They also must become involved at high levels in their local and national societies if they wish to climb the academic ladder and be successful. They get noticed by publishing positive outcomes; the more positive the result, the better for them. It is also very frustrating to spend a lot of time on research and find that your intervention does not work. What is more, it is difficult to get negative outcomes published.

There are many ways to creatively turn a negative result into a positive one. All you have to do is either alter your data or selectively include or exclude data so they show what you want to show. These strategies can be conscious or unconscious, but either way they pose a problem for those who rely on the literature to make decisions. One tactic is to find ways to conveniently eliminate those who don't respond to the treatment from the study group. Another is to bias inclusion criteria so those included have a better chance of responding. The problem is that when researchers consciously exclude nonresponders from outcome data, potential patients suffer. I once had a patient who was involved in a study of a new type of minimally invasive spine surgery. Postoperatively, his pain was much worse. He never did get better and, many years later, committed suicide because of his intractable pain. I found out that he was excluded from the study results because he was taking "excessive pain medication," even though he was taking more medication because the procedure had failed. Excluding patients of this type clearly made the procedure look more effective than it really was. However, technically the investigator was not guilty of fraud because he did list this as an exclusion criterion in the fine print of the study. If you only read the abstract, though, which is what most physicians do, you missed it and would overestimate the value of the procedure.

Bias of this type is not always so intentional. As much as we long to deny it, there is inherent subjectivity in any clinical study. For example, part of my practice is electromyography, or studying patients' nerves electrically. When a patient is first referred to me, I review the chart and examine the patient. I then create hypotheses and pretest likelihoods that I test. All too often, as I proceed through the test, I am confronted with data that challenge my pretest impressions, my preconceived notions. For example, patients with hand pain are often referred to me. The surgeon and the patient hope I can give them a diagnosis that promises a "quick fix"—for example, a pinched median nerve at the wrist, also known as carpal tunnel syndrome (CTS). The referring surgeon often attempts to "sell" the patient to me by emphasizing the CTS-like symptoms and minimizing those that conflict. However, as I test the patient, I may find that she has pain without numbness, which is usually caused by a different condition that is not amenable to such an easy solution. When this happens, I have the option of accepting the conflicting data and challenging my hypotheses, or ignoring or altering my data. With a very subtle shift of a cursor, I can eliminate the conflict. Doing so satisfies my need for a nice, easy solution. It also satisfies a surgeon's need to justify an operation and the patient's need to "just fix it." My dilemma is amplified because the patient and surgeon are relying on me to provide information that will satisfy those needs. They are all too willing to go elsewhere if I don't do so. In fact, one electromyographer told me he willingly altered results to "keep my surgeons happy." So if I am honest, I lose patients and income. If I am not honest, the patient undergoes an inappropriate operation. The urge to be dishonest is quite hard to ignore.

Change the setting to one where you, as a researcher, are studying a clinical problem. After years of effort developing a "promising" new drug or surgical implant, more than a few patients are showing unwanted side effects or not responding as well as hoped. Big brother in the form of your funder is watching. You have staked your career on the outcome of this research. Fame and fortune, academic security, await you. All you have to do is "eliminate the problem." Just as the surgeon described above found a way to eliminate my patient from his study, so too, a researcher can easily figure out how to eliminate a subject by embellishing or creating exclusion criteria for that individual.

Academic honesty is heroic. Too often it does not pay. Big brother is not limited to the university hierarchy and big business. The media also participate. They only wish to show results that are newsworthy. Negative results do not sell papers and attract readers to websites, whereas positive results do. Therefore, the media seek the positive and avoid the negative. While this is most apparent in the lay press, it also exists in the medical literature. As a result, the public only hears about promising treatments.

The same phenomenon occurs at professional meetings, where the keynote speakers are often those who have made some wonderful discovery, while the negative results are relegated to the poster presentations, if the researcher has the guts to present the data at all. That said, I did once attend a national symposium whose keynote speaker actually questioned the academic honesty of pain researchers and encouraged a more honest stance toward research.

Readers of these studies display the same bias. When I scan a journal, my mind tends to look at the positive studies, those that give me some new way to treat a difficult problem. I conveniently ignore those studies that question my current practice. In this I am no more honest than those presenting the data.

It should be possible to give equal weight to positive and negative studies—at meetings, in the literature, and in the universities. While it is intellectually difficult to take a step backward, when you are lost you need to recognize the importance of retracing your steps. In this regard, a negative study is intellectually more important than a positive one.

The problem of bias is complicated by the discrepancy between the laboratory and the real world. Academicians function in a laboratory where treatments work much better on rats than in the world where humans live. Too often, researchers flood clinicians with information obtained from mice, wowing them with scientific terminology and descriptions of complex chemical pathways. Too often, I leave such meetings excited that someone has a solution. Too often, I send patients for such treatments, only to have my patient and myself discover that while the mouse is alive and well, the press releases were premature, and the patient continues to suffer.

Still another problem involves the practice of peer review of research before it is published or presented. Most journals have relatively large boards of individuals who serve this purpose. In theory, this practice should ensure academic honesty. Theoretically, you would be less likely to cheat if you knew you were going to get caught. In reality, this is not always true. It is apparent that if you have a "name" in a particular field, you will have a much easier time getting published. Whether you deserve that fame or not is another story.

Of more concern, in this media-crazy world, is that some researchers use the media to do an end run around peer review. They create a therapy, publish a limited outcome study that may or may not satisfy the needs of scientific rigor, and then pitch the therapy to the media. The media then create a public demand for the product. This is especially a problem with therapies that involve an off-label use of an existing FDA-approved technology. In such cases, the researcher may dispense with the accolades of the scientific world in favor of those of the population at large. He is seeking notoriety and wealth, too often at the expense of the patient. This issue has been huge since producers of medical technology realized they could profit by marketing directly to a naïve public. While physicians are not as knowledgeable as we would like to believe they are, they are still in a much better position to assess the relative merits of a technology than patients. I believe that this type of promotion is dangerous, and it should not happen.

In general, the desire to be recognized and finish first practically forces individuals to cheat. It is rather like an intellectual ingestion of steroids. It would be nice if academia adopted a different attitude such that all work together to solve a problem, and all share in the satisfaction of a job well done. Competition is good, and it drives us to be better, but there should be limits.

One way to define those limits is to create significant repercussions for academic dishonesty. The academic world needs to more effectively recognize when it is going astray and police itself when that happens. As I mentioned, when I first began my career in spine care, it was not unusual to see a researcher promote a 90 percent success rate with a specific intervention. Because of these astronomical claims of success, academic spine physicians clearly felt pressured to come up with such results if they wished to compete with their colleagues, even if they had to cheat or lie to do so and even if doing so was, in the end, harmful to the patients. They weren't fooling anyone. Everyone knew these outcomes were bull except, perhaps, for the young, naïve, and inexperienced like myself. It should not take great courage to stand up and challenge such results, and physicians should be encouraged and rewarded for having the audacity to do so.

I have come to admire honesty and humility more than any of the other virtues. The pressures on us to lie, to fabricate, to deceive in order to promote our standing in society can be great. However, when we deceive, we do harm someone—whether ourselves or another person. I have been blessed to learn from so many wonderful teachers who have had the courage to do what they thought was right, no matter the consequences. Someone who readily and honestly acknowledges not just what he or she knows, but what he or she doesn't know, is in fact an expert and, perhaps, a hero. I long for a system that encourages this type of expertise.

NINE

The Workplace and Entitlements

Creating "Inability" out of "Disability"

Nothing is more dangerous than discontinued labor;
it is a habit lost. A habit easy to abandon, difficult to resume.
Victor Hugo, *Les Misérables*, 4.2.1

Entitlement programs are designed to provide financial and other assistance for those in need. While we do not state that all citizens have a *right* to such assistance, we do see it as a social *responsibility* to help those who cannot fend for themselves.

Entitlements are a form of charity, and through entitlements, we acknowledge the needs of these individuals as all encompassing and offer shelter, fuel, food, money, education, and health care through subsidized housing, fuel assistance, food programs, "welfare," Social Security Disability, scholarships, tuition assistance, vocational rehabilitation, Medicare, and Medicaid. These programs offer assistance for current needs while providing people with opportunities for a better, more independent future.

By referring to these public programs as entitlements, we imply that our citizens have an inalienable right to them. Whether this is a right or a gift is an important distinction I will discuss later. A society cannot function without both rights and responsibilities, and many entitlement programs acknowledge this by expecting recipients to pay the gift back either financially or through public service. For most recipients the services are supposed to be only a safety net, and the assumption is that they will take the responsibility of working hard to again achieve self-sufficiency. For this reason many of these programs limit the amount of services that can be received. Others have no limits. Some programs, such as Medicare and Social Security for the elderly and disabled, are a payback for prior contributions over the course of a lifetime. In providing these services, we acknowledge that misfortune can visit all of us. In an instant, a lifetime of accomplishment, accumulation, thrift, and savings can be erased, leaving a previously independent individual or family destitute. Such is too often the reality of the pain patient.

This chapter discusses separately entitlements for pain related to occupational injury and for pain not related to occupation, since the programs that address these two categories are quite different. In both cases, however, as workers increasingly find themselves disenfranchised, our economy functions in deficit and recession, and our population ages and becomes more disabled, our ability to supply such assistance grows more and more limited, magnifying the problems the disabled face. Chapter 10 will cover private health and disability insurance.

The Notion of Work in America

When I moved to public school in fifth grade, I was a chubby, shy kid, disabled by seasonal asthma. I was actually a decent athlete, better than most kids in my class, but I certainly didn't look like one. On one of the first days at my new school, we gathered at gym class to pick sides for dodgeball. I watched in uncomfortable silence as my fears came true . . . I was the last one to be picked. Nobody treated me with contempt. Nobody called me names. Nobody threw balls in my face or broke my glasses. They didn't need to. The selection process alone shattered my self-esteem. I felt terrible.

When the game started, I was a nervous wreck. I needed to prove that I was good, that I was valuable. I was afraid of screwing up and confirming to my new classmates that I deserved to be the last one picked. I was lucky. I never had played dodgeball before, but I proved to be good at it. My skills at dodgeball did not translate into every other activity, but it didn't matter. The fact that I was good at something guaranteed that I was never picked last at anything again. Still, I never forgot the pain and wondered what would have happened to my self-esteem if I wasn't good and was perpetually picked last.

In adulthood, ability on the dodgeball court is replaced by ability in the workplace, and it is from this "court" that the pain patient is too often excluded, and in effect, degraded. Whether the exclusion is explicit or implicit, the message is that the patient is not worthy. In effect, the pain patient is assaulted with yet another injury, this one to the psyche, and perhaps even more painful than the original physical insult.

To understand how exclusion from the workplace affects the pain patient, it is important to understand the American concept of work, which is qualitatively different from that of most other cultures. On my first trip to Europe, I had some preconceived notions. I had always thought of Germans, for example, as meticulous and driven. So it came as quite a shock when a German I befriended during a week there informed me that Germans believed Americans to be the hardest working people in the world. We aren't like Europeans. We don't take siestas. We don't sleep eight hours every night. We don't take long vacations.

That concept seemed funny to me because I was so used to hearing fellow Americans complain about people in our country who freeload, "entitled" people who don't do their share. And pain patients who receive entitlements are among those stereotyped as lazy. I began to wonder whether we weren't setting our expectations so high that what is considered normal in other places seems unacceptable to us. To conform, to meet expectations, to be hired, one must be willing to meet this high bar. Those who can't are functionally excluded. These expectations are fueled by our competitiveness. We are not satisfied with a job well done or merely being as good as others. We need to be better than others, no matter the effect on our physical, psychological, and social health.

Hard work means long hours. As a physician, I am fully aware of this warped sense of values. I once rode up the chairlift at a local ski area with a seventy-year-old physician who bragged about his 70-hour workweek. It did wonders for his self-esteem, but left little time for his family. I still brag about the 80- to 130-hour weeks I worked as a resident. I shudder in fear that other doctors may find out I work only 50 hours a week now—supplemented with 10 to 20 hours of volunteer work, work around the house, and my writing, though! I pride myself that I get only six hours of sleep a night, usually collapsing on Friday nights from exhaustion. I recall an older surgeon chiding me for not starting my day until 8:00 AM. He started his at 5:00 AM, as "real men" do.

We brag that we don't take time off for sickness. How many times have you heard people brag that they have "never taken a sick day"? One of my colleagues actually bragged that he came in to work *and operated* with a temperature of 104° F. I wondered how his patient would have felt if he or she had known. Fortunately, with the arrival of such mysterious and frightful diseases as swine flu and H1N1, we finally realized that maybe it was better for all if we stay home when we are sick.

Americans' whole sense of identity is tied to our work, which is more than a means of making a living and supporting our families. It is a source of pride. We work weekends. We take work home at night. Some of us work *two jobs*. White-collar workers carry their work everywhere, thanks to the smartphone, the laptop, and the Internet. Blue-collar workers brag that they use and abuse their bodies. There is something very reassuring in knowing we have such an identity, that we work hard and *contribute*, and we will do whatever we need to do to maintain that identity. Losing it can be devastating.

When Pain and Disability Interfere with Work Ability

> No country, however rich, can afford the waste of its human resources. Demoralization caused by vast unemployment is our greatest extravagance. Morally, it is the greatest menace to our social order.
>
> Franklin Delano Roosevelt, Fireside Chat, September 30, 1934

Americans, the biggest consumers in the world, are also the biggest creators of waste, whether garbage, toxic chemicals, sewage, or nuclear by-products. Our excessive expectations of work also create a waste of humanity. Too often, those who can't meet the standard are left to the human waste heap. Just as there is much nutritional value remaining in the food thrown out by restaurants as damaged and not worthy of being served, there is also much productive value remaining in people deemed not worthy of the American workplace and too often referred to as "damaged goods."

Both in human and financial terms, this problem is daunting. According to data from the Centers for Disease Control, 35.8 percent of all reported disabilities are due to painful conditions (back, spine, arthritis, rheumatism).[1] It is clear that persistent pain has significant financial as well as nonfinancial consequences. The inability of a substantial percentage of our population to support themselves creates a financial challenge for the whole country. Consider the following:

Over fifty-one million Americans (18 percent of the population) are
   classified as disabled.

Three in ten Americans entering the workforce today will become
   disabled before they retire.

Accident or illness will force one in five employees to miss work
   for at least one year before they turn sixty-five.

One in seven Americans can expect to be disabled for more than
   five years.

The average long-term disability lasts two-and-a-half years.

Nearly seven million workers currently receive Social Security
   benefits. Almost half are under the age of fifty.

Most Americans are not prepared for such a challenge to their
   income: 44 percent spend more than they earn, more than
   50 percent have no pension, 33 percent have no retirement
   savings, and 71 percent live paycheck to paycheck.

Three-hundred-and-fifty thousand bankruptcies are blamed
   on injuries and unexpected illnesses.

Nearly 50 percent of all mortgage foreclosures are caused
   by disability.

Only 10 percent of all disabling accidents and illnesses are work
   related and covered by workers' compensation.

Over one hundred million workers are without private disability
   insurance.

Seventy percent of workers in the private sector have no long-term
   disability insurance.[2]

Like everyone else, pain patients seek to meet the American work standard, but fail because their pain does not allow them to work a forty-hour
week, or an eight-hour day with a half-hour lunch and two fifteen-minute
breaks, or to work overtime. It does not allow them to lift occasionally,
frequently, or repetitively; to bend, twist, squat, or kneel; or to drive for
long periods. They cannot use a computer or otherwise use their hands or
feet repetitively for long periods.

A change in ability often forces injured workers to look for other employment, but here they come up against other barriers. First, employers seek "unblemished workers." Second, very specific skills are required to perform increasingly more specialized tasks. Such abilities sometimes require time-intensive and expensive training. Skills that may be of great value in one occupation often are not transferable to another. Such specificity makes movement from one trade or job to another more and more difficult, especially for those with a disability.

This problem is compounded as people age. Training requires an investment that assumes a worker will be with the company for a long time. Older workers with a limited work life do not justify such an investment. To add insult to injury, the concept of what is "old" for the workplace keeps growing younger, even as our life spans lengthen.

Those who run businesses, who design or operate machinery, and who educate are valued. But those who have worked physical jobs and become limited by pain are extremely vulnerable if they lack the education or ability to transition into a desk job. When they can no longer use their backs to earn their bread, they are lost. So are the office workers who suffer from repetitive trauma and can no longer punch a keyboard all day. We are developing an increasingly skilled waste heap of damaged workers who have much to offer, yet languish on entitlements because they cannot fit into the American workplace. They suffer not only from physical pain, but also from the pain of exclusion. They are effectively being put out to sea on the ice floe.

Based on my twenty-eight years of experience, I have identified five types of injured workers:

1. *Those who suffer a devastating injury and cannot work.* Some believe there is no such thing as a person incapable of work. While that may be true in the abstract, it is not true in reality. Clearly there are people who cannot do enough work in a competitive workplace to support themselves or their families. An ability to support one's self and family is the definition of meaningful employment.

2. *Those who are injured, suffer from pain, and want to work, but do not have transferable skills that would allow them to find competitive, meaningful employment.*

3. *Those who do have transferable skills and are able to find work that brings in an income similar to what they had before.*

4. *Those who do find employment, but earn less than they did previously.*

5. *Those who are just seeking an easy way out of their responsibility to support themselves.* They exaggerate their inabilities in order to avoid work and obtain entitlements.

Rather bizarrely, we assume that most injured workers are of this fifth type. They do exist and are a burden to our system, but my impression is that they are more the exception than the rule. Many pain patients on entitlements would do anything to contribute, but have neither the knowledge nor the ability to fit into the American workplace. Many worked very hard before their injuries and would do so again if they could. Many lament the loss of self-esteem that comes with an inability to contribute. Many identify with the work they can no longer do. They see themselves as washed up, no longer valuable.

I am reminded of a senior claims adjustor who suffered from chronic hand and wrist pain. She readily admitted that the only reason she could still work was that at her level she did not need to use her hands as much as a junior claims adjustor. She kept her job only because of her experience. She worked because she had to, but she suffered. Like many others with pain, she was quite aware that she could never make as much money, live her current lifestyle, or support her family on an entitlement. Most who suffer from pain must make a daily cost-benefit calculation, weighing their economic needs versus their health needs. Most only stop working and resort to entitlements when the latter exceeds the former. Often the choice is made for them. When their pain limits their productivity, they are let go.

Too often, the door of termination is one-way. Reentry is difficult or impossible. Finding a new job within one's abilities is a challenge. Many start out with self-confidence, but lose heart as each successive door is slammed in their face. Many learn to lie about their disability. They claim they can do more than they can, merely so they can be productive. They find ways to hide their limitations, living in fear that their ruse will be discovered.

As business washes its hands of the pile of unproductive, damaged human goods, it unwittingly shifts responsibility to support those in pain to society as a whole, straining our entitlement systems and our ability to satisfy our obligation to help those in need—many of whom would help themselves if they could.

Defining Disability and Impairment in the Context of Pain

The concept of pain as a unique disability worthy of charity is relatively recent. In the past, it was assumed that pain was ubiquitous and similar from person to person and merely an accompaniment of another disabling condition such as a broken leg or a spinal cord injury. The disability was measured not by the pain, but by the extent of the underlying condition. In the same way, abilities and expectations were measured merely by assessing that underlying condition. When that condition resolved, any residual pain was not considered a disability, and the sufferer was expected simply to suck it up and get on with life. These assumptions still remain among those who have never really suffered from pain in general, or chronic pain in particular, or lived with someone who suffered that pain. Experts have only recently come to appreciate the complexity of pain and to acknowledge that all pain is not alike. This new understanding has profound implications for the concept of pain as a disability in itself, an issue that is further complicated by the way we have chosen to explain, measure, and compensate disability.

The first and perhaps most important problem is deciding whether pain in itself is a disability that deserves entitlement. Despite the fact that pain creates disability, there is surprisingly no agreement on this question for several reasons. First, as I have explained, there is no consensus on what pain even is. Many fail to acknowledge that it is not a single entity, but rather varies from person to person and situation to situation. Failure to understand and accept this variability will influence whether a person accepts pain as a disability. What is more, acute pain, chronic pain, and neuropathic pain are all totally different entities neuro-immuno-psychologically, and this difference has dramatic ramifications on a sufferer's abilities and disabilities. It is not unheard of for a football player to play an entire game with a fracture, yet require crutches to walk when the game is over. Nor is it unheard of for a football player to suffer through innumerable injuries throughout a career, yet be totally disabled from more mundane occupations when his career is over. What is disabling, the fracture or the pain? What is disabling, the cumulative injuries or the pain these injuries create? Pain is considered a part of football; therefore, one willingly plays through it, at least up to a point. Pain is not supposed to be a part of life, or so we are led to believe; so once the fans and the thrill of the game are gone, the player is less willing to accept it.

Second, pain tolerance is variable. Some people can tolerate severe pain for long periods, while others can do so for only minimal periods. Some people can tolerate severe pain, others not even minimal pain. These are unique characteristics of the individual, with both nature and nurture playing a role. There are cultural, racial, and sex-related differences in pain tolerance as well.

Third, pain tolerance and associated disability vary over time. I was being questioned once during a deposition about the severity of a patient's disability. To illustrate what it was like, I put a "Spock hold" on the questioning lawyer and asked if it hurt or if he found it disabling. He said it was uncomfortable, but he could deal with it. So I challenged him to think how it would affect his sleep, his physical activity, his mood, his sexual function, his enjoyment of life, and his work function if I put a clamp on the same area and locked it in place, leaving it there for eternity with no chance for removal. I suggested that what started out as a fairly trivial discomfort would after a while cause profound disability. He said he understood and asked me to remove my hand. In the same way, patients who struggle valiantly to work despite a painful disability will suddenly become unable to work when their hope of cure disappears, and they must confront the reality that their pain will accompany them for the rest of their lives.

The following discussion refers to impairment as well as disability. *Impairment* is defined as what is wrong with a person, whereas *disability* is how the impairment affects the person functionally. For example, a broken leg would be an impairment, and inability to walk because of the break would be a disability.

These concepts have been used by many entitlement systems to help decide whether an individual is truly in need of services. Although naturally we want an objective system that can definitively differentiate those in need from those who are not, such a system does not exist, nor will it ever. That does not stop us from trying to create it. Each entitlement system has its own objective criteria that it uses to determine whether someone is qualified to receive services. For physical and neurological disabilities, systems based on impairment are generally used. The most commonly used system is the *American Medical Association Guides to the Evaluation of Permanent Impairment.* The AMA was charged with the impossible task of simplifying the complexity of impairment into a single number, a percentage of the "whole person," which in theory allows us to compare one person to another. Based on this number, the guide enables us to assess first whether or not a person is entitled to receive assistance and, second, how much assistance she or he can receive.

To my knowledge, nobody has ever assessed the validity of an impairment rating, our current gold standard. However, it is quite clear that this measure is not accurate or valid. It is even clearer that it is not reliable, since there is a huge interobserver variability in the number obtained. Nevertheless, we persist, merely because an impairment rating is a number and we like numbers. Numbers are simple, even if what they measure is not. The problem is that a faulty number is fated to produce erroneous conclusions and poor decisions. When we use an impairment rating to simplify a complex problem such as disability created by pain, blatantly ignoring the individual's actual pain in the process, we are guaranteed to make mistakes in our assessment, which in turn are guaranteed to create adverse consequences for those in pain.

When we measure impairment in order to determine the need for entitlement, we overlook several facts. First, to most people, impairment is irrelevant. They care less about the name for their problem than they do about their limitations. I have a friend with quadraparetic cerebral palsy (meaning all four limbs are affected). There is no doubt in my mind that if his impairment was objectively assessed, his rating would be quite high. Still, throughout his nearly sixty years, he has been very functional. He drove and walked. He held a very responsible, important job his entire life. Then he began to have pain in his hip. This pain, had it been measured, would have added little if anything to his impairment rating. His motion had not changed. What had changed was that he couldn't walk very well. He started falling and having secondary injuries. This man, who despite his many limitations had lived a very "able" life, was suddenly disabled, not by cerebral palsy, but by pain. That creates its own problems of bias (further discussed in chapter 10). Because of the biomedical bias of our antiquated health-care system, in the past pain was considered a disability, subjective and therefore not measurable and not considered directly when making determinations about entitlement. The creators of the AMA guides assumed that pain was assessed indirectly through its effects on the range of motion of a particular joint, the chosen method for determining orthopedic impairment, and its effects on strength and sensory loss, the chosen methods for determining neurological impairment. It took five revisions and thirty-seven years of the guides before anyone realized that these premises were false. As the writers continue to tinker with the guides, and even though pain specialists finally have some input into their design, pain is still considered a disability, not an impairment, and thus is not directly measured.

Non-Work-Related Pain

Imagine, for an instant, that you have a college degree, you have a job, and you live in a nice neighborhood. You are married with two children. You have worked hard to get where you are, and your efforts have paid off. To maintain your position, you continue to work hard. Life is good.

Then, one day, through no fault of your own, everything changes: you develop a painful disease, or you are involved in a car accident. Suddenly, you have limitations you never had before. You seek treatment, but there is no cure. You are left with pain. Overnight, things you previously found easy to do become difficult, if not impossible. You can no longer sleep at night, engage in sex, play the sports you enjoyed, or play with your children. Most important for our discussion, you can no longer work as well as you used to. Your identity is shattered. Your nest egg is threatened.

Your pain is not work-related, so you get no workers' compensation. You may or may not have a disability policy. If you do, it provides substantially less income than you were making previously.

If you have a "nice" employer, he or she may put up with your lost productivity for a while. In theory, if your company is over a certain size, it is required to provide you with "reasonable accommodations" (whatever that means) to stay at your job. The reality is that when it becomes apparent you will never be the same, when you can no longer contribute to your company in a meaningful way, you will inevitably be let go. The workplace is not a babysitting service. If you have a less-than-altruistic employer, he won't wait so long.

Quite soon a financial crisis develops. Bill collectors show you no sympathy. You fail to pay the heating bill, the mortgage, the electric bill. You must choose between food and other necessities to survive. You seek another job, but struggle to find an employer willing to take a chance on you. You lose your health insurance. Now you are unable to afford the care you need, and your abilities decline even further. Marital stress builds. Your "able" spouse is forced to take on more responsibility.

To compound your problems, others question the legitimacy of your pain. Even though you have worked hard all your life, people assume you are "dogging it" and can do better. Eventually, their prophecies become self-fulfilling. You begin to question yourself. You wonder if this pain and the limitations it creates are all in your head.

Your self-esteem is battered and bruised. You have lost everything that is important to you. With your tail tucked firmly between your legs, you are forced to do something you swore you would never do. You ask for help. Already humiliated by your trials, you find little consolation in the public assistance system, which inherently dehumanizes. You despise what you must do, but you do it in order to reverse the downward spiral you find yourself trapped in.

For some, there are happy endings. Although their lives will never be the same, the safety net they fall into gives them enough support to find the help they need to return to a productive lifestyle of some sort. Others, though, have either fallen too far or their situations are too hopeless for them to be helped. Their support network falls apart, and they sink further and further into despair.

There is nothing abstract about this scenario. In my pain management practice, I see it played out daily. I am reminded daily of the cruelty of such an unpredictable world, which creates a sense of great impotence in me. As I see it, the problem is that the safety net is set so low that people can fall a long way before they get help.

We expect those citizens who can to support themselves. Like Mr. Smith, many who are disabled by pain want to work, and many could if the work were tailored to meet their limitations. The question then arises: while Americans have a *responsibility* to support themselves, do all capable Americans have an inalienable *right* to work? If so, how do we go about ensuring that right?

AMERICANS WITH DISABILITIES ACT

In a sense, we already have answered those questions with the creation of the Americans with Disabilities Act of 1990 (ADA). This civil rights law prevents discrimination against the disabled in employment, in public facilities including transportation and accommodations, in commercial facilities, and in telecommunications. The law states that "covered entities" may not discriminate against a qualified individual with a disability and must make reasonable accommodations to include him or her.[3]

Needless to say, there are many legal hurdles to enforcing this law in a competitive workplace. First, "reasonable" and "qualified" are not defined. Second, if two people apply for a job, one able bodied and one not, the law cannot be used to force the company to hire the disabled, and it is rare to have only one applicant for a job. A person who is employed at the time of the injury is somewhat protected, but only if any modifications required are "reasonable." The law does not apply to small businesses below a certain size, which as it happens, make up the bulk of our economy. In times when the supply of labor exceeds the demand, then, the law has little clout.

The law does limit what information a disabled person must share with a prospective employer. The person does not need to identify the nature of her disability or show any medical records. Any hiring decision must be made based on qualifications. The litmus test is that the individual must be qualified to perform the job.

The problem is that no matter how we try, we habitually make judgments about people we don't know based on their appearance. These judgments are shaped by cultural and other experiences. Thus when we see a person with a limp, a speech defect, or another physical "defect," we don't think "disabled." Rather we think "unable" or "invalid." When we are hiring for our business, we immediately think this person is not worthy, and it takes great conscious effort to defy that impression.

At the same time, it requires very little conscious effort to find ways around the ADA. First, some disabilities, including pain-related ones such as a limp, a grimace, or a stumble, are obvious. If there are other "qualified" individuals, such physical signs may be enough to disqualify that individual. Second, some businesses require drug screens prior to hiring. Patients on opioids or benzodiazepines are then, for all practical purposes, forced to state why they are taking such medications. Such patients cannot obtain commercial driver's licenses or pilot licenses, in effect restricting them from these fields and others.

Third, many pain sufferers have been terminated because of their pain or have lost considerable work time. Others have been out of the workplace for a long time. It is understandable that an employer searching for a reliable employee will ask the individual the reason for such absences. The law does not prevent this, and such a revelation may be enough to disqualify that individual, especially when there are others who are as qualified.

It is also important to note that when the ADA went into effect, pain itself was not considered a disability. Technically, then, those who suffered from disabling pain were not covered by the law. At the time of its passage, despite my profession, I never even considered that it might have any role in helping pain sufferers find a job or keep one. It came as quite a surprise to me and others how quickly personal injury lawyers began using the law to "assist" their clients. While the net effect of their actions was helpful in supporting those with pain, and they did succeed in getting the spirit of the law extended to include those disabled by pain, their hidden agendas were less than altruistic and created more problems than they solved. The new law created a whole new avenue for potentially lucrative lawsuits lawyers could use to enrich themselves, exploiting their clients' disabilities in the process. While attorneys benefited from these actions, they succeeded only in getting prospective employers to view people with pain-related disabilities as an even greater potential liability.

In the end, while the ADA clearly has helped improve community access for the disabled and has made a statement that the disabled can contribute, with respect to helping people disabled by pain find work, it has been effective only when the supply of labor is low relative to demand and anyone with a pulse is valuable.

SOCIAL SECURITY DISABILITY INSURANCE AND SUPPLEMENTAL SECURITY INCOME

When people disabled by non-work-related pain cannot find work, if they are not covered by private disability insurance they must resort to an entitlement program that forces them to prove they are disabled, a process that is often dehumanizing. It is basically begging. In the end most find either that the safety net is set so low that they cannot come close to supporting themselves in the manner to which they were accustomed, or that the benefits they receive are only temporary. Still, something is better than nothing; and that something gives them great disincentive to seek work, since if their job search is unsuccessful, they risk losing everything. The downward spiral may be arrested, but it is not reversed.

There are two programs intended to assist those in need due to disability, Social Security Disability Insurance (SSDI) and Social Security Insurance (ssi). ssdi is funded through payroll taxes; its recipients have worked for a certain number of years and made contributions to the Social Security trust fund. ssdi candidates must be under the age of sixty-five and have earned a certain number of "work credits." After receiving ssdi for two years, a person who is blind or has a disability is automatically eligible for Medicare. ssdi benefits are paid after an individual has been disabled continuously for five months. The benefit amount is based on the past earnings record, much like the regular Social Security retirement benefit.[4] However, people rarely receive benefits this quickly. The application process may actually take months to years, though once approved, benefits are paid retroactive to the time the disability began. That may be of little consolation if the individual has exhausted his life savings and become destitute while waiting to be approved. Even more problematic, many people who are truly disabled never receive services.

ssi, by contrast, is strictly need-based and is funded by general fund taxes. Candidates must have limited income and resources. The monthly payment is based on financial need and varies up to the maximum federal benefit rate. Some states add money to federal ssi payments. Approval generally takes three to six months and benefits are paid retroactive to the date of application. In most states, beneficiaries are automatically eligible for Medicaid.[5]

Social Security Disability, in particular, is subject to horrific abuse. It has become customary for attorneys to take a percentage, usually 25 percent, of an individual's claim. On paper, it should be unnecessary for a claimant even to need an attorney. But the system is designed so that it is nearly impossible for a claimant to "win" without one.

The process begins with a definition of disability that is outlined in a guide used by the individual who reviews the applicant's file. Technically, if the person meets that definition he receives ssdi. If not, he receives nothing. The individual has the right to appeal twice, for a total of three reviews. The first two decisions are made by a clerk, who applies the terms in the guide to the individual. Most often the patient is rejected both times. If he appeals, the decision is turned over to an administrative judge. The person can plead the case himself or have an attorney present. The stakes are high—perhaps the difference between eating and starving—so the desperate claimant turns to an attorney. In my experience the odds of success are much greater for someone with legal representation.

Work-Related Pain and Workers Compensation

Workers' compensation covers people injured in the course of their work. This safety net is set much higher than that for non-work-related pain, at least in theory. It is instructive to look at why and how the workers' compensation law was developed, how it is supposed to work, and how it really works.

Like many contemporary systems, American workers' compensation law has its origins in antiquity. The basis for such laws has always been the assumption that an employer has a responsibility to care for and compensate an employee injured in the course of employment. In 2050 BC, the Code of Ur-Nammu in ancient Sumer provided for monetary compensation for specific injury to a worker's body parts. The Code of Hammurabi from about 1750 BC provided a similar set of rewards for specific injuries and their implied permanent impairments. Similar systems existed in ancient Greece, Rome, Arabia, and China. All consisted of schedules based on specific injuries.

Such schedules were replaced in the Middle Ages by arbitrary compensation based on the wishes of the feudal lord to whom a serf was bound. That culture assumed that an honorable lord would care for his injured serf, but he was under no legal obligation to do so. In the late Middle Ages and early Renaissance, English common law replaced the arbitrary system, much to the detriment of the injured worker, who was now required to prove injury through an expensive tort system. The likelihood of success was impaired by the cost of the process and by what was referred to as the "unholy trinity of defenses." The first, "contributory negligence," meant that if the worker was in any way responsible for his injury, the injury was not compensable. The second, the "fellow servant" rule, provided that the employer was not liable if the injury resulted from the negligence of another employee. Third, the "assumption of risk" meant that an employee who accepted a contract was aware of any inherent risk of the job and could not be compensated for any injury caused by it.[6] Remnants of common law persist to the present. Although we no longer recognize the "unholy trinity" of employer defenses, we still require the injured employee to prove that the injury occurred at work, which too often entails great time and expense, aggravates the underlying pain issue by delaying treatment and rehabilitation, and creates an unpleasant adversarial relationship between employer and employee and their representatives. This scenario is a common experience for those who suffer from chronic pain created by work injury.

Needless to say, common law created a very uneven playing field between employer and employee, clearly favoring the former and creating the potential for a hazardous workplace. To rectify this imbalance, all subsequent workers' compensation laws have attempted—often unsuccessfully—to level the playing field by giving the worker the right to compensation without undue expense. At the same time, the laws sought to minimize potential financial stress to the employer.

The first attempt to make such changes occurred in Prussia under Chancellor Otto von Bismarck. Like many politicians, he was motivated less by altruism than by a pragmatic need to maintain a stable base of political support, specifically the working class, which was increasingly being courted by the political left. He therefore created the Employers' Liability Law of 1871, Workers' Accident Insurance in 1884, and finally, Public Pension Insurance. Most systems currently in place mimic these laws. Bismarck's system created compensation for injured employees, with the greatest compensation for those injured on the job. In a visionary move, the system also provided for rehabilitation. Employers were protected by a provision stipulating that they could not be sued in civil court by an injured employee, thus creating a "no-fault" system. Compensation for injury, rehabilitation, and tort protection are all part of current workers' compensation programs.[7]

The United States left the creation of workers' compensation laws to the states. In 1911, Wisconsin passed the first state law. By 1948 all states had passed some form of workers' compensation legislation.[8] Except for federal employment, workers' compensation law in the United States remains governed by each individual state. While statutes vary, they share much in common. Each system is modeled after the Prussian system described above. The central tenet is "no fault" insurance that accepts industrial injury as a fact of life. Employers participating in the system have the benefit of tort exception for injuries covered by workers' compensation, although employees may sue a third party felt to be responsible for their injuries. If they do and are successful, the proceeds from such suits must first go to reimburse their workers' compensation carrier.[9]

All American workers' compensation programs are employer funded, either through purchase of commercial insurance or through self-insurance. In most states, participation is optional, but most employers participate, and 80 percent of the American workforce is currently covered under some form of workers' compensation insurance.[10] In most states, a state compensation board handles claims, although decisions can be appealed to the state court system. In five states, claims are taken directly to the state court system, but special state agencies exist to help process claims.[11] In most states, compensation is paid both as wage replacement, usually at about two-thirds of salary, for the period of total disability and as a lump-sum payment for any permanent partial disability. Employers, through their insurers, are also liable for any medical and rehabilitation costs.[12] To create an incentive for companies to hire already disabled employees, many states also have "second injury funds" run by the state that private insurers contribute to. These funds are used to make up the difference when a second injury proves to be incapacitating only because of a prior injury to another body part.[13]

Employees actually enter the system when they begin employment, before any potential injury has occurred. The job they assume is examined for any potential hazards, and preventive measures are taken. The Occupational Safety and Health Administration (OSHA) oversees this process; it issues and enforces health and safety standards for the workplace. Every employer in the United States is held accountable to OSHA. The goal is to prevent injury. This is accomplished through the inspection of job and workplace design (ergonomics).

Nevertheless, injury still happens. It can be either sudden or cumulative. In either case, once an injury is recognized, it is up to the employee to report the injury to the employer and fill out an incident report. The report is then submitted to the state labor board and to the employer's insurance carrier. If the insurance company deems the injury compensable, all future medical care, reimbursement for lost wages, and rehabilitation are compensated. In effect, workers' compensation serves as both health care and disability insurance. It also serves as a form of life insurance when an individual dies as a result of an industrial accident. In such an event, the employee's estate is compensated. The decision about whether an injury is compensable can be quite complicated, especially when the injury is due to repetitive trauma or is unwitnessed. Even when the injury is witnessed, the witness may be reluctant to come forward and support the claim.

In general, once an incident report is filed, the initial treating physician must make a decision about work-relatedness. If the doctor does not feel the injury is work-related, the employee may seek another opinion. If the employer does not feel the injury is related, she too can seek another opinion. Disputes are brought to the state labor board. Such disputes naturally create an adversarial relationship between parties, delay treatment, and forever adversely alter the employer-employee relationship.

In most states, once an injury is accepted as compensable, health-care and work ability decisions are made by the employee's treating doctor; and the employee has the right to choose his or her own physician. If the employer questions these decisions, she has the right to obtain a second opinion (independent medical examination, or IME). In some states, the insurer or the state must approve a plan of care before treatment can commence. This also can create delays in treatment.

Disability can be considered partial or total. If the treating physician feels the employee has a partial work capacity, the ADA mandates that the employer must provide "reasonable accommodations" for performing a "light-duty" job. Again, small businesses that employ fewer than thirty employees are exempt from this requirement, although their insurance carrier may require such accommodation as a part of the insurance policy. If the light-duty employment is full-time, it is assumed the employee will be paid at the level of previous wages. If it is part-time, it is assumed the insurance carrier will make up two-thirds of the difference between part-time pay and pre-injury pay. If the treating physician believes that the employee can fully perform all duties of his or her job, then the employee has a full duty work capacity. The employee still has the right to receive reimbursement for all medical expenses related to the injury, wage reimbursement for any work time missed because of treatment, and a lump-sum settlement for any permanent partial impairment.

The employee is considered totally disabled if the treating physician believes the employee cannot work or if the employer is unable to provide reasonable accommodation. In this circumstance, the employee is compensated by the insurance carrier at a rate set at two-thirds of the pre-injury salary. The purpose of setting compensation less than salary is to give the employee an incentive to return to full productivity. It is important to note that compensation is not subject to income tax; and therefore, in effect, the employee is being compensated at a level higher than two-thirds. It is theoretically possible for high-end earners to receive compensation almost identical to their pre-injury salary.

The goal of the system is to work with injured employees to help them heal and return to work as quickly and safely as possible. It is recognized that the longer an injured worker is out of work, the less likely it is that he will return. This is true for several reasons. For one, the more severe an injury, the longer it takes to heal, and the more likely it is that there will be a permanent disability to some degree, which will impair an employee's ability to work.

In addition, the longer we are away from work, the more mentally deconditioned we become. We feel alienated from our workplace, and increasingly fear our return to a place where we previously felt comfortable. We recall how we viewed other injured workers when we were at work and assume that our fellow employees will feel the same about us. We feel a sense of guilt at having let others down. As time passes, it becomes increasingly challenging to reenter the work environment. During my own two-month disability when I was an intern, I struggled with the notion that I was letting my coworkers down. I felt so guilty that I feared seeing them again. I was fortunate because they did treat me well. What would have happened had they not? I would have been permanently ostracized from a place where I had previously felt comfortable.

Workers also fear re-injury. Once we have been injured, we seek to avoid activities that aggravate or re-create our pain and the mental anguish the pain creates. The more severe or long lasting the pain is, the greater the fear, especially if the pain is persistent or permanent. In a very real sense, this is a posttraumatic stress disorder, which accompanies all significant injury. While we always encourage a fallen rider to "get back on the horse" as quickly as possible, a newfound fear will always accompany it; and the more severe the trauma, the greater the fear, and the greater the likelihood one will avoid the activity altogether.

How the employer treats the injured employee also plays a major role in how quickly the employee returns. To some extent, the employer's behavior will be dictated by his pre-injury relationship with the employee. However, that is not always true. No matter how much an employer valued the employee, an injured worker is still a financial liability. She creates lost productivity and unforeseen cost. Working at a mandated light duty, while quite useful in helping an injured worker return to full productive employment, creates an unfavorable cost-benefit ratio for the employer. In other words, it costs more to keep the employee than she can produce. A compensable incident also may cause the employer's insurance premium to rise. Businesses large enough not to be exempt from the ADA are more able, but sometimes unwilling, to support the cost of injury and light duty. The larger the employer, the more impersonal it is likely to be. In a large corporation, the injured worker becomes a threat to the bottom line. Decision makers have no previous relationship with the injured worker, and they find it easier to exclude her. The longer a worker is absent, or the longer she is on a relatively nonproductive light-duty status, the less welcome she may be. No matter what the law says, it is difficult to return to an environment where one is not valued, and the law cannot change that.

How an injured worker is treated also depends on the supply of labor. If the supply is limited and the cost of finding a new employee and training him or her high, the injured worker will be more valued. If the supply is high, especially if the cost of training is low, the injured worker will be less valued, and it is less likely he will return. The longer the employee is away, and the more the cost of his absence rises, the less valued even a previously valued employee will be. To protect the injured worker's rights, most states mandate that the employee's job must be held for a certain period of time, usually one year. An employee who cannot return to full employment within one year can be "terminated."

Over time, the injured worker progresses through treatment algorithms, and he eventually comes to a point of "Maximal Medical Improvement," or MMI, when all involved determine that there is no further medical intervention that is likely to yield more functional improvement. Any further treatment will only serve to "maintain" the employee's current condition. At this point, several things can happen, varying from state to state. What always occurs is a determination of work ability and permanent partial impairment. Based on work ability, the employee will return to previous duties, return to the previous employer at light duty, seek alternative employment, or be considered permanently disabled. If the individual is unable to return to previous duties, the insurance carrier must help her find new employment at a similar or less remunerative job. If less remunerative, the insurance company must cover a percentage of the difference in income for a specified period of time.

At some point, a settlement is considered. In some states, a settlement ends any relationship between the employee and the insurance company. In other states, if totally or partially disabled, the employee may continue to receive income, coverage for maintenance medical services, and rehabilitation services. In all states, the settlement includes a lump-sum payment for a permanent partial disability, the amount of which is based on a schedule. The treating physician or a designated physician calculates a permanent impairment percentage based on some reference, usually the *American Medical Association Guides to the Evaluation of Permanent Impairment.* The employer or employee may get a second opinion on the percentage. The information is presented to an "impartial" third party, and a dollar amount is awarded. In some states, the employee also may receive a lump sum against future wages. If this is done, the employee waives the right to receive further compensation for lost wages. In some states, a lump sum also is included for future medical costs, and the employee will receive no future reimbursement for medical expenses for this injury.

Rehabilitation is a part of the process from start to finish. The sooner the employee begins focusing on the future, the better. It is assumed that all parties will participate actively and responsibly in this process. Realistic goals and time frames are set. It is important to get the employee back in a work setting of some sort as soon as possible. As healing occurs, the level of activity is increased. When the point of MMI is reached, and the long-term goal involves finding a new job and acquiring new skills, the insurance company will assist with this process. Again, it is important to note that the insurance company is only responsible for helping the injured worker find a job that pays an amount similar to his or her previous job. For example, it would never be expected to help an injured nurse go to medical school. Throughout this process, the insurance company is represented by a claims adjustor, who assigns a nurse to oversee medical management and a rehabilitation nurse or vocational specialist to oversee rehabilitation.

In theory, all have the injured employee's best interests at heart. Nowhere in this ideal process is there a need for a lawyer. The problem is that the way the system is supposed to work and how it really works can be quite different, often with negative ramifications for employer, employee, and society. This is especially true in cases of chronic pain, where treatment outcomes refuse to follow the expectations of health-care providers and the schedules of claims adjusters. For the chronic pain patient, the system falls apart in predictable places, much to the detriment of his or her long-term mental and physical health. To explain how this happens, I want to look in more detail at three critical points of the process:

What are the important issues in the workplace before the injury
  happens?

When an injury happens, how is it determined to be compensable?

What happens when the duration of disability exceeds what is
  "medically reasonable"?

BEFORE THE INJURY: WORKPLACE DESIGN
AND EMPLOYER ATTITUDE

Studies have suggested that the most important factors determining
whether an injured worker will return to work are how much the person
likes the job and how much the job likes the person. This last statement is
a much more complicated concept than it might seem. How the workplace
is designed speaks volumes to employees about the employer's attitudes.

Let me share two examples. Bill was injured while working at a small
company. I don't recall the nature of his injury; but I remember that when
it occurred, his employer stopped what he was doing, brought Bill to the
hospital, and stayed with him, leaving someone else to supervise the job
site. He stated openly that his employee's health was his major concern,
checked frequently to see how Bill was doing, and assured him that a
place would be there for him if and when he was able to return to work.
The employer had designed the workplace ergonomically, adapting each
job station to the needs of the person using it. He got to know each of his
employees and treated them with respect. He set up a plan of task rotation
so employees would not overuse any one particular muscle group. When
employees had concerns, he listened.

The second example is a low-level supervisor for a large company that
owned many factories. His injury was mostly attributable to poor workplace design and poor safety inspection. Management had virtually no
contact with its employees and showed little concern for their welfare,
knowing that each could be easily replaced. Tasks were highly repetitive,
with minimal break time; and overtime was expected, including weekends and holidays. There was no task rotation. Workstations were neither
ergonomic nor tailored to employees' needs. Injuries were frequent, but
employees lived in fear of reporting one, knowing they would be ostracized,
more by the management than by fellow employees. They also were quite
aware that as soon as they returned from their convalescence, they would

be fired and replaced. Most employees of this company had limited skills and knew they had few other job options. While taking advantage of the employees' desperation, this company enticed them with good benefits. No matter how poorly they were treated by the Scrooge-like management, they worked through pain until they dropped and were too often left with a lifelong problem.

This supervisor came to me with a rotator cuff tear that would heal in time. More important, though, I needed only to look into his eyes to see he had suffered a head injury as well, and its ramifications never went away. His short-term memory was compromised, and he could not function in a noisy, complex environment. While his shoulder soon healed, his cognition did not. His rehabilitation nurse told me that the company would accommodate his limitations. I explained what they were and then approached the patient about returning to work on modified duty. He refused. When I asked him why, he said that one of his duties as a supervisor, dictated by management, was to promptly terminate any injured worker, no matter the circumstances, once he or she was released from workers' compensation. He was sure that he too would be terminated the minute he returned, and he would lose all of his benefits with little hope for future employment.

Bill was injured in a legitimate accident. His employer showed his concern not just by accepting responsibility, but also by setting up an environment that was a pleasure to work in. The second worker's injury was preventable and due to employer negligence. Despite this, the employer never showed compassion and never accepted responsibility. Instead, while running a modern-day sweatshop that hired only the desperate, it threw out injured workers like some would throw out the trash, creating a culture of fear.

These examples provide two extremes on a spectrum. Most companies fall somewhere in between. But in my experience too many lie toward the end where employees are treated as dispensable. It is true that no matter what an employer does, some employees will be perpetually unhappy. However, in my experience these people are the exception. It is unfortunate that our behavior as employers (I am a small business owner and employer) toward our injured workers too often assumes that they are "milking the system." Employers also too often assume that how they treat their employees does not matter. That is not true. How an employer sets up a workplace and how he treats an injured worker will go a long way toward creating an incentive for the worker to heal and return to work. People will go the extra mile for those they respect. They will seek vengeance on those who abuse them.

It is essential that an employer do all she can to set up a congenial and safe workplace. While this may entail a cost in the short term, it saves money in the long term. This is where the science of ergonomics comes in. Ergonomics is hardly an abstract science. It is mostly pure common sense. Every factor that affects workplace function, from the color of the room to its smells and sounds, the ventilation, the fit of the workstation to each particular individual, and the rotation of tasks must be considered.

Most managers have never performed the jobs they oversee. Too often, when an employee complains, they dismiss the complaint as whining. Would it not be better for them to attend to the concerns? Would it not be reasonable for them to actually try out the job—for eight hours a day, five days a week? The best ideas come from the "trenches," from those who actually do the job. Management must be willing to listen to their advice. Respecting the concerns of those performing a job not only improves job quality and prevents injury, it also conveys a sense of caring. That, too, is common sense.

DETERMINING WHETHER AN INJURY IS COMPENSABLE

Once a worker is injured, the compensation system should be mobilized, but too often it is not. Artificial barriers are set up: by the system, employers, the insurer, the court system, and the worker himself. I have observed that when the system victimizes the injured by failing to recognize their needs, it actually sows the seeds of a chronic pain problem. As I have explained, when we victimize we alter the neurophysiology of pain, and can create or contribute to a chronic pain state.

Two assumptions I discussed in earlier chapters affect how those involved in the system treat workers with persistent pain. The first is the assumption that there is an objective explanation for all pain, which as we know is incorrect. The second is the assumption that we can understand another person's pain in terms of our own experiences and expectations, which are shaped by those we accept as experts. That too is incorrect.

System-Created Barriers   The first set of barriers is created by the system as a whole. Often systems are designed to prevent the worst possible outcome, even if that outcome is uncommon. In the workers' compensation system, the worst possible outcome is a fraudulent claim. Most involved in the system believe that this outcome is infrequent and that most injured workers have a legitimate claim. Still, to prevent fraud, such a worker must prove his disability. This, in effect, punishes the many for the actions of a few. Think of a time you were hurt. How would you have felt if instead of compassion, you were treated with contempt and disbelief? Too often I have heard my patients say that if that they had known how poorly they would be treated, they would not have reported their injury in the first place. That is not how the system is supposed to work, but often it does.

It is amazing to me how well-intentioned efforts by patients, their families, and their providers can be undone in a few seconds by unkind words directed at them by those who control the purse strings. Those who interact with individuals seeking assistance, whether a workers' comp claim adjustor, a welfare worker, an employer, or a Social Security worker, need to be trained to be compassionate. They must be taught that it is not a sin to be disabled, to suffer from pain, or to be destitute. The worker at the insurance window is the face of the system. How she responds to the person seeking help has significant ramifications. A kind word can go a long way. Workers need to understand that these patients are desperate, and desperation creates demanding behavior. Shutting a window in that person's face only aggravates the problem. Acknowledging the desperation while communicating that they are there to help and will help is therapeutic and healing.

Worker-Created Barriers   While the system may be set up against the pain patient, one would assume that patients would advocate for themselves. Often they don't. Surprisingly, injured workers often set up their own barriers to care. The first barrier is denial. Often I am amazed by what workers are able to deny. Every day, patients tell me their work injury actually happened months before, but they assumed it would get better if they kept pushing through it. Some injured people work for months, even years, with the effects of their injury before reporting it. This behavior delays treatment, which we assume works best when done early. Although there is minimal literature to support this statement, it probably has some truth. Denial also delays the filing of a claim. Most states allow a grace period of up to two years to file a claim after an injury. However, the more time that elapses after an injury, the more suspiciously the system views it. The injured employee must prove that the problem occurred on the job. Many things happen over time. Did the injury really happen at work? What about that time the person lifted the lawnmower at home? Could that or some other injury have caused the problem? It is all too easy for the insurance company representative to find alternative explanations.

Such delay also poses problems for the treating doctor, who must determine whether the problem is work-related. Since the workers' compensation safety net is set much higher than that for non-work-related disability, there are clear incentives for a person with a legitimate injury, even if not work-related, to claim workers' compensation. This is a type of secondary gain. How is the physician to make a decision in support of the employee when the only evidence of injury is the employee's word, and the injury is old? There is often little objective data that can be used to make that decision, and the physician is forced to choose either to trust the employee or not. When confronted with such a situation, I decide whether what I have been told is plausible or not. Then I make a decision, knowing I am going out on a limb.

Another barrier facing an injured worker is fear. As I have noted, workers fear how their fellow employees will view them, based on how others have been treated. If someone is ridiculed for reporting an injury and "making it hard on everyone else," then others will have a disincentive to report it when they too become injured.

Workers also fear the employer's reaction, again based on past experience. If they have witnessed others being treated harshly, they will be reluctant to report their injury. They fear losing their jobs, especially if they have limited options. This problem is acute if it means giving up a job identity they may have worked years to obtain.

Many fear the workers' compensation system itself. Horror stories abound in which injured workers share their inhumane treatment by the system. I hear and witness such stories every day. We base our actions on assumed risk. If we assume the risk of being treated badly is high, we are more likely to live with our problem or find other means of taking care of it.

Sometimes it is not fear or denial that stands in the way, but ignorance. Most of us don't know what our rights are in general, and many injured workers don't know theirs. They don't know what to do when injured or whom to turn to for help. An unfriendly system, employer, or even fellow employee is often of no assistance. They face a grossly uneven playing field, where they must fight for their rights against those who not only understand the laws better, but also know how to twist and manipulate them in their own favor. This leaves the worker without a sense of control. When we lose control, overwhelmed by sensory and legal overload, we take the path of least resistance, which is to give up or never try.

Employer-Created Barriers   Employers too often deny the existence of a problem, although for quite different reasons than the employee's. An injured worker creates an increased insurance risk and decreased productivity, two things that threaten the bottom line. Employers are also human, and often they deny for the same reason anyone else does. They don't want someone to be hurt. They definitely don't want to be seen as being responsible for causing the injury, especially if the effects are permanent. As long as they deny the severity of the injury, it doesn't exist. This does wonders to massage the employer's comfort level. Often employers acknowledge the person's injury but actually place the blame on the employee in order to avoid responsibility, falling back on the standard notion that the injured is at fault.

Employers may combine denial and blame by trying to eliminate the problem, for example, by firing the employee before she has a chance to file a claim. Or if that isn't possible, they may find a creative way to release the employee after the claim has been filed. Some employers take the injury personally, believing the worker is out to get them, and react defensively, in effect denying any responsibility.

While these techniques may be effective in the short term, eventually the chickens come home to roost. Denying, blaming, eliminating, and personalizing only anger the worker, unnecessarily creating an adversarial situation and motivating the worker to fight for his or her rights. Then a lawyer comes knocking on the employer's door. When this happens, the cost and complexity of the problem are magnified logarithmically.

Worker injury creates other problems for the employer: the cost of making modifications to the job and decreased productivity resulting from the loss of a worker. Employers are graded by job site safety. An injury adversely affects their safety record, with potential ramifications for their insurance premium. They fear repercussions from regulatory agencies that may find fault with the way the job site is run and either assess fines or demand expensive modifications. These are all incentives to muffle injured workers' claims.

Employers may have unreasonable expectations of their employees, especially in labor-intensive industries. No employee should expect a job to be painful. However, many employers believe that pain is part of the job and that a worker should expect it. There is a difference between a sore back and an injured back, however, and too often, an employer may be oblivious to the difference. When a worker reports an injury, some employers assume it is a natural part of the job. Employees want to be valued by their employer. By effectively communicating to the employees that pain is part of the job, they are giving their employees a disincentive to report an injury.

I frequently hear of injured workers who are subject to ridicule by their employers, especially if their recuperation entails some light duty on the job site. In effect, the employer is holding up the injured employee as a bad example for all employees to see. I have had patients who were so afraid of being subjected to such treatment that not only did they not report an injury, they did everything they could to hide it.

As we have seen, when an injury occurs, the worker initiates the workers' compensation process by filing an incident report. This report is then sent to the insurance company, where a decision is made as to whether the injury is compensable. The employer plays a role in this process by sharing information with the insurance company. To the extent that the employer ridicules, denies, or blames the worker for the injury, he adversely affects the acceptance of the claim. Injuries that are witnessed have a greater chance of being accepted, so employers may want to tilt the scales in their favor by eliminating the witness. I have seen cases where employers either explicitly or implicitly threatened potential witnesses, causing them to change their stories out of fear for their jobs.

Sometimes employers outright lie. We often accuse those seeking entitlements of being motivated by secondary gain. But secondary gain is not limited to the worker. For an employer, a low injury rate is a significant secondary gain, and she may be motivated to do whatever it takes to keep that rate low and deny injury. I have seen employers fabricate stories, claiming the worker was injured elsewhere, as a means of trying to avoid responsibility.

Insurer-Created Barriers   Like any business, insurance companies try to maximize the bottom line. They do this by increasing their stock sales and sales of their insurance products, and by minimizing payouts for losses. While they claim that their reason for existing is to aid the injured worker, their real goal is to satisfy their investors. This is not a totally selfish premise. You can only satisfy your stated goal of helping those in need if you satisfy those who fund you. The problem is that the goals conflict. Paying out large amounts in compensation has an adverse effect on profits, and stockholders will take notice. As a result, insurance companies have every incentive to minimize payouts, and they do this in a number of ways, effectively creating barriers to access.

First, all claims are viewed with some degree of suspicion. In effect, the insurance company sets up a wall to protect itself against potential claimants, and this wall is defended by the claims adjustor, who takes the position that the claimant is guilty until proven innocent. In my experience, claims adjusters believe that fraudulent claims are a much bigger problem than is really the case, and they often seem to assume a claim is fraudulent until proven otherwise. I believe that claims adjusters are actually taught this and come to believe it. It becomes a paradigm that must be defended. This attitude not only restricts access to the system, but also affects the mental health of the claimant.

What strikes me as odd is the degree of randomness in this process. Some clients with a weak case are accepted without question, while others with an airtight case are ignored or abused. I almost have come to believe that adjusters spin a "wheel of fortune" to decide how they will treat a claimant. Does every adjustor's office employ a "Vanna"? I hope not, but I have no better explanation.

Often it is open to question whether an injury even occurred, or that it occurred at work. Employer and employee may have different perspectives on this, and it is up to the insurance company to decide who is factually correct in a situation where objective facts are few and it's essentially a case of "he said, she said." In such a case, the insurance company has every incentive to take the employer's point of view, and often that is what they do. Often, however, employer and employee agree on the injury. Instead of accepting the claim in the face of such overwhelming evidence, the insurance company may deny it, leaving employer, employee, physician, and just about everyone else scratching their heads.

Adjusters have a range of presumably legitimate reasons to deny a claim. Aggravation of a preexisting condition is a great one. For example, the MRI showed some "arthritis" in the joint. That must be the problem, not the lifting injury. It doesn't seem to matter that the person never had a problem before the incident. Or the repetitive injury wasn't caused by the employee's typing at work, but the quilting she did on Saturdays. If physical reasons don't suffice, the adjustor makes up mental ones: the person is somatisizing, or converting, or whatever. Use a big word to explain the reason for the denial, find an "expert" to verify it, and you're golden!

At this point, the struggle becomes employee versus insurance company. The employer, subservient to its insurance company, plays a reduced role. I have been surprised to hear employers speaking of frustration over how poorly the insurance company treats their employees. And in this respect, the employer really is relatively helpless. He certainly has the right to take his business elsewhere, but often he doesn't have a lot of other options, giving the insurance company excessive leverage. Even if the employer does have another option, that won't help this particular employee. Once a claim is filed with an insurer, it stays there. The employer discovers that he has made a pact with the devil and has no ability to control the outcome.

In the world of "he said, she said," the notion of repetitive trauma provides fertile ground for creative denial. Repetitive trauma occurs not from a single major incident, but rather from repetitive overuse over time. It is common sense that anything, if overused, will eventually fatigue and fail. If someone lifts all the time, eventually the back will degenerate and fail. If one types all the time, the fingers and the wrists will rebel. And while the body has some recuperative abilities, these are not perfect. Repetitive use occurs over a long period of time, and not all incidents that contribute to it happen in the workplace. All of us use our hands repetitively or lift at home.

When a sudden injury happens at work, no matter what outside factors may play a role, the incident is usually considered work-related, no matter how absurd that may be. For example, we know that herniation (protrusion) of a spinal disc is the endpoint of a repetitive process called the "degenerative cascade." The final event that creates the herniation can be quite trivial. Sometimes it is a sneeze. However, if the event happens at work, it is considered, without question, work-related. One of my patients suffered a permanently incapacitating disc herniation when she leaned over to get her purse out of her desk drawer. The claim was accepted. But if there is no such identifiable incident, if the trauma is minor and cumulative, how does one judge work-relatedness? Such uncertainty allows the insurance company almost infinite leeway in making their decision to accept or refute. The incentive to deny is inescapable.

Another problem is that adjustors and their supervisors rarely have any medical knowledge. I once performed a nerve conduction test (NCS) on a woman to assess for possible carpal tunnel syndrome (CTS). As we talked, it became clear that she had no idea what "NCS" meant. She later identified her occupation as senior claims adjustor. I was stupefied. I asked how she decided whether to accept a claim for CTS if she didn't know what an NCS was. She said that she just accepted whatever her expert said. Note that she was a *senior-level adjustor* who supervised others! Is it surprising the system is so dysfunctional?

In making decisions, adjustors rely on several sources. First, and probably most important, they rely on their preconceived notions. If adjustors have negative assumptions about claimants that are either taught by superiors or reinforced by them, they are likely to create a barrier-driven culture. Second, adjustors rely on the claimant's incident report, which they interpret through the mental filter of their preconceived notions. Third, they rely on information from the employer with its own inherent problems outlined above. Fourth, they rely on a set of manuals that outline different injuries, how debilitating they may be, how long the disability may last, and how much each should cost. These manuals are based on statistics summarizing the experience of the general population. If a person's experience is different from the majority, he is considered abnormal, or the exception. Too often, that is where the chronic pain patient resides.

Finally, adjustors rely on "experts" who are actually consultants with varying levels of experience and preconceived notions of their own that affect the quality of their advice. They are often paid well for their services. To keep the gravy train going, they have every incentive to see things the insurance company's way. This creates an inevitable bias in their recommendations.

Complex problems often result in varying opinions on causes, effects, and solutions. Thus a chronic pain patient's evaluation is subject to a clash of opinions. As I have said, people generally choose a point of view that is beneficial to their own bottom line. So an insurance company will typically select experts who see things their way. To the extent that an adjustor relies on skewed information as a result of preconceived notions, inaccurate information from employers, skewed manuals that do not acknowledge the reality of chronic pain, and biased information from "experts" who may not have any knowledge about those they are judging, the adjustor will tend to deny services to those who deserve them, creating a major barrier to care for those in need.

Court-System-Created Barriers   When the inevitable disputes arise, the injured worker or the insurance company has the right to seek mediation. In most states, this is performed by the labor board, where the evidence presented essentially boils down to "he said, she said." It is true that—short of out-and-out corruption (which probably also occurs)—the board is not influenced by financial incentives as the insurance company is. Still, those who sit on the labor board have their own preconceived notions. Most judges have little to no medical knowledge. In most states, to counter the biases that may arise, boards usually are composed of an odd number of individuals of varying backgrounds. As in any court, each side presents evidence, and the panel makes a collective decision. Decisions are binding, but may be appealed. One of my patients appealed his case all the way to the New Hampshire Supreme Court. He had a chronic problem that required "maintenance care." The insurance company argued that it was only responsible for care necessary to bring his condition to the maximal medical endpoint. If my patient won at any level of the judiciary, the precedent would have dramatic ramifications for the bottom line of all insurers in our state, so the insurance company had great incentive to fight my patient's claim. The Supreme Court found in my patient's favor, and ever since, the State of New Hampshire requires that any and all maintenance care for a work-related injury be covered in perpetuity.

While TV shows present the courtroom as a stage for wonderful drama, it is not a place for the faint of heart, and that is where the main barrier to this process lies. Claimants have already been injured, and their pain persists. Instead of receiving compassion, they have been further injured by the contempt of their fellow employees, their employer, and the insurance company. In this "kill the guy with the ball" game, they have sometimes even experienced contempt from their families and friends. Their only solace has come from an attorney whose own motives may be open to question. Still, they must trust someone. Together, attorney and claimant face an open court where the opposing attorney will use every fact and fantasy at her disposal to discredit the plaintiff. This is a world of only black and white, right or wrong. Blow after blow is directed at the self-esteem of the claimant, further battering an already tortured psyche. Many find it easier just to give up.

The nature of the courtroom creates still another barrier. The motivations that make for a good insurance expert allow such a person to thrive in the courtroom. The motivations that make for a compassionate provider destroy such a person. Therefore, patients experience difficulty in finding experts willing to support them. In fact, workers' compensation patients have trouble even finding providers willing to care for them and the legal baggage they bring. While it is generally thought that patients who receive compensation have poorer outcomes with specific injuries than patients who do not, this is frequently assumed to be because there is a secondary gain of money and freedom from responsibility. The truth is that in such cases rehabilitation often is hampered by the secondary loss of belittlement by the system, and that is a loss a provider is unable to manage. I do not recall being told that such care was part of the practice of medicine. I was taught to be a patient advocate, but I was never told that this included legal testimony.

In such a frightening world, a lawyer becomes a necessary evil. Certainly there are wonderful, highly skilled attorneys out there who put the needs of their clients equal to or ahead of their own. I have had the privilege of working with many such. There are also many exemplary defense attorneys who know whom they represent, but seek, as much as possible, to inflict no further harm on the patient. In the true spirit of the law, they seek truth and a reasonable settlement. Unfortunately, they are not the rule. Insurance companies have deep pockets, and they can afford to hire skilled attorneys who see things their way. These are, in effect, legal sharks who have a goal in mind and will destroy all who cross their path, no matter what the cost to that individual.

Injured workers have a limited ability to decide who is best to represent them. Often they must rely on the ads they see in the phone book, on the city buses, or on television. The system allows these attorneys to charge up to one-third of any settlement. This creates several problems. First, injured workers with small claims struggle to find any attorney to represent them, especially when the injury results in full recovery with virtually no lump-sum settlement. Second, many attorneys do not wish to get involved until a settlement is pending. Then they ride in on their white horse and take one-third of what the patient probably would have gotten anyway. Third, attorneys have every reason to increase the cost of the claim, since that affects their take. In order to do this, they must exaggerate the disability. This frequently results in a greater use of health-care services at a greater cost and a delay of rehabilitation and return to a productive lifestyle. In fact, returning to a productive life harms the patient's legal value. This is why plaintiff's attorneys often act as a barrier to rehabilitation.

Patients' legal and medical needs don't disappear when the settlement is over. But once their one-third is in hand, the plaintiff's attorneys frequently disappear, leaving the patient alone and vulnerable. Now the insurance bully sweeps in and takes advantage of the patient's vulnerability. The insurer commonly denies care, forcing the patient to either go back to court or give up. Battered and bruised, instead of standing up for his or her rights, the patient usually gives up.

I consider much of what I have described so far to be corruption, which to me means putting the needs of the self over those of one who suffers, and worse, taking advantage of that person's plight. It is clear that there also is corruption in the more conventional sense. Judges are bought off and panels manipulated. In states where insurers are few and hard to find, they hold considerable political clout and are able to manipulate the legal and judicial systems to their benefit. (Chapter 11 discusses the legal system in more detail and offers general suggestions for reform.)

WHEN THE PATIENT DOES NOT GET BETTER

Let us now assume the claim has been filed and accepted. Care has been rendered. If all parties are on the same side and function as a team focused on the needs of the patient, things go well. This is usually the case with patients who recover function quickly or those with an obvious physical disability. Although the discussion above might suggest this is unusual, the team often does work together. But what happens when the patient turns out to be one of the 10 percent who do not get better—who dare to defy the expectations of the providers and the insurance company manuals and develop a chronically painful and functionally limiting problem?

Every time I admit a patient to the hospital for pain control, I know a shudder runs up and down the spines of all the staff. I swear that when I announce to central booking that I am admitting a patient, the floor leaders draw straws, and the short straw gets stuck with my patient. Perhaps that is why I find myself on a different floor each time.

Each staff member is well aware of the problem lying ahead: a person in pain who did not respond to conventional treatment. Everyone has a different idea of what the problem is:

"It's not in the back, it's the piriformis!"
"It's not in the piriformis, you idiot, it's a bladder problem!"

"I remember when my cousin had the problem, and it turned out to be a tumor!"

"There is no doubt this person is milking the system!"

"That's stupid. The problem is an unresolved oral phase of development spurred on by an overbearing mother and an unavailable father!"

"Huh?"

"She needs an MRI!"

"She needs a CT!"

"She needs a consult!"

"She needs a psychiatrist!"

"She needs a priest!"

"She needs a swift kick in the ass! When I hurt my back, I worked through my pain!"

Everyone is convinced their idea is right and everyone else is wrong. Nobody is acknowledging their limitations. Worse, nobody is actually listening to or acknowledging the needs of the patient. Inevitably, this behavior "splits" the staff. When the team does not work together, it does not work at all, and care suffers. Rather than take responsibility, they blame the patient.

Let us now place that same patient in the world of workers' compensation. The hospital staff at least share a common knowledge base, preconceived notions, and bottom lines. They also work together. But in the world of workers' compensation, the knowledge bases are extremely variable. While we would like to assume physicians are the most knowledgeable, that often is not true. As I have explained, most physicians receive little to no education about chronic pain, and their responses are based less on fact than on misperception. And as we've also seen, often physicians can't even agree on what they don't know. Nonphysicians, who must rely on physicians for information, don't know what to think. This allows adjusters great leeway.

To complicate the situation, each party has preconceived notions about the knowledge and motivations of the others. An insurance company views a physician with a contradictory view in favor of a claimant as a "patient whore." A physician who is a patient advocate sees a physician who provides contradictory expert testimony for the defendant as an "insurance whore." There is no discussion. Combatants choose sides and prepare to do battle.

The courtroom is the battleground. Assaults are launched from each side. The pain patient is caught in the crossfire.

At the same time, the pain patient is not purely a passive victim. Despite his injury and limitations, he can take responsibility for adapting to his condition. He doesn't have to blame others for his predicament. But often what happens is that he grieves and gets angry at a health-care system that he believes has failed him and at insurance companies who refuse to accept his problem as real or pay for his needs. He is angry at losing the ability to support himself and angry at God or fate or whatever for allowing a "bad thing to happen to a good person." And part of this picture is a very real sense of entitlement that leads to the assumption that others will resolve the problem. With such a preconceived notion, there is no need to take responsibility.

It is no surprise, then, that the system becomes dysfunctional and random, and the costs in dollars and human misery mount unnecessarily. When the lawyers and doctors retire to the golf course, and the claims adjustors and other insurance executives to the comfort of their homes, the injured worker is left to deal with the pain and the disability alone. Nothing has been solved.

Principles of Successful Rehabilitation

A desire to surmount a barrier is only fueled by incentive. While there are many incentives for the system as a whole to change, there are few for the individual participants, except the pain patients. Thus the status quo remains, much to the detriment of those in pain. The concern is that the system may collapse on itself, which, in the end, *will* affect everyone. More specifically, the cost of work injuries and entitlements is astronomical, increasingly straining our corporate and government budgets. The human cost is also high.

The following discussion refers frequently to the "team." The team consists of all the individuals who, in theory, work to help the patient recover from her injury or adapt to it: health-care providers, insurer, lawyers, employer, and so on. The patient and her family are a very important part of the team. Ideally, since all share the goal of helping the patient return to her highest level of function, all should work together as an inter- or multidisciplinary team. In reality, they rarely do.

Most of us are motivated by money, but my impression is that compassion saves money. Think of two patients we have already met: Jane, in the prologue, and Bill, in this chapter. Bill was injured at work. No one ever questioned the legitimacy of Bill's problems. Bill did everything he could do to return to work, knowing he had a desirable job to return to, where he would be valued. Eventually he did return, albeit at a lower level of function, largely because of the support he received from everyone: his employer, his caregivers, fellow employees, and the insurance company. He never felt a need to hire a lawyer. His employer's actions not only saved a life, they saved everyone a lot of money.

Jane also was injured at work. She required three operations, but she never was able to return to her previous job because of her pain and limitations. In the beginning, people did listen to her and treat her compassionately. Jane did her best to adapt. She took online courses to learn computer skills. She volunteered to use these skills to create an at-home employment opportunity. She could not work eight hours a day without breaks; but she could work at her own pace, and she could do her job from home. This is the point where the system ceased to be helpful. A little thinking outside the box was all that was needed, but instead all those involved in trying to help her vocationally told her that what she needed was beyond their capabilities. Instead of adapting, they kept trying to force her into traditional employment, which did not fit her abilities. At this point, her medical needs and costs were minimal.

When Jane's physical state deteriorated further and she needed someone to care for her, the nurse manager questioned her integrity, even though nobody else in the system was doing so. The nurse manager's actions assaulted Jane mentally and emotionally. What had been an easy pain problem to handle was magnified dramatically, and with that change came a substantial increase in the cost of Jane's care. If that wasn't bad enough, Jane became unemployable. Before the arrival of this nurse manager, Jane was employable, having been creative and figured out how she could work from home. Before, she had had a stable marriage. Afterward, she became difficult to live with, and her husband, who had stuck with her throughout all her problems, could no longer handle the stress and left her. A quack, meaning a bad health-care provider, had made a crock, meaning an unmanageable patient, at great cost to the entire system.

If we are to maximize the human potential of those who suffer from pain, it is critical that we seek to break down the barriers to care. First, we must lay down some ground rules.

CORE PRINCIPLES

The solution begins with the following two *core principles:*

Compassion for those who suffer. Let us agree not to violate, degrade, or exclude. Instead, let us support, build up, and include, following the Golden Rule. Let us make the needs of the sufferer at least as important as our own needs. Let us not let our own bottom line get the best of us. It is absolutely crucial that we do nothing to aggravate the sufferer's mental and physical torment.

Take responsibility for our actions, whether we are a part of the system or the person in pain. The goal is to bring all participants together to help the injured rejoin the workforce in as swift and safe a manner as possible. Each member of the system—doctor, nurse, insurer, employer, fellow employee, family member, politician, lawyer, judge—should share that goal, not just because it is good for the bottom line, but because it is good for a fellow human being. I don't wish to trivialize the effect on the bottom line. Taking time to care for someone in need may cost time and energy in the short term, but in the long term it saves everyone money. It saves businesses unnecessary expenses on insurance and legal fees, it saves excessive costs to insurance companies, and it substantially reduces entitlement costs to our society as a whole. Taking time to care also increases the likelihood that the sufferer can return to function and contribute positively to society at some level. I would add that there is an additional benefit in knowing that you have helped another person in need. In giving, one receives satisfaction. There may not be a way to put a price tag on that, but it is a clear benefit that can be communicated to stockholders and other third parties. Advertisements that claim "we care" are only effective if that is really true. Showing compassion, listening to the needs of the injured, and accepting their experience as real communicates caring, and the injured will be more likely to take action to help themselves because of it.

It is the responsibility of the injured to find a way to accept what has happened without being distracted by anger, guilt, and vengeance. The focus must be on the future, not the past. One cannot change the past, but one can work to make as good a future as possible. That needs to be the focus of intervention from day one. This does not mean that one cannot grieve a loss of function. Grieving is normal and expected. However, we cannot allow it to paralyze the sufferer. We have come to understand that the longer one stays off a sprained ankle, the harder it is to rehabilitate function in that ankle. Similarly, the longer one stays out of the workplace, the harder it is to get back into it. The sufferer needs to keep her eyes on the future, lest she turn into a deconditioned and functionally useless burden to society.

The role of the other participants is to assist and encourage the sufferer in this process. Sometimes that will not be easy. Each member may need to practice "tough love." Tough love is demanding; it requires participation and a sense of obligation and responsibility from the sufferer. In the short term, it may aggravate suffering, but in the long term it will bring the sufferer to a better level of function. This is especially difficult when the goal is not totally clear. Still, one only improves by expending effort. It may be emotionally difficult to push someone to make this effort, but make no bones about it—it is love. And there is nothing loving about enabling a pain patient to rest and wallow in self-pity. Tough love is most effective when communicated in a way that says: this is painful for you and for me; but through it all, I will be there for you and with you. There is no abandonment.

If only one team member seeks his or her own personal agenda, the system falls apart. So it is critical that all agree on the core principles.

Self-Awareness

The next step required to solve any problem is to analyze our own motivations. To begin, we must take a step back, take a deep breath, and then to the best of our ability assess our goals for this individual, understanding that these goals are uncertain, constantly changing, and must be categorized into long and short term.

We also must be willing to acknowledge what we know and what we don't. When a problem does not respond in a reasonable time frame to the typical ministrations, we must acknowledge that for whatever reason, chronic pain will occur in an almost-fixed percentage of those who suffer from virtually any injury. This does not necessarily represent a character flaw in the injured person or in those who care for him. It is a reality we have a limited ability to understand or change.

Given this reality, let us not resort to blame. Several years ago, a friend, who happened to be one of my employees, began to complain of work-related pain. Like many other injured workers, she had expected it to go away and in her denial did little about it. Initially, she only experienced the pain at work. Months later, when she finally told me what she was feeling, the symptom was affecting her whole life, and the cause became apparent. Unfortunately, in assessing her situation, I wore three sometimes conflicting hats: friend, doctor, and employer. As her friend, I was upset that she had ignored the problem, perhaps aggravating something that might have been treatable had she attended to it earlier. As her doctor, after listening to her and checking out her workstation, I acknowledged that the problem was related to her work. What frightened me was my initial gut reaction that my practice would be adversely affected by an injured, valuable employee. Although her problem had been created by me as her employer, rather than accept responsibility for seeing that she was properly cared for, I blamed her for her problem and refused to accept that her job was the cause. I just assumed she was trying to take advantage of me as her employer.

Interestingly, she did not blame me. She only wanted to feel better. Embarrassed by my initial reaction, I took a deep breath and acknowledged my feelings as irrational. Only then could I react more appropriately to her needs.

There was no happy ending to this story. She did not get better. While in the end, after much introspection, I chose to believe her, others in our workplace did not. However, my belief in her was powerful and therapeutic. That was apparent each time I saw her. It was also apparent how destructive others' lack of belief was. Each time that issue arose, I could see her anger build, her muscles tense.

I tell this story to make it clear that I fully understand why employers tend to blame and deny. When I was in their shoes, I did the same, at least at first. It took great introspection for me to acknowledge my feelings and react appropriately. I am supposed to be an expert on this type of thing. I was also the employee's friend. If I have to struggle so hard to be accepting, I can imagine how hard it must be for an employer who is neither an expert nor a friend. Still, employers must take that deep breath, examine their own feelings, and listen to the injured. That step is critical in the healing process.

SHIFTING THE GOAL FROM CURE
TO REHABILITATION: FIVE FACTORS

As soon as it is apparent that a pain problem is not getting better, *we must agree to shift our goal from cure to palliation and rehabilitation.* Palliation means that we do whatever we can to minimize the pain. This means more than just medical and physical therapies. It also means relating to the patient with compassion and putting his needs above our own, lest we unnecessarily do him harm.

Rehabilitation means helping the patient find meaningful function in all aspects of her life, not just the workplace. It must start the minute treatment starts. I believe there are five important factors in successful rehabilitation of the chronic pain patient: acknowledgment, acceptance, honesty, forgiveness, and communication.

The team working with the patient must *acknowledge* the patient's pain and limitation and at the same time promote residual function. While we must compassionately understand that the injured person grieves, we should not allow the grieving to keep her mired in the past. "Candor with hope" must be our mantra. We must be honest about what we can offer and acknowledge that, at some point, things may be better, but we must focus on what we can do now. In taking this direction, it is reasonable to allow some hope.

The patient needs to come to a sense of *acceptance* and an understanding of his limitations. That does not necessarily mean giving up hope for a cure or dramatic improvement. Difficult pain problems do sometimes go away. However, searching for a cure without trying to maximize function within one's current limits is akin to finding oneself in quicksand. The more one struggles, the more stuck one becomes. The more one focuses on the pain, the harder it is to adapt.

In chapter 2, I described Jill, a patient whose pain I had been unable to cure. I thought she felt I was failing her, but when I encountered her years after she stopped coming to see me, she told me that my belief in her had actually helped. She explained that she had learned to live with her back pain, which had not diminished in the intervening ten years. What did change was that she acknowledged the pain and her limitations and took control of her situation. She figured out what she could do and what she couldn't, found a job within her limitations, and was doing very well. She had stopped seeing me not because she was upset with me, but because she had come to an acceptance of what her future would be and what she had to do. She added that she would love to hear me say I had discovered a magical cure since I last saw her. But when I said there was no such thing, she was not disappointed.

Jill's story taught me that sitting and waiting for a cure that may never come merely aggravates the problem. In my experience resolutions like hers only happen for people who persist, who move forward and begin to plan an alternative future. I would love to say this is easy. It is not. Grieving is a very active process, and only with great energy and insight, and a little help from others, does one come to the conclusions that Jill came to.

Honesty is a two-way street. All members of the therapeutic team, patient included, need to be honest regarding their beliefs about what is going on with the rehabilitation plan, the outcomes of the various treatments, other options, and the goals for the future. They must communicate these beliefs to everyone involved, with the joint goal of helping the patient achieve his goals in life. If someone disagrees with the plan, she must say so to the team, and these concerns should be discussed. Holding those feelings inside does a disservice to the team. It is not that unusual for one person's honest observation to change an entire treatment plan for the better.

Providers must also be honest about what they can and cannot offer and not merely keep providing therapies in an attempt to delay the inevitable acknowledgment that they have done everything realistically possible for the patient's pain. At one meeting I attended, a neurobiologist concluded his talk by informing the audience that *there are no major pharmacological cures for chronic pain on the horizon in the near future, if ever.* I found this comment inspiring. For the previous four days, I had listened to speaker after speaker tout the virtues of their various therapies, often promoting outcomes I could not possibly believe. The one thing all these therapies had in common was that if they helped at all, the effects were only temporary, and all they did was delay the inevitable return and persistence of the pain. I wondered if the only reason we offer therapies is to palliate the patient while she goes through the grieving process.

The problem is that all these therapies cost a great deal, as well as give the patient a false sense of hope that delays adaptation. Until the patient and the providers accept the pain for what it is and honestly convey this awareness to each other, the patient cannot take control of his life and adapt. I have observed that *when patients do take control, they don't need all our therapies.* I have seen dozens of patients function just fine without pain medications. I have seen many patients turn off their spinal cord stimulators, stop getting injections, and do their exercises on their own, without the benefit of the watchful eye of the physical therapist, and not only do well, but sometimes actually thrive. That neurobiologist's honesty was liberating for me and changed my practice; for example, I started talking people out of getting expensive injections. This wasn't easy. Honesty in the face of suffering is difficult, but it is tough love, and necessary.

Throughout this process, we cannot allow vengeance to intrude. Persistent anger perpetually eats away at those who fall prey to it, aggravating their suffering and rarely, if ever, succeeding in punishing those upon whom they seek vengeance. *Forgiveness,* while difficult, is liberating. It brings teammates together, while vengeance divides them.

Inherent in all these factors is the importance of *communication.* Imagine a football team trying to function without communication. If a wide receiver zigs instead of zags, the quarterback will throw the ball to the wrong place. Often it is intercepted. The play fails and the team suffers. Exactly the same thing happens among the patient's treatment team. Rehabilitation is successful only when all members are on the same page, constantly communicating. Again, the patient and her family are an important part of this team.

FACILITATING THE RETURN TO WORK: EDUCATION AND INCENTIVES

In treating thousands of individuals who were injured and had to adapt to a change in, if not a worsening of, their work capacity, I have been struck by the critical role played by educational level in their ability to adapt. One of my patients was highly educated and highly motivated. He ran a company in which he was not just the owner, but also a worker. The job was physical. After an injury, he could no longer perform the physical tasks the job required. Unfortunately for him and his company, he could not delegate his physical work to others, so the company went out of business. Almost immediately after his injury, he acknowledged his limitation and began planning a new career path. Because he was well educated, he had multiple options. Soon, he was busy in a new job, having required virtually no assistance from anyone else in making this transition. All he needed to hear from me was what the options were for his care and an honest appraisal of the likelihood of success of each.

I also have worked with many poorly educated people who dropped out of school to take well-paying but physically demanding jobs. When they got hurt and couldn't return to work, they struggled because they had no other marketable skills. Too often, lost and unsure how to proceed, they gave up while still very young and became permanently disabled, forever a burden on the system. These observations have shown me the critical role played by education in enabling people with disabilities to return to a productive life.

The spark must come from within, and education can provide it. Young people have an obligation to learn and to develop varying skills involving both mind and body. Then, if trouble happens, they will be able to adapt and fit back into the workforce in some other way. That said, it is never too late to learn, and sometimes an injury and a change in functional ability provide the opportunity for an individual to learn new skills within his physical and mental abilities. Therefore, education and reeducation are an important part of the return-to-work process.

For the most part, rehabilitation is common sense. Those who possess both motivation and common sense adapt with little to no assistance. When motivation and common sense are lacking, the process is much more challenging. To help provide motivation, the employer and the health-care provider must give the employee incentives to return to work. A welcoming environment and financial incentives are crucial. If it costs more to try to return to work and fail than it does to stay out, there will be little incentive. I believe it is reasonable for injured workers to be paid a percentage of their original salary when out of work. This gives them an incentive to return to productive employment. There should be a reward when workers try to return: the percentage of pre-injury income they receive should be increased on a graded schedule. When they return to work on full duty, they should receive the same income they received prior to the injury. If they try and fail, their income will fall, but never to zero. If workers risk losing everything, they have little incentive to keep trying.

No employer should ever terminate an employee merely because of injury. As I have said, employers often wait until the employee returns to full-duty work and then fire him or her. This not only creates a great disincentive for other injured workers to make the effort to return, it is also downright inhumane, especially when someone worked hard to return.

Those injured outside the workplace need other incentives. First, *we must raise the safety net so that nobody needs to become destitute before they receive help.* Stop the downward spiral an incapacitating injury creates before it veers out of control. While we should subsidize injured workers, we should also expect them to contribute to society in some way. This may involve participating in a meaningful vocational rehabilitation program. It may mean volunteering in a community organization. It may mean working part-time. However, there cannot be a free lunch. Again, this is tough love, but we see the problems created by an overly entitled society in terms of both lost productivity and skyrocketing entitlement costs that strain our ability to support them. Workers also must show some effort to actively resolve the problems they face by complying with their treatment.

At the same time, no subsidy should be "all or none." As an individual returns to work, she should not risk losing everything. Her return to productivity should be monitored; and if she seems to be failing, she should not have to go to the back of the line to reinstitute her subsidy.

Employers need incentives too. If they won't hire injured workers, all the rehabilitation in the world is useless. *In order to encourage businesses to hire disabled pain patients, we must change how we define meaningful work.* This can be done in several ways.

First, we must acknowledge that many people can be productive, but not in a setting that requires travel to a workplace where they must work in a defined period of time. Many patients with pain can work, but need to do so at their own pace. Many can work forty or more hours a week in this manner. In our computerized world, it is increasingly possible to work at home at one's own pace, resting as needed.

Other injured workers can work part-time, or in a sheltered setting, where they are producing and can earn an income. But such an arrangement must not result in a loss of subsidy. If the individual earns a paycheck, it is reasonable to reduce the subsidy, but total pay should never be less than the pre-return-to-work subsidy—two-thirds of pre-injury earnings. People should be able to exceed this amount through greater productivity. This would give them a reason to get up in the morning, doing wonders for self-esteem. It also would lower entitlement pay. Since people will only act against their self-interest if they are appropriately motivated, businesses can be encouraged to participate in such programs through either a subsidy or a tax break. Possible liability can be handled by maintaining or expanding secondary injury funds.

Finally, *we must have the courage to be creative:* in care, physical rehabilitation, and vocational rehabilitation. Each patient's pain problem and life situation is unique. Therefore, each solution will be unique. Stereotypical solutions do not work for pain-related disability, waste money and other resources, and harm patients. If Jane had been offered an opportunity tailored to her abilities, she probably would be working, she might still be married, she would be less depressed, and she would be costing society a lot less money.

Solutions

We must acknowledge pain as a unique disability, not merely an accompaniment of another disability, and strive to find creative, valid, and reliable ways to measure its functional effects on ability. We must eliminate the useless concept of impairment.

In assessing disability, we need to recognize the balance between an individual's abilities and disabilities and how they relate to the specific tasks that particular individual needs to perform on a daily basis.

We must be willing to step in and aid people in the early phases, well before the downward spiral, well before they become destitute. It is much easier, less expensive, and more compassionate to resolve a problem early on than when it has spiraled out of control.

Entitlement systems must be more compassionate and user friendly. It is critical that those on the front lines provide a kind, compassionate face for the system that encourages those in need to ask for help, and more important, not feel embarrassed in doing so. People don't need help when all the forms have been filled out in triplicate and multiple hearings have been conducted over months or years. The system must respond to an applicant's needs in days.

Private organizations and volunteerism provide a substantial percentage of charitable care. Whether from businesses or individuals, such care is crucial. The importance of these valuable services should be recognized, encouraged, and supported. One way we already do this is in allowing such entities as nonprofits to be exempt from taxes. We can be more creative, however, and encourage government to partner with or defer to such organizations when a valuable need is being met. As I have said, large organizations are unable to be sufficiently responsive to the needs of individuals; small, local organizations may be much more effective. Rather than inefficiently duplicating services, it may make more sense for government to "privatize" services to organizations that have an incentive to be efficient and to show results in a cost-effective manner. It is clear that this process requires oversight, which is critical for creating accountability.

Large organizations may provide an economy of scale, but they inevitably lose focus by their inability to see the faces of those affected by their decisions. The less impact the worker in the trenches, who sees the plight of the disabled on a daily basis, has on decision making, the less empowered she is to assist those in need; and the more incentives she has to be responsive to the needs of her supervisors, the less effective services will be. That is why I believe large organizations such as federal and some state governments are incapable of responding to the needs of those they serve. Government should oversee and support, but not provide direct services. That should be the role of local government and private organizations.

Creating a more responsive system will enable us to raise the safety net before a disability spirals out of control. In doing this, we must recognize that disability is relative, and so is lifestyle, and therefore it may not be appropriate to set a dollar amount on when to initiate services. It makes sense to provide some amount of prorated assistance early on for finding new options for employment before people end up in the line at the local soup kitchen, homeless and devoid of self-esteem. We have set our safety net so low that some people become destitute before they qualify for services. The net effect is to push a person so far into a hole that it is nearly impossible to climb out.

Entitlement systems must involve expectations. We recognize that an entitlement is a gift. However, we also recognize the moral poverty that is created when a gift is given with no expectations, no strings attached. The problem arises when the recipient no longer sees the entitlement as a gift, but as a right. It is easy to see how this could happen, because such a belief is implied in the very word "entitlement." Too often we have no expectations of the disabled. Instead we reward disability, and the more we do so, the more disabled people become. In this way the system creates and reinforces a sense of need that actually robs the recipient of meaning and self-esteem and perpetuates his sense of uselessness. This is how we actually create "inability" out of disability.

The entitlement provides the recipient with an opportunity to be excused from the financial and vocational responsibilities of life for a time so she can heal mentally, psychologically, and socially. Her responsibility is to use this time to confront the barriers that the new disability has created and find a way to return to the labor force so she can again contribute to the society that has cared for her.

Why don't we pair expectations with entitlement? I asked a policymaker this, and he told me that doing so is too hard and too expensive to enforce. I question that conclusion. To the extent that the current system actually *promotes* disability by rewarding it, in the long run it is probably more expensive than a system that clearly promotes expectations.

A better gift is opportunity. It is critical that entitlement be coupled with immediate expectations and opportunities for the recipient to create a better future. We all have something to offer. We should make no value judgments on how much each individual contributes, only expect that each does contribute. What is greater, one who gives much of what little he has, or one who gives little of the great amount he has, even if the latter is much more than the former?

An example of an immediate expectation might be that in exchange for assistance the individual is expected to perform a community service and also attend a vocational assessment and retraining program. Community service is not a punishment. Rather, it should enable the individual to actively transition off entitlement and back into a socially functional role. Constructive community service actually may serve as a form of vocational retraining, with the potential to open new opportunities. When designed in this manner, service is bound to be much more meaningful for the individual, while also being cost-effective for society.

However, in creating expectations and assigning service tasks, we must acknowledge each individual's physical, mental, psychological, functional, and social limitations and individualize each recipient's program. Our expectations should not burden the person with excessive hardships. It is never appropriate to tax someone beyond his capabilities. We also must acknowledge the multiple roles people play. For example, when assessing a single mother of two children who is limited by back pain and lives in a house, the evaluator must determine the permanence of her condition, the time required for medical treatment, the nature of her transferable skills to other less physically taxing employment, the needs of her family, and the financial and physical needs of her home before creating expectations. Her commitments to her family and her treatment may not leave enough time for vocational reeducation and community service. A value judgment must be made as to which is more important at this time.

As the process of entitlement, service, and retraining proceeds, participants should be expected to progress toward independence. As this happens, the entitlement should be reduced commensurate with the independent income the person generates; but as I said, she should never have to take too big a risk in order to succeed. Our current system effectively punishes participants for trying to become independent by cutting or eliminating their benefits, but a properly designed entitlement system can encourage initiative by cushioning the falls that are bound to happen.

Some people never will be totally independent. Disabilities do pose limits, and many will reach a limit short of total independence, necessitating a lifetime of entitlement. This does not mean that expectations cease, though they may be modified.

Because each person's financial needs are relative, services should be prorated accordingly. Needs are constantly changing, and therefore, the entitlement amount must be reassessed on a relative basis. The system must be flexible in other ways as well. Pain, and the disability it creates, can vary greatly over time. Many pain patients function well for weeks or months, and then are stricken by flare-ups. For others, flare-ups may be daily or weekly, necessitating a change in expectations or an increase in entitlement. For many pain patients, this variability is a part of life and can be built into the system by creating flexible schedules. For example, an individual may be expected to work so many hours in a month, rather than so many per day. A pain patient may be able to work 120 hours in a month, but be incapable of working four hours every day. On some days he can work eight hours, and on others he cannot work at all. Such people still can be quite productive, just on their own schedule, not someone else's. The Internet allows many creative opportunities for remote employment.

Pain should be defined as a disability covered by the ADA. Then we must creatively reward businesses for hiring those disabled by pain, through subsidies or other means. Sheltered workshops already provide this opportunity for the mentally disabled. Such programs should be expanded to include the physically disabled, especially those suffering from pain, who may be the largest group of those who suffer disability.

Our entitlement system is broken, and our budgets are paying the price. The system must change. But change begins with compassion. We need to understand that the needs of our fellow humans are more important than our bottom line. If we take this one step, the next few are so much easier. Mother Teresa has shown us the way:

In her apostolate Mother Teresa was full of initiative. The difficulties and challenges in her work often provided opportunities for innovation. Such was the case of Jacqueline de Decker, a Belgian nurse and social worker who wished to join the Missionaries of Charity but could not because of poor health. Mother Teresa came up with the solution: since Jacqueline could not work with the poor in Calcutta, she would share in the apostolate by becoming Mother Teresa's "second self"—a spiritual twin who would offer to God her prayers and suffering for Mother Teresa and the fruitfulness of her work. Mother Teresa in turn would offer her prayers and good works for Jacqueline. Jacqueline and others who could not join directly in the work ("the sick and suffering co-workers," as they were later called) would join efforts with the sisters in fulfilling the common aim of satiating the thirst of Jesus. *Mother Teresa believed that finding a purpose in their sufferings would give them a new incentive to carry on:*

"Love demands sacrifice. But if we love until it hurts, God will give us His peace and joy . . . Suffering in itself is nothing; but suffering shared with Christ's Passion is a wonderful gift. . . .

"You see the aim of our Society is to satiate the thirst of Jesus on the Cross for the love of souls by working for the salvation and sanctification of the poor in the slums.—Who could do this better than you and the others who suffer like you? . . . Therefore you are just as important and necessary for the fulfillment of our aim.—To satiate His Thirst we must have a chalice—and you and the others—men, women, children, old and young, poor and rich—all are welcome to make the chalice. In reality, you can do much more while on your bed of pain than I running on my feet, *but you and I together* can do all things in Him who strengthens us. . . .

"Everyone and anyone who wishes to become a Missionary of Charity—a carrier of God's Love—is welcome, but I want specially the paralyzed, the crippled, the incurables to join . . ."[14]

If Mother Teresa could find a place in her "workplace" for the disabled—a place that required much time, energy, and dedication—why can't America?

TEN

Health and Disability Insurance

The Law of Unintended Consequences

There is only one difference between a bad economist and
a good one: the bad economist confines himself to the visible
effect; the good economist takes into account both the effect
that can be seen and those effects that must be foreseen.
Frédéric Bastiat, "What Is Seen and What Is Not Seen"

We now understand that our country's insurance system is broken
and in need of repair, and in 2010 Congress passed the Patient Protection/
Affordable Care Act (PP/ACA) as a means of beginning this process. The
debates about this law still rage. In chapter 3, I described my 2010 trip to
Washington to ensure that funding was appropriated for the Pain Care Policy Act (PCP), and my discovery that the health-care experts for our senators
and representatives knew little not only about the problem of untreated
pain, but also about the PP/ACA itself. Considering that their bosses had
just voted on that bill, with dramatic ramifications for the country's future,
I was dumbfounded.

I went home more cynical than ever about our nation's priorities. We can
land a man on the moon, but we can't treat pain efficiently, nor do we want
to. In my training, I had learned that by managing pain aggressively in the
acute phase, one could prevent the development of chronic pain. The cost
savings of doing so are huge—not only medical but also insurance costs,
entitlement costs, and lost productivity. Shouldn't our representatives
understand this as they create policy?

The two central problems of our insurance system are *cost* and *access*,
which are hardly mutually exclusive. The challenge is to control or reduce
cost while simultaneously increasing access in a nation that demands free
choice. More specifically, how do we allow access to those most in need,
who are also the most expensive to treat, such as the disabled and those
in pain?

This chapter explains how and why legislation addressing these issues is created and passed by people who are often ignorant of the effects it has on many who suffer. It discusses both commercial private health-care insurance and disability insurance, including employer-offered group disability insurance and individual disability insurance. I will briefly outline the history of these insurances in order to better understand how we got where we are. I will then look at the problems these insurances pose for chronic pain patients and how the PP/ACA may help or harm them, and then conclude with suggestions for how these insurances may better serve people with pain.

How Health Insurance Came to Be

In 1910, a pivotal study of American medicine known as the *Flexner Report* was published.[1] Abraham Flexner, charged with investigating the state of medicine in America, concluded that it was "deplorable." The knowledge base of the typical doctor was limited, the quality of medical education poor, and the use of basic scientific method inconsistent. In a nutshell, many doctors were "quacks," albeit friendly ones. Flexner recommended an overhaul of American medical education. His recommendations resulted in a dramatic improvement in the quality of medicine in the United States.

But as treatments improved, the cost of care increased. Before the 1920s, health care was affordable and no insurance was necessary. In the 1920s, however, rising costs threatened the availability of care for those who needed it most. To resolve this problem, the Blue Cross system was developed as a nonprofit insurer serving local community organizations. Blue Cross did not discriminate; it charged everyone the same premium. This arrangement was due to a curious mix of philanthropic dedication to serving the poor and a desire on the part of hospitals to sell insurance in order to guarantee a parade of patients.

For-profit insurers, who had previously considered medicine an unpromising market, noticed the success of the Blue Cross system and entered the market, creating a new problem: they began to set premiums based on relative risk and tended to avoid insuring the riskiest customers. This "cherry picking" effectively funneled the care of the riskiest groups—the aged, disabled, and poor—either to the nonprofit providers, or worse, out of the system altogether. The for-profit insurers thrived, while nonprofits increasingly struggled to fulfill their self-imposed pledge to provide for the needy.

A new dynamic emerged during the industrial boom that followed World War II, when labor became relatively scarce. Large companies began to offer health insurance as a "perk" in order to attract workers, who were typically young and healthy. The result was a worsening of the funnel effect. People who really needed health-care insurance could not afford it and often could not get it. To resolve this issue, Medicare and Medicaid were created in 1965, offering government-run health insurance to 20 percent of the population—and at the same time providing an instant catch basin into which for-profit insurers could further divert the poor, elderly, and disabled. At the same time, Medicare and Medicaid, chronically under-funded and overregulated, created a burden many providers did not wish to shoulder. Many practices, citing excessive overhead, refused to accept patients covered by these insurances. Such patients either were diverted to providers who would accept them, or worse, received no care at all.[2] (This problem persists today, as we will see.)

As health-care costs continued to climb, the insurance industry sought ways to counter this trend. It created Health Maintenance Organizations (HMOs), which proliferated and were successful. History now repeated itself. In their early phase, HMOs were largely nonprofit organizations. In 1981, only 12 percent of the insurance market was served by for-profits. By 1997, the number was closer to 65 percent. The result of this shift was a further decrease in access to insurance for the poor and infirm; a greater burden for Medicare, Medicaid, and nonprofit insurances; and an increase in the denial of various treatments, while private insurers and hospitals became more profitable. Moreover, with the dramatic shift of for-profit insurers and hospitals into the health-care "market," the bottom-line men-tality began to invade health care.

An HMO sought to control health-care costs in many ways. It contracted with providers, agreeing to pay an up-front lump-sum reimbursement. This incentivized physicians to treat fewer people; the fewer the interventions they prescribed, the more they pocketed at the end of the year. The HMO further "encouraged" participating doctors to cut costs by withholding a certain percentage of their fees, which was only reimbursed if the physi-cian's total charges fell within specific guidelines. Chronic outliers risked being eliminated from the pool of participating doctors; my physician friend, described in chapter 6, was fired from such an HMO because "he spent too much time with his patients." Insurers often negotiated contracts with large groups, effectively limiting, or even eliminating, private or small-group practices.

To control the perceived excesses of specialists, primary care doctors were forced to serve as "gatekeepers" who controlled whom the patient could and could not see. Costs incurred by referrals to specialists affected the primary care doctors' bottom line, giving them every incentive not to refer.

In this way HMOS directly shifted a substantial portion of the burden of cost-containment to physicians. They assumed the rest of the burden themselves by effectively rationing more expensive treatments, such as MRI scanning. While routine and preventive care would be covered with little question, expensive and specialized care was subject to review and could be denied. The days of unlimited care were over, but the results were not all bad; the rate of health-care growth as a percentage of GDP slowed. Preventive care and healthy behaviors were rewarded. Patients were encouraged to take charge of their own health care.

However, physicians struggled, facing the dilemma of doing what they deemed necessary versus controlling their bottom line. Worse, they risked losing their livelihood if they too often chose the needs of the patient over those of the practice. In many parts of the country, HMOS grew quite powerful. Many physicians, out of fear of losing their practices and believing they had few options, reluctantly joined, sacrificing their autonomy and perhaps their ethics.

Needless to say, patients with complicated and expensive problems suffered too, restricted by limited access and limited coverage. Newspapers ran stories of cancer patients being denied care. Their stories made good headlines, but the difficulties of others with chronic problems such as pain went unnoticed.

To remain sustainable, many practices shifted costs to those who could pay. They did this by overcharging private payers and private insurances. Private insurers then began to negotiate. The actual fee the doctor charged was almost never paid. Negotiations cost time and money, increasing the cost of practicing medicine. Private individual payers, who had no negotiating clout, had to suck it up and pay the whole inflated bill, unless the health-care provider was willing to adjust the fee.

There were other costs. Lawyers began to see medicine and malpractice as a fertile field for lining their own pockets. The lawsuit, previously uncommon, became a feared accompaniment of medical practice. Defensive medicine and risk management, two concepts that didn't even exist when I completed medical school in 1985, began to control physician behavior, resulting in unnecessary and expensive testing and care and causing costs to skyrocket. Simultaneously, the computer invaded medicine, and previously unimaginable technologies established a very expensive presence. Armed with such weapons (too often without a clear understanding of how to use them efficiently), medicine began to promise wonderful outcomes, many of which it could not produce. Patients expected perfect outcomes, no matter the cost, and that expectation drove further cost increases.

Facing this increasingly unfriendly environment, physicians fought back by forming bigger and bigger groups, such as PAS (professional associations), PCS (professional corporations), and PPOS (preferred provider organizations), which had negotiating clout. Many physicians, overwhelmed by the business aspect of medicine, sold out to hospitals and other corporate entities, leaving the business side to them. This trend is called the *corporatization* of medicine, and its root cause is physician fear of such complexities as the excessive costs of technology, regulation, and risk management. The number of physicians estimated to be in private practice was 66 percent in 2005.[3] By 2014, that number was estimated to be only 25 percent.[4] In selling out, physicians were forced to choose between masters: the insurance company or the new corporate entity to which they belonged. To most, the corporate entity was preferable, offering at least the illusion that their own needs would be considered. And these entities did wield clout. However, organizations of that size required managerial talent, something few physicians possess or have the time or energy to pursue. Businessmen took over. Alien words such as "product line" and "market share" invaded.

The focus of treatment shifted from overall management of a medical problem to piecemeal attention with emphasis on procedures. It is naïve to believe that complicated problems can be resolved by whittling away at a portion of them with a knife or needle, when the deeper issues driving these problems are not addressed. Treatment of chronic diseases such as pain must be holistic. But holism does not pay, and therefore goes largely ignored. Constantly changing insurances and provider contracts further disrupted primary care, fracturing any semblance of continuity. With nobody clearly at the helm, care became increasingly fragmented and inefficient. Despite my mother's rheumatoid arthritis, she lived to the age of seventy-nine, way beyond her life expectancy for such an illness. In large part this was because she had the same rheumatologist for thirty-five years. In the current medical model, such continuity is becoming extinct, and the ramifications for those who suffer from chronic illness are huge.

Things were at this point when the Clintons proposed the health-care reforms of 1993. Although their intentions were valid, their method of reform was faulty. By systematically excluding physicians, they turned them into opponents who, together with insurance companies, fought the plan and killed it. Their proposal had created a threat, and the threat created a fear, which fueled the progressive melding of medicine and business, with negative consequences for both patient and doctor, as well as the entire the health-care system.

As I write this, over two decades later, despite all the attempts at reform detailed above, things are worse. The rise of health-care costs is strangling personal, corporate, and government budgets. Bottom-line behavior increasingly disrupts effective health care. Legal risk creates excessive fear among health-care providers and eliminates certain specialties, such as obstetrics, from many areas of the country. Primary care doctors are disappearing, and in their absence health care becomes increasingly fragmented and inefficient. The health-care dollar is shifting to those who specialize and away from those who manage. The poor, the disabled, and those in chronic pain struggle more to find care and constitute a substantial portion of those with public insurance. While insurance companies, their stockholders, a certain percentage of citizens, and medical specialists thrive in this environment, the system as a whole is sick.

Chronic Pain and the Insurance System

Inaccessible, costly, inefficient, fragmented health care not only affects the viability of the entire health-care system but also worsens the quality of life for those who already suffer from chronic pain. How common is chronic pain? How well is it treated? How much does it cost us? The answers are somewhat nebulous since they depend on how one defines the condition. The 2011 Institute of Medicine report estimated that about one hundred million Americans (roughly one-third of the population) are affected by chronic pain at a cost of up to $635 billion in medical care and lost productivity.

This estimate does not include potential costs for those who have no access to care, nor the unquantifiable costs that the disabled incur, such as loss of self-esteem, loss of avocational function, and family stress and breakup (secondary losses). A more recent study's conclusion that persistent pain affects 39.4 million adults in the United States is dramatically lower than the IOM estimates. The authors of this study state that differences in the operational definition of "chronic" explain the discrepancy.[5] Still, even the lower figure accounts for a substantial percentage of the population and a substantial cost.

In 2012, the Agency for Health Care Research and Quality reported that 5 percent of the U.S. population uses 50 percent of the health-care dollar, and those who make up this 5 percent remain remarkably stable from year to year.[6] They include the elderly, the disabled, and those with chronically painful problems. While this statistic does not measure the specific cost of chronic pain to society, it is clear that people in pain contribute significantly to the overall cost. Thus, the problem they pose is large, and the potential cost is huge. To resolve this problem, we must identify the factors that limit these people's access, and then summon the will to address them.

Addressing a problem requires acknowledging it, and the first factor, as I have explained, is that we don't recognize chronic pain as a problem. It is not taught in medical schools and rarely addressed at non-pain-related medical conferences. The stance of our entire medical establishment, including organized medicine, insurance companies, and the government, toward this problem boils down to "piecemealing," "cherry picking," or sweeping it under the rug.

To the extent that insurance companies do acknowledge the problem of chronic pain, they find creative ways to avoid covering it. They put up a wall guarded by untrained and unsophisticated claims adjusters armed with books and charts created by "experts," which allow them to decide what should and should not be covered. These "experts" often have skewed their recommendations toward satisfying their own needs. While "interventional" procedures with limited support in the literature abound and are covered, mental health services, comprehensive pain services, vocational services, and true multifactorial, holistic services are not covered. The system forces patients to beg for care, which as we know damages their sense of self-esteem and further aggravates their pain.

I was once confronted by an eighty-year-old woman struggling to find someone who would merely be willing to prescribe pain medicine for her. She could find plenty of people willing to needle her and cut her open, but she wanted someone to care for her! She was astute enough to realize that needles and knives pay, but care doesn't. She challenged me by saying that she knew she could get what she needed "on the street" if she had to, and at her age, she refused to needlessly suffer her pain and the assault on her dignity. If the insurance companies, the doctors, the police, and the DEA did not like it that was tough. I wondered what I would do in this woman's shoes, or what any of us would do. Very likely, we'd make the same demands.

The barriers only begin with limiting care, for that can be done only to those already inside the door. Not letting someone in that door by denying insurance to high-risk patients is much more effective. Our system allows companies great leeway to decide who and what they will cover. Preexisting conditions, conditions not covered, and excessive risk are all creative ways to deny care. Even though insurance companies are subject to government oversight, they function as virtual monopolies, able to control for whom they provide services and what those services are. One of my semiretired patients who had HMO insurance paid a premium of $1200 a month and had a $10,000 deductible, yet his insurance company still challenged every medical intervention that his doctors recommended. The company's cadre of paid-off "experts" would conclude that his proposed plan of care was not medically reasonable and necessary. It is true that the denial came with instructions on how to challenge the decision (in tiny print), but challenging the bully is never easy. Even though states provide insurance boards as patient advocates, most patients do not have the will or the way to bring such a challenge. And so the insurance companies continue to behave in this manner, because it is cost-effective. The larger they are, the more control they have, and the freer they are to do this.

And can we blame them? The role of the officers of any company is to maximize profits. Most executives are paid to produce short-term results and have little incentive to consider the long-term effects on those they serve, or refuse to serve, not to mention society at large. In fact, they have every disincentive. The problem is that their short-term benefits have created long-term problems for all. Access to care, especially for those with costly medical problems such as pain, remains a problem despite the PP/ACA. Can the government, influenced by powerful lobbies, provide effective oversight?

While insurance companies limit access directly, excessive costs limit access indirectly. Cost may be a bigger problem than access, but it is one that all parties have the power to influence. I was able to discuss the PP/ACA with my state's former governor, who asked what I thought the problems were with the law. I rattled off my list of concerns, and his response was simply that the basic problem was that the law did nothing to control cost. Our three-party insurance system (consumer, health-care provider, and insurance company) gives insured consumers what amounts to a blank check to purchase medical services in any way they and their providers deem reasonable. I have already detailed the major factors responsible for excess costs. I believe, however, that the fundamental factor underlying all the others is the extent to which all parties act in their own self-interest and not in the interest of the whole. We may complain about an insurance company's tactics, but it is trying to control costs, albeit for its own benefit. How we go about controlling costs while allowing access will determine whether and how the system can be sustainable. As Hillary Rodham Clinton has stated, "The present system is not sustainable. The only question is whether we will master the change, or it will master us."

Any architect knows that a structure is strongest when it has a stable base. A pyramid is most stable when its base is on the ground. Who would build a pyramid with the tip on the ground? It seems foolish, but as I explained in chapter 6, that is actually how our health-care system is constructed, with specialists dominating the top of the pyramid and those who manage pain and other medical and psychological problems as a weakened base. While some patients may benefit in the short run, overall the system and those it serves suffers. Instead we must strengthen the base of the pyramid.

Cost, Access, and the ACA

The ACA attempted to address both cost and access. Prior to its inception, our health insurance system did allow those who could afford it access to care, and roughly 80 to 85 percent of Americans were insured or could afford needed care. Over time, the number of people with such access shrank, leaving an increasing number without insurance, and these individuals are now being covered by public insurance, mostly Medicaid, at great cost to both the state and federal governments. Perhaps the most important pillar of the ACA is the requirement that all individuals have some form of health insurance or pay a fine. In theory, that should resolve the problem of access, although in practice this is not likely to happen.

For the purpose of this discussion, I divide the population into three groups: the poor, the middle class, and the wealthy. The wealthy already have insurance and can afford the plans and the deductibles. Many very rich people choose not to buy insurance at all; as one such person said, "Why should I buy health insurance when I can afford whatever care I need without having to deal with the restrictions of an insurance company?" These individuals would hardly notice any fine they had to pay. However, since what they pay in fines is substantially less than what they would pay for insurance, their choice represents money lost to the health-care system as a whole.

The ACA addressed health care for the poor by broadening the definition of who is poor, making more people Medicaid eligible. The problem is: who will care for them? Increasingly, physicians are not accepting Medicaid because reimbursements are insufficient to cover costs. A 2014 study of fifteen U.S. cities showed that only 46 percent of doctors accepted Medicaid.[7] Medicaid is funded by tax dollars and provided by the individual states with federal subsidies. Increasing its budget would strain both state and federal budgets at a time when most are well in the red.

As for the middle class, the law requires this group to buy insurance if they do not get it from their employer, further stressing their limited resources. The ACA expects more of insurance companies in terms of services provided and increased regulations. Such costs are being passed on to consumers in the form of higher co-pays and deductibles. (In this and other ways, detailed in chapter 15, the PP/ACA not only does not lower health-care costs; it does much to increase them.) The HMO-insured patient I referred to earlier paid $28,000 out of pocket for health-care costs in 2013. Few in the middle class can afford this level of expense. Already financially pressed by other increasing costs (heat, housing, food, electricity), they face a barrier to care that the ACA did not remove.

Another problem was that a large percentage of the uninsured were healthy people who made a conscious assessment that the benefits of being insured did not outweigh the costs, and the fines were insufficient to offset this disincentive. But for the insurance system to be viable, the healthy must pay in.

The PP/ACA is in its infancy, and it is too early to make any judgments about its efficacy. But with respect to its effect on those who suffer from chronic pain and chronic disability, I have many concerns. At this writing, individual and overall system costs are higher than expected, while it is not clear that accessibility has improved. Fragmentation seems to be increasing. I was reminded of this by a Christmas card from a long-standing patient. I saw her and her husband for complicated pain problems resulting from their time in a concentration camp in Bosnia, but I had not seen them in quite a while and was concerned enough that I was planning to call them. The one thing they could count on prior to the PP/ACA was continuity of care. Now, I learned from the card, their new insurance, created by the PP/ACA, did not include our medical group, so they had to find care elsewhere and were having difficulty doing so. That problem was not created by the PP/ACA; it had been present for several years. However, the PP/ACA was supposed to fix it. Not only has this not happened, but in my experience the problem is worse. Any new contraption, whether a new model car or a health-care system, requires a bit of tinkering before it achieves its maximal outcome. The PP/ACA needs quite a bit of tinkering if it is to be truly helpful for those who suffer from complex medical problems.

Health Insurance Solutions

For a broader discussion of reforming the entire health-care system, see chapter 15. Here I offer solutions to the problems posed by those with chronic pain.

EDUCATE

The 2011 IOM Report emphasizes that we cannot make rational decisions with imperfect information. Certainly we cannot rely on biased "experts" who are bought off to see a problem the way their employer wants them to see it. Instead physicians, insurers, government officials (regulators), and the public all need to be educated about chronic pain. Pain physicians must take the lead on this, and indeed that is happening. Such education must include the following:

> *Setting realistic expectations.* I am not aware of any reliable way
> to quantify this, but I am certain that we spend a substantial
> amount of money trying to *cure* pain when our goal should

be to *ease pain and suffering*. The focus of this entire book is eliminating unnecessary suffering, and it is quite clear to me that our ignorance of the issue of pain creates unreasonable expectations on the part of patients, families, and employers, which only magnifies the patients' suffering.

Changing the notion that chronic pain is a character flaw. Substantial resources should be devoted to this. Name calling assaults patients' integrity and magnifies the problems they face.

Educating the writers of the manuals that adjusters use to accept or deny treatment, and gaining access to the system about chronic pain so that these manuals better reflect the realities of chronic pain as currently known. As I have said, knowledge of chronic pain is a moving target, as we learn more each year; and the manuals must reflect both what we know and what we don't. But the current manuals are based on statistical assessments. For example, 90 percent of all back problems get better in three months. Does that mean we should deny care to the other 10 percent because they fall at an arbitrary point of abnormality in the bell curve? That is what happens now.

CREATE CONTINUITY OF CARE

I see many patients who are cared for by a local community health center staffed largely by residents whose training includes two to three years of managing outpatients. At the end of their training, the care of their patients is transferred to the next resident. I am struck by the tremendous variability among residents in attitudes about chronic pain. Patients who are cared for by a resident who cares for them thrive. But too often, that resident is replaced by another with a dramatically different, often negative, view toward pain. This transition can be extremely traumatic, and the patient, often low income, has few other options and in effect suffers a two-year punishment while hoping the next resident will be better.

The same problem exists in the health-care system as a whole. Doctors are retiring earlier, fewer are going into primary care, insurance is constantly changing as are the physicians each plan supports, and fewer physicians accept Medicaid and Medicare. The need to find a new doctor every two to three years is common now among all my patients.

The solution to this problem is to strengthen the two levels of primary care referred to in chapter 6 that manage problems, whose members include primary care doctors, psychiatrists and other mental health professionals, and physical medicine and rehabilitation professionals. We can do so in two ways:

Make managing care financially viable by diverting financial resources from those who piecemeal care to those who manage it, either by subsidizing those who provide management services or by changing fee schedules.

Provide incentives to medical students to go into these needed fields, such as education subsidies or subsidies to help them establish practices once they complete their education. I am not naïve enough to believe that every doctor has the mental and physical makeup to manage chronic pain, which is a very challenging field. Yet there is virtually no financial incentive for any physician to do it, and that must change.

REVERSE THE TREND TOWARD THE CORPORATIZATION OF MEDICINE

My father practiced medicine until he was sixty-five, my father-in-law until he was eighty-three. But now physicians are retiring much earlier. While this may reflect a general social trend, many say they retire because of loss of autonomy, excess complexity, and excess regulation of medical practice. These are social trends that my generation did not face when we went into medicine, and many of us do not like them. Perhaps younger physicians, who never practiced in the laissez-faire manner of my generation, can adapt and thrive in this new world, and my concerns are misplaced. Still, I believe anyone functions much better when she controls her own destiny. The ramifications for the patients are important. My mother's rheumatologist practiced until he was seventy-five, and she died shortly after he retired. While there were many reasons for her death, it was clear that the transition to a new doctor, who did not really know her as a person (as opposed to an illness), was traumatic for her and played some part.

I believe it is critical that we give physicians incentives to stay in practice and also strengthen private practice. Physicians must at least have that option. We can do this by reversing the incentives to sell out to larger entities such as hospitals, HMOs, and other corporate providers. Some have suggested subsidizing those in private practice, an idea that I think has merit. But we also must make practice simpler, for example, through management and technology cooperatives that private practitioners share. A few years ago, our state medical society outlined a series of goals for health-care reform. One was to return joy to the practice of medicine. An important aspect of making this happen was allowing the physician to care for the patient unencumbered by the needs of a corporate structure or bottom line. Such patients would receive better care, greater access, and less fragmented care.

MAKE CARE MORE EFFICIENT

As costs rise and reimbursements fall, health-care providers seek to maintain profits by seeing more patients in less time. The twenty-minute visit becomes the ten-minute visit, and so on. While this trend might seem to improve access to the system, it actually doesn't. For one thing, much of that time is spent on such tasks as documenting and ensuring appropriate reimbursement. It is impossible to take care of all of a chronic pain patient's needs in that ten-minute spot. Instead, care is piecemealed. Each patient is allowed only one complaint. If she has others, she must come back for another ten-minute slot. One of my friends was cited by her office manager because she treated a patient for a urinary tract infection. The patient's presenting complaint was something else, and she just happened to mention the urinary symptoms as they talked. Apparently, it was outside the office's code of conduct to take care of a simple, unrelated problem. It may sound totally absurd, but that's what happens when businessmen dictate health-care practice.

As I have noted, we are reasonably confident that providing fast, efficient care can prevent the development of chronic pain. So what is the typical path for pain patients? They may wait weeks for an initial assessment of their problem, which may last only ten minutes and only scratch the surface of what is really ailing them. They are then referred for a service such as physical therapy and not reassessed for a few months. At this time, if there is no improvement, they are farmed out to a specialist whom they must wait weeks or months to see. That doctor orders tests requiring prior approval. Once the tests are done, the doctor recommends a treatment that also requires prior approval. One of my patients had a simple problem, a torn cartilage in his knee. He waited months to get approval for an MRI and more months for approval for his surgery. Meanwhile, he developed all sorts of secondary problems from walking funny for nearly a year. I was seeing him for back pain, a problem that never would have occurred if his initial problem had been addressed in six weeks, as was entirely possible. Many other chronic pain issues also are preventable.

In order to eliminate such inefficiencies, the system at every level must be much more responsive. Here are three critical suggestions.

Spend the Necessary Amount of Time with Patients   Instead of setting arbitrary limits to time spent with patients, the length of the consultation should be determined by the patient's needs, and billing and insurance reimbursement should be directly related to the complexity of those needs and the time spent. I will never accept the necessity of a ten-minute visit. Doctors should be given the incentive to spend time with the patient. One practice I know honored a provider for all the money she brought in. How did she do that? She saw only the simple problems and refused to see complex ones. Her less-honored colleagues saw those patients. That needs to change, and it will only happen if the incentives are in place.

Change Documentation Requirements   The dictum "document, document, document," taught increasingly in medical schools, results in much time wasted and diverted away from the patient. This level of documenting is unnecessary. It is done to satisfy Medicare, Medicaid, and the insurance companies. In order to participate in Medicare and Medicaid, health-care providers must use electronic health records. As I have explained, EHRs are expensive and do not convey useful medical information; frequently they even do not say why the patient is seeing the provider. I often must ask a new patient why she has been referred to me, because the information is either not in the EHR or is so buried in useless data that it is impossible to find. This is only one component of the time-consuming and expensive burden of unnecessary documentation that distracts from the doctor-patient interaction.

These documentation regulations were developed by public health officials and government bureaucrats looking at the overall public health picture. Their goals included trying to make sure the government was not getting ripped off by providers, creating a public health database, and assessing outcomes of the health-care system as well as of individual hospitals and care providers. These are useful goals, but this macroeconomic point of view can do great harm on the individual level. Yet doctors must follow the regulations in order to survive financially.

I would eliminate EHR requirements. EHR should be optional and unrelated to reimbursement. This change alone would dramatically reduce the cost of individual practice. But providers would have to rise in unison and refuse to accept Medicare and Medicaid until the change is accomplished.

Increase the Role of Health-Care Extenders   "Health-care extenders," such as physician assistants and nurse practitioners, do not have the training to provide the services a physician provides. But they can spend time with the patient at a lower cost. I hear many patients complain that their doctor does not spend enough time with them. To a point I can accept that. But I cannot accept it of a physician's assistant or a nurse practitioner. The importance of their services must be recognized. It is exciting to see many of these practitioners going into pain management. But their work is not adequately reimbursed relative to their surgical counterparts. In my opinion, their services are more complex and their level of responsibility greater than those even of surgeons. By doing a great deal of time-consuming case management without physician oversight, they play a major, cost-effective role in minimizing fragmentation and advocating for patients. Increasing their reimbursement to reflect their function will incentivize them to go into needed fields and improve access while decreasing cost.

MAKE INSURANCE PORTABLE

Many of my patients are elderly people who relocate to be near their children. They are covered by Medicare, the only truly portable insurance. Other patients relocate to New Hampshire or away from it to find better job opportunities. Their medical care is complex, and their success in their new environment depends on access to health care. Still others do not relocate, but face problems when their employer or their state changes insurances. A new employer plan may deny preexisting conditions such as pain outright. The second problem occurred when our state outsourced some of its Medicaid system, creating several plans that provided very different access to care for those with chronic pain. This was how my patient from Bosnia was denied access to my services.

For care to be effective, it must be fully portable, with no denial for prior conditions. All providers must be included in all plans. The PP/ACA addressed this issue, at least in part, by limiting exclusion for prior problems such as chronic pain, increasing competition by creating exchanges, and lowering intrastate limitations on out-of-state insurers. But portability remains a problem, for reasons I will discuss further in chapter 15.

IMPROVE PATIENT ADVOCACY

Patients need an advocate. State insurance commissions are supposed to do this, but they are often ineffective. In my experience, when denied care, most patients are not even aware that they have this option, or they lack the will or knowledge to access it. Many feel their problem is unique and they are alone, and it is hard to take on a bully by oneself.

In this area there are some grounds for optimism, as chapter 3 explained. A number of organizations, such as the American Academy of Pain Medicine and the American Pain Society, try to serve this purpose; and their collective efforts have resulted in the Pain Care Policy Act and the subsequent IOM report. Although the changes have been slow, they are coming. If we can change the perception of chronic pain in America, we can create a united force that can better advocate for those who suffer and hopefully improve insurance company behavior.

Disability Insurance

When I developed a depression in the midst of my medical training and was unable to function, I had to take two months off from work. At first I thought this disability would only last a short time. My coworkers encouraged me to "get well." I didn't. As days turned into weeks and one hospitalization turned into another, I became more and more discouraged, not because of the suffering my illness created, but because I thought I wasn't of use to anyone and felt guilty that my coworkers had to work harder to cover my absence. Even worse, I feared for my future. I had worked so hard to get to that point in my life, and I saw all my accomplishments and my hopes for the future slipping away.

I was fortunate. I made a full recovery and returned to work, arguably better than ever. After this experience, I was better able to appreciate the vicious cycle of disability initiated by an illness or injury. I learned that only a strong person can climb out of such an abyss alone. Most of us need help. I was lucky to have support from friends, family, and most of all my coworkers. If not for their kindness, I doubt that I would have recovered. However, while kindness is an elixir that stimulates and heals, it is not sufficient for survival. We also need money. I was quite fortunate that my residency program had a good disability insurance policy.

In order to examine the problems our current disability insurance system faces, it is informative to look at its evolution over time.[8] Commercial disability insurance began with communities of independent artisans, mariners, and others who gave willingly to funds that would support one of their own who became disabled. They were compassionate in that they were willing to help someone who was in need. At the same time, they were safeguarding their own vulnerability should they become unable to work. Over time, commercial ventures of independent underwriters replaced the system of informal, small community funds and became the earliest insurance companies. With this change, the concept of transferring risk from the individual to the group shifted from a community venture to a business venture.

With the Industrial Revolution came an increased risk to workers and an increased likelihood of disability. Disability policies written at that time were restrictive, covering only disability from accidental injury, not sickness. Most policies could be canceled and premiums could be raised at the insurer's will. In addition to these problems, these policies often were unavailable to those who needed them the most, specifically, those in high-risk occupations.

With the creation of government-mandated workers' compensation programs, commercial disability insurance began offering broader benefits so insurers could attract more customers. To minimize the risk of malingering, the benefit paid was related to the insured's actual earnings. Riders coordinated benefit options so benefits could not exceed the person's prior income, eliminating any disincentive to return to work.

Beginning in the 1980s, insurers began to focus their attention more on professionals and white-collar workers, who presumably were at lower risk, and those more likely to return to work. Commercial insurers abandoned lower-income, higher-risk individuals, who were better served by government programs. Among higher-income segments, the need for disability insurance is greater than ever today, and commercial insurers are targeting these groups, especially the self-employed, for whom a loss can be devastating.

Short-term disability generally covers a period of up to twenty-six weeks. If the individual is still disabled at the end of this time, coverage shifts to the long-term plan, which covers her until she can return to work, or until she reaches the end of her expected work life, usually age sixty-five. This assumes that the individual or the employer has purchased both short- and long-term disability policies, which often is not the case. There is a waiting period. You cannot collect benefits until you have been disabled for a certain period of time. Typically, the higher the cost of the plan, the shorter the waiting period will be.

Like entitlement plans, commercial disability insurance does not fully cover the disabled person's previous income. Typically, for short-term disability you can expect to receive 50 to 70 percent of your income, while for long-term disability you can expect to receive 50 to 80 percent. The more you pay for the policy, the higher the percentage you get. Plans are structured in this way in order to give the individual an incentive to return to work. Most plans will take into account other sources of disability income so that total benefits from all sources do not exceed the percentage in the plan.

Policies may specify disability from "any job" or "own job." In a competitive insurance market, policies tend to require disability from the individual's own job as sufficient to warrant a benefit. Policies that pay only for total, as opposed to partial, disability tend to be less expensive and therefore more attractive to the consumer.

Employers who purchase group plans have the incentive to purchase the lowest-cost plan that will cover the generic needs of all employees. It may be enough for some, yet not enough for others. Those not covered by an employee plan, or not sufficiently covered, can purchase an individual plan tailored to their needs and their ability to pay. But many choose not to. The cost of disability insurance is high, and the perceived risk is thought to be low. In fact, the actual risk of disability is high, and most people have not saved sufficiently to cover it. Those without the foresight to protect their income by anticipating a potential disability create a substantial burden to the country in terms of direct cost for income replacement and health insurance for disabled workers and their families, and indirect costs in terms of lost productivity.

There are a number of reasons why 70 percent of American workers have no long-term disability insurance, but one is total denial. While we feel sorry for friends who become disabled, we fail to acknowledge that there, but for the grace of God, go we. A disabling illness or accident happens in just a moment, as it did for me. It is a moment that can change our lives forever. I never thought I would have to worry about becoming disabled. Had it been up to me, I would never even have thought of getting disability insurance. I am thankful my employer felt differently.

Aside from the need to prevent disability in the first place through employer attention to creating a congenial, ergonomic workplace, already discussed in chapter 9, the biggest problem with private disability insurance, as with public programs, is access to the system once a worker is disabled. Problems with access include lack of education on the part of insurance consumers, cost of policies, constrained personal budgets, constrained corporate budgets, restrictive underwriting, difficulties in defining and proving disability, fraud, and details of the fine print.

Even if I had been gifted with the foresight to buy my own disability insurance, I would have been clueless as to how to sift through all the different policy options and fine print. Whom do we trust to purchase a policy from? Insurance salespeople are in business to sell. It is to their benefit to maximize their client's satisfaction, as doing so will provide more customers. Still, charlatans abound who are your best friend when they sell the policy, but are nowhere to be found when you need to file a claim.

So whom do we trust? The answer is nobody. An educated consumer will research all policies and interview several possible insurers, in effect soliciting bids. This process requires more time, energy, and knowledge than most of us possess.

Disability insurance policies are not cheap, especially high-end policies with short waiting periods that cover disability from one's own occupation and offer a relatively high percentage of lost income. It is estimated that an individual should expect to pay between 1 and 3 percent of his income for disability insurance. For those living on the financial edge, this can be prohibitive. When combined with our inherent denial of the possibility of becoming disabled, it is easy to see why many choose not to purchase insurance.

Employers too increasingly face constrained budgets. They also seek to lower costs, and one way to do this is to reduce or eliminate perks such as disability insurance. They may provide only long- or short-term disability insurance, but not both. They may purchase less expensive, more restrictive policies. They may choose not to offer disability insurance at all, and they are under no obligation to offer it. When costs are high, sales are low, and the supply of labor exceeds demand, employers have little incentive to spend a lot on such perks. As a result, like health insurers, disability insurance companies are funneling poorly educated people in high-risk, physically intensive jobs to charitable organizations and governmental programs.

Once injured or ill, a person must prove her disability. In my experience this is less difficult with private insurance than with workers' compensation. Still, a problem exists. Insurance companies require a physician's assessment of disability before they will distribute benefits. One would like to think the personal physician's assessment is final, but it is not. The insurance company can still deny coverage in several ways. They may choose to interpret a less than carefully worded doctor's statement as insufficient to justify disability. They may rely on an expert's second opinion, which may contradict the personal physician's and is very difficult for the disabled person to challenge (see chapter 10 for more on such experts). The patient does have the right to appeal to the state board of insurance, but the process is lengthy and expensive and favors those with deep pockets, that is, the insurance company. Often it devolves into a "he said, she said" situation, where the decision is based less on logic than on the judge's personal bias.

Insurance is restricted by the fine print. Policies may pay out only if the insured is totally disabled from all occupations, or only for injury but not illness. Waiting periods may be long. Certain conditions may not be covered. Benefits may be insufficient to meet one's needs. Premiums may be open to change, and policies may be cancelled without notice.

Some underwriting is fraudulent, but so are some claims. An individual may submit a claim even though there is no disability, or there may be an injury or illness that is not sufficient to produce disability, but is exaggerated in order to get a benefit. There is also a question of secondary gain. For example, it is well known that the biggest predictor of disability is job satisfaction. A dissatisfied employee may embellish symptoms in order to escape an unsatisfactory work environment, yet still receive financial support.

Although such fraudulent behavior is likely infrequent, the system is structured to minimize and control fraud, creating excessive barriers to those who really require services.

Disability Insurance Solutions

In my experience, the problems with disability insurance are less onerous than those of health insurance. Still, they exist, with great cost to our society. The primary goal is to maximize access and limit the burden to social programs.

EDUCATE CONSUMERS

We should begin by educating consumers so they understand the costs and risks involved. In our office we have regular meetings about 401K policies and health-care options. It would be helpful for companies to offer similar educational sessions on disability insurance so employees can make educated decisions. Perhaps we should start such education in school, before employees enter the workforce, and make education about risk and insurance part of what used to be called "home economics."

ELIMINATE FINE PRINT

Insurers should not only describe restrictions clearly in writing in policies, but also verbally explain the ramifications of those restrictions.

CLARIFY ASSESSMENT OF DISABILITY

We need to better define what is disabling and streamline the process of accepting or rejecting disability. Certain disabilities, such as spinal cord injuries, are clear. Others, such as back injuries, are less so. When conflicts and questions arise, a truly disinterested third party can be helpful. It is doubtful that this should be an "insurance doctor." Instead, I recommend independent panels of the sort I describe for criminal and civil court cases in the next chapter.

PROVIDE REHABILITATION

Rehabilitation should be part of every disability policy, with the goal of making the disabled able. While it would make sense to offer vocational rehabilitation as part of disability insurance services, this is often not done because of the assumption that the cost of providing the service exceeds the potential benefit of getting someone off disability and returning him to the workforce. However, this may not be true, and I believe this service should be offered initially. The patient can be motivated by a stepped process that rewards him for achieving each step—perhaps financially, but more important, by enabling him to move to the next step. It is critical to success that the client not be abandoned when he finds new employment. Currently, when someone finds a new job, disability benefits cease. If he fails at the new job, he must reinitiate the entire process. This creates an excessive fear of failure and gives the financially desperate no incentive to try to return to work. Instead, there should be a window of time, perhaps six months, when the client tries out the new employment. If he fails because of his disability, he can again receive his previous benefits with little question.

INSURE HIGH-RISK OCCUPATIONS

Commercial insurers will not insure certain high-risk occupations, which unnecessarily exaggerates their risk and creates disincentives for people to enter them. The list of uninsurable occupations varies from company to company, and any occupation can be insured for the right price. However, the hazardous occupations generally considered uninsurable include heavy manual labor and those that bear a high risk of accident or environmental hazard, such as jobs involving explosives or heights. Creative solutions, such as business partnering with government through subsidies and tax breaks, could lessen the risk to insurers yet provide coverage for those who are currently uninsurable.

ADDRESS FRAUD EFFECTIVELY

Fraud does exist, and we need to address both insurer and consumer fraud. However, we are so focused on eliminating malingering that we overstate its occurrence and treat everyone as guilty until proven otherwise, which limits access. The solution begins with changing the perception of chronic pain among insurers so that they understand that while it may represent a statistical aberration on the bell curve, it is real. Adjusters' manuals must reflect this awareness.

I was struck by how easy it is to accomplish this perceptual shift when I gave a talk to a large group on "Managing Chronic Pain: Destigmatizing the Stigmatized." Several adjusters were in the audience, and several said that I had changed their whole perception of chronic pain. What bothered me was that many had been in the business for years. An effective tactic is to make people think of someone they know who suffers from chronic pain, as I do when I describe my mother, who was disabled but still was able to do things. Some say making the issue personal in this manner risks losing objectivity, but I believe it is critical.

Eliminating fraud also requires medical experts who are truly unbiased. In the next chapter, I recommend creating a pool of independent experts for the court system. A similar pool, paid a reasonable rate and funded by insurance companies with the money they already use to pay their experts, can evaluate disability cases. The pool must consist of physicians who are knowledgeable about chronic pain. As doctors become better educated about pain, this pool will grow. For denials, there must be an easily accessible and not onerous appeal process. A second opinion from another member of the pool who is blind to the initial opinion should suffice. If the two experts disagree, their opinions can be submitted to a judge of some sort. Over time, if the insurance company feels the client's actions are fraudulent or the client believes she is being unfairly treated, either can appeal to this judge.

It is unacceptable that four out of ten working-age Americans are unable to contribute to society. By acknowledging the problems people with chronic pain face, rather than blaming them, we can develop creative solutions to ease their suffering, reinstate them as productive members of society, and lower the social costs they create. Once again, the solution begins with compassion.

ELEVEN

The Legal System

Disorder in the Court!

I will treat all persons whom I encounter through my practice
of law with fairness, courtesy, respect, and honesty. . . .
I will never reject, from any consideration to myself, the cause
of the defenseless or oppressed.
Excerpts from the Colorado Attorney Oath of Admission

In preparation for this chapter, I researched many attorneys' oaths for different states and chose that of Colorado for simplicity. All of these oaths admonish attorneys to treat all parties with respect and never reject the cause of the oppressed or defenseless. The pain patient certainly fits into this category. If members of the legal system lived up to their honorable calling, there would be less of a problem for those who suffer. But often they don't, and the legal profession has created a system that further victimizes these very oppressed.

Patients usually become involved with the civil courts as plaintiffs, through Social Security Disability, workers' compensation, personal injury claims, and divorce. Occasionally, a patient may become involved in a criminal court. This is less common and is preventable.

The legal system pits the plaintiff and the defendant, representing two opposing realities, against each other. Usually both plaintiff and defendant need to hire an advocate, generally a lawyer. The presentation is a debate, which functionally is a cross between a boxing match and a poker game. The lawyers slug it out verbally, and a judge, judges, or a jury determine the winner.

How the Game Is Played

Each side bolsters its position by collecting evidence. Is there objective evidence of injury? Did the injury happen where the patient says it did? Is it as severe as the patient says? Are the treatments provided medically reasonable and necessary? What is medically reasonable and necessary for an injury of this type? Does the policy cover these treatments?

The evidence is the cards the attorney has been dealt. Once he reviews the evidence, he decides if he wishes to play the hand. If he does, he creates a point of view, which he defends at all costs, whether it is based in reality or not. To support it he emphasizes corroborating evidence while suppressing evidence that casts doubt on it or refutes it. The attorney thus seeks to change the colors of the entire tapestry of the case into black and white in order to tilt the scales of justice in his client's favor.

Each lawyer's job is to play her hand as well as possible and win the game. A lawyer is judged on how often she wins. Thus there is an incentive to win at all costs. Although one side is not allowed to withhold information from the other, bluffing and manipulation of the information is fair. Each lawyer eloquently attempts to persuade the judges that her side is right. A poker face and persuasive skills are valuable and may in fact be more important than truth.

In the middle of this game is the patient, who has been hurt and is suffering. The complex rules, which even most lawyers struggle to understand, bewilder him. Bewilderment creates fear. Fear triggers a fight or flight reaction, which generates anxiety. Anxiety, as we know, amplifies pain.

Right from the start, the patient realizes that the legitimacy of his complaint is being questioned, usually by the defendant, but sometimes by others. That comes as a shock to most patients, whose pain makes them feel justified in seeking compensation—especially since the law or their insurance company says they are entitled to it. When this is questioned, their integrity is threatened. They become defensive, angry, shocked, sad, anxious. They want to lash out at those who question them, a reaction that, curiously, the court perceives negatively. The angrier a patient is, the worse she does as a witness or plaintiff. It is hard to stifle righteous indignation. Meanwhile, all these emotions increase her pain.

Once all the evidence and the experts are assembled, the game begins, though not necessarily in the courtroom. Frequently it begins in the hallway or on the golf course, where the case is discussed and settlements are suggested. Most often the client is not present. Each side tries to frighten the other into settling and seeks a mutually acceptable solution. If they find one, the patient receives a financial "award" as a settlement, of which the patient's attorney receives a share, usually at least one-third of the amount. Since the client is not involved in this negotiation, the lawyer has to convince him or her that the settlement is the right choice. Sometimes this involves effectively blackmailing the client by telling him that if he refuses the settlement, he could end up getting less than the agreed-on amount from a jury. For a patient who may have waited years for this moment, the thought of getting less than two-thirds of the negotiated settlement—all of which would be inadequate to cover his needs—is hardly palatable. However, under effective persuasion, he learns to fear the alternative and reluctantly accepts.

Sometimes the case goes to trial and is heard before a jury, a single judge, or a panel. For the patient, this process involves tremendous fear, since she has an incredible amount to lose. Throughout the trial, her integrity is supported by her own attorney and assaulted by the opposing counsel. A criminal defendant is supposed innocent until proven guilty. In civil court, the patient is treated as guilty until proven innocent. The degree of victimization this involves directly contravenes the therapeutic goals for the patient. Some patients never recover from the insult. Some have told me that they felt more assaulted by the legal process than they ever felt from the injury. Others develop a clear posttraumatic stress disorder from their experience. Even watching a legal proceeding on television is too painful for them.

Win or lose, the result is often appealed, forcing the patient to continue to live in the past, unable to create a new beginning. The process goes on indefinitely. For a patient with a workers' compensation claim in a state that allows medical compensation for the life of the individual, the game goes on forever. The claims adjustor, the doctor, and the lawyer can escape the stress merely by going home at night. The patient is stuck with it.

THE LEGAL LIMBO

Lawyers frequently encourage patients to avoid moving on with their lives, sometimes explicitly, but more often implicitly. The lawyer may suggest to the patient that "ringing up large medical bills" will make the potential settlement larger by increasing the value of the claim. This makes the patient more valuable to the lawyer but harms the patient by delaying rehabilitation. Patients with low-value claims have trouble finding representation. In many states, even though a claim may be settled, the patient can still make future claims on the insurance company, for example, in a workers' compensation claim. However, once the settlement is reached, attorneys can expect little further income, and they become harder to find. This leaves the patient at the mercy of the insurance company, creating a sense of helplessness, which creates fear, and so on.

Patients can remain in a legal limbo for years with no clear predictable outcome. Endlessly facing the unknown, especially with one's financial well-being at stake, creates fear that further amplifies the pain. Meanwhile, being in limbo prolongs the anger phase of grieving and unnecessarily delays active rehabilitation. Until patients are over this phase, it is difficult for them to accept rehabilitation, which requires accepting an altered future. While it is unclear precisely how much of a role litigiousness plays in impairing rehabilitation, it is quite clear to most practitioners that it poisons the process. It is also clear that once patients settle a claim, they rarely show a dramatic improvement in function. Is this because they would have had the same outcome anyway, or is it because the delay has caused damage and rehabilitation is futile at that point? Timing is everything in rehabilitation. Does the legal process adversely affect the timing? We don't know the answer, but the question is on the table.

The stress of the legal limbo, with no clear goal to work toward other than the possibility of a future payout, also does tremendous damage to the patient's family. It is not unusual to see a spouse who "can't take it anymore" walk away. Then it's on to divorce court and another lawyer.

THE DOCTOR ON TRIAL

Sometimes it is not the patient who finds herself on trial, but the healer. While some acts performed under the guise of medicine are egregious, most of those brought to the courtroom are not. The results of a well-intended treatment have turned sour, and the patient, or society, blames the physician. Usually these proceedings occur in civil court. Occasionally, they occur in criminal court. Here I will discuss the former; chapter 13 discusses the latter.

Early in my career, I met a patient with a fairly straightforward problem. She had a herniated disc with radicular pain (arising from the irritation of the nerves that branch out from the spinal cord). The MRI confirmed the finding. I told her surgery was an option, but there was a conservative path to follow, which was somewhat new at that time, at least in New Hampshire, but well accepted nationally. She chose the latter. She was treated with epidural steroids (delivered by injection directly to the spinal nerves and the disc) and physical therapy, and she got better.

Several weeks later, her herniation increased, something that happens in 15 to 20 percent of people who have surgery for this condition; we don't know what the rate is for successful nonoperative care. She came to our office with a recurrence of symptoms similar to her original ones. I was away, but my colleague saw her and treated her appropriately with oral corticosteroids and analgesics. That night, her symptoms progressed, and she developed an acute *cauda equina* syndrome, which resulted in temporary paralysis in her legs and difficulty urinating. She went to the emergency room and eventually underwent emergency surgical decompression of the affected nerves. Her neurological symptoms improved, but she was left with chronic pain. She later herniated again above her surgery and needed another surgery.

This patient then sued me, contending that had she been sent for surgery right away, she would never have needed any more surgery, would not have had chronic back pain, and would not have had a second disc degenerate. By convention we speak of the "plaintiff's" case, but there is no doubt that these contentions were shaped by her attorney. She later justified her suit with the assertion that her neurosurgeon had said that if he were she, he would get an attorney. The neurosurgeon denied ever saying that.

While all this was going on, I talked to the patient's husband, who thanked me for everything I had done for them. He later denied saying that. In fact, I had been there for her at every turn. I had given them my home phone number. I had explained the rationale for my recommended treatment program to them. The unfortunate reality was that she had a rare syndrome that could not have been predicted. Given her failure to respond to treatment, and the fact that she required further surgery for disc pathology, it was likely that she would develop chronic pain.

I will never forget my feelings when the sheriff arrived to hand me the notice that I was being sued. After the talk with the patient's husband, I had assumed they were comfortable with everything I had done for them. I was blindsided. Waves of shock, anger, fear, and sadness ran through me for a long time. I had done nothing wrong. I followed the textbook and did what I thought was right. I felt bad that she was suffering, but my attorney quickly told me not to publicly acknowledge that; it wouldn't look good in court.

I was angry at my patient. After all I had done for her, why would she seek retribution against me? I was angry that I could no longer feel compassion for someone I had cared for and who was suffering. I feared the courtroom. It was a neat place to watch on television, but I had no interest in being a member of the cast, especially as the accused.

I now also feared this patient. My attorney told me that juries tended to view patients with paralysis sympathetically, even if it was only temporary. Having treated spinal cord injury patients for years, I knew he was right. These patients always found someone to blame for their infirmity, whether or not that person bore any responsibility for their condition, and they usually won in court.

I was suddenly afraid of all my other patients. I had done my best for another human being, and she had turned on me. Who would be next? I was now afraid to practice medicine.

I feared the plaintiff's attorney. She was from a high-powered Boston law firm, primarily because the patient couldn't get a New Hampshire firm to take her case. Even though I know it is irrational, I can't help feeling that everything Boston is better than everything New Hampshire. I feared that my attorney would not be able to stand up to the Boston attorney and feared how she would portray me.

I feared the loss of respect that losing would entail, especially within my medical group. I feared being tagged with the scarlet letter of being registered in the national registry, which I would have to report every time I filled out any medically related application. I feared being considered a loser, or worse, a bad doctor subject to the world's judgment.

It was during this case that I learned how the legal system works. Each side collected evidence and then experts to support its claims. I found sixty-five scientific articles in peer-reviewed journals that justified my actions. My attorney retained as experts the heads of spine surgery at Massachusetts General Hospital and Johns Hopkins, the latter recognized as one of the world's foremost authorities on *cauda equina* syndrome. Two people I greatly admired were coming to my defense. I should have been happy, but I wasn't.

I felt I was losing everything. Never motivated by money and prestige, I had become a doctor to help people. To do my job, I needed to have faith in what I was doing and in my patients. The legal process severely challenged that faith. The joy and honor I had felt in being a doctor were being taken away from me, as was my humanity.

I became suddenly, painfully aware of what my patients went through when they entered the legal fray. For many months, the stress ate away at me. I wondered how a patient with fewer resources than I had could possibly deal with all this. I wondered if God was teaching me a lesson. All bad experiences are opportunities. I tried to look at this as an opportunity to learn and to mold my future behavior. This may have been an honorable goal, but it did not make the process any easier.

A few days before the trial was to start, our legal team ventured south to Boston to depose one of the experts testifying on behalf of the patient, a semiretired neurosurgeon from a small town in Pennsylvania. My attorney was able to get him to admit that I had done nothing wrong. With some satisfaction I watched the opposing attorney lose her composure as her case unraveled. Her other expert had no credentials in spine pain and was much less credible. As we drove north, for the first time in months I felt confident that justice would smile on me.

The next day, both sides met in court for jury selection. I watched with mixed emotions as my former patient hobbled into the room on crutches, her lawyer taking great pains to show prospective jurors how disabled she was. I fought to maintain my composure as I watched what I could tell was my patient's obvious embellishment of her disability. I consoled myself in knowing that not only my own two experts but my patient's as well had stated categorically that I had done everything right. Jury selection was still in progress when we left for the day. I was prepared for battle.

The battle never came. I received a call that night that a settlement had been reached. In exchange for dropping the charges against me, my medical group agreed to pay a sum that, although much less than the patient was looking for, was still substantial. In my mind, a dollar was too much. I also learned that the patient's attorney received $100,000 as payment for her incompetence. I was furious. Being an idealist, I wanted to fight the honorable fight, but my attorney told me the decision to settle was a no-brainer. No matter how good a case you have, he explained, a person in obvious pain evokes great sympathy from a jury, who are more likely to vote with their hearts than their minds.

I learned that my experience was hardly unique; this scenario plays itself out every day in our courts. Plaintiffs' attorneys often choose to take a case based not just on its merits, but also on the potential payout. As a bargaining tool, they try to scare the defendant with a huge potential settlement and a "black mark" in the national registry. There is supposed to be a penalty for frivolous lawsuits, but it is nearly impossible to prove this. Consequently, a plaintiff's attorney faces little risk in bringing a suit and has the potential for a very large gain.

While this system clearly benefits attorneys, particularly the plaintiff's attorney, the damage to society is considerable. In particular, the ramifications for medical care are huge. While the total payout for judgments in favor of the plaintiff may be relatively small as a percentage of the total cost of health care, the cost of defensive medicine is extremely high.

First, most physicians carry malpractice insurance, which for some specialties and in some places can exceed $100,000 per year. It is the rare practice that can absorb the rising costs of insurance. Consequently, it is becoming harder and harder to attract qualified people to high-need specialties such as obstetrics, creating a shortage felt in many parts of the country.

Second, the prospect of potential lawsuits sends physicians into defensive mode. It is not the lawsuit that creates the cost, but rather, the *fear* of the lawsuit. Fear, perhaps irrational, dictates behavior. The fear is that the one "t" not crossed may come back to haunt the physician. So paperwork must be filled out in greater detail. Tests, sometimes unnecessary, must be obtained to CMA (cover my ass). To manage the paperwork, more time is spent and more people are hired. Time is taken away from the patient and devoted to the paperwork. All this creates higher costs. Somebody has to pay these costs, so the cost of medical care rises. In fact, the vast majority of lawsuits are found for the physician, and no dollars need be paid out to the plaintiff. But the physician still incurs a substantial cost from the expense of defending the suit and time lost from the office. There is also the emotional cost, which forever changes the way a physician looks at a patient.

It is clear to me that the quality of the doctor-patient relationship suffers from a lack of trust. Because of all the factors listed above, the doctor begins to treat the medical record more than the patient. The patient truly becomes a piece of paper. High-risk patients are feared, especially pain patients. The legal ramifications of treating a pain patient are profound, whether it means documenting care, ordering defensive tests, standing up for a patient in a civil court, protecting oneself from regulatory scrutiny from government agencies, or protecting oneself from a potential lawsuit.

Whenever I attend a pain meeting, I am told that the solution for all my problems is to "document, document, document" all my actions. I am sorry, but I have a busy practice. I went into medicine to "heal the sick," not "buff the chart." I do not have time to "document, document, document." I refuse to put the needs of the chart ahead of the needs of my patient, and I refuse to live in fear of my patient.

Who in their right mind, in this world of cost-containment, would ever want to take on pain management? Many physicians don't. Many try, but throw in the towel. Some physicians have taken a passive-aggressive stance. They "go naked" and refuse to carry malpractice insurance. They do not bill insurance carriers. Instead, the patient pays the fee up front, and then submits the bill herself to her health insurer. In this way the health provider can cut costs by a third or more and minimize the hassle of practicing medicine today. Such providers long for the glory days of medicine when patient care was their first and foremost concern. Is the risk of going without malpractice insurance and relying on a less-certain income stream paid directly by patients worth it for the doctor? For some, yes; for others, no. But if we could cut health-care costs by a third, it would be worth it to society.

Lest we forget, someone must pay the cost of the courts. The more trials there are, the more judges and stenographers and policemen and court-rooms we need. Who pays for that?

The Medico-Legal Expert

> The greater the ignorance, the greater the dogmatism.
>
> Sir William Osler, MD, *Montreal Medical Journal* (1902)

After completing my residency in physical medicine and rehabilitation, I began my first job in New Hampshire, at the Easter Seals center. I was under the impression that my primary role would be to help newly disabled people adapt to their acquired physical challenges. I saw myself working with people suffering from myriad disabilities, such as stroke, head injury, amputation, neuromuscular diseases, or spinal cord injury. I had some idea I would be seeing pain patients as well and was pleased to know I would be prepared for that. Since my residency had done little to prepare me for pain management, I had spent a lot of my free time learning about it.

I was unaware that New Hampshire physicians thought of a physiatrist simply as someone who specialized in managing difficult pain problems. In fact, they were seeking a convenient way of offloading a problem they didn't want to deal with. Soon I found myself doing almost nothing other than treating chronic pain. As much as I advertised my other skills, the local physicians took little notice.

Looking over one of my early schedules, I noticed that someone was scheduled for an "IME."

"What's an IME?" I asked a colleague.

"It's an independent medical evaluation," he responded.

"Oh. What's that?"

"It means they want you to comment on the management of the patient and offer suggestions."

"Wow," I thought, somewhat naïvely. I was out of residency for only a few weeks and someone already thought I was an expert! Still, knowing how poorly prepared most physiatrists were for managing musculoskeletal pain, I thought it odd that I was being asked to comment on an orthopedist's management of a patient, especially since he had been in the field for years and had spent his whole career studying this area. I was unaware that I was overrating both the insurance company's motives and the orthopedist's abilities.

Over the next year or so, I did several IMES a week. During this time, my partner and mentor, Paul Corcoran, taught me that the IME is an opportunity to look at the problem in a different way and offer suggestions that might help both the physician and the patient. He felt it was crucial that the physician include the patient at all stages of the evaluation and share her thoughts with him, both verbally and by sending him a copy of her report. Being both naïve and idealistic, I wholeheartedly agreed with this approach, and still do. No matter how the patient enters my office, whether by insurance company referral for an IME or otherwise, he is still my patient, and the Hippocratic Oath guides my actions. I also had been taught to believe in my patients; so unless otherwise apparent, I always gave the patient the benefit of any doubt.

One day I saw an elderly woman and was quite impressed that at her age she was still working. She had been injured, and the insurance company wanted to know if I thought she could do an alternative job as a night watchperson in a relatively seedy area of a small city. The job required her to watch monitors and periodically walk the premises. It was clear that she could do the job physically, but not mentally or emotionally. She was in utter fear of this job, a fear I shared. She was my mother's age, and the thought of my mother being forced to do such a job infuriated me. I wrote as much to the insurance company, and her attorney was more than happy to use my report to his advantage.

A few days later, I received a call from an insurance company representative who wanted to talk about my report. He said I had caused them great embarrassment, and they had been forced to settle her case at a time when they really didn't want to. He added that he recognized my need to be an advocate for patients, but he would appreciate it if I would periodically "see things our way." He seemed to miss the point that having a job meant a great deal more to this woman than a paycheck. It was an opportunity for her to get out of her house, remain productive, and feel alive—an affirmation that she was still important.

I asked if he would let his mother do that job. He refused to answer, saying it was irrelevant. I said it wasn't. I told him I would continue to do what was best for the patient. I never received another IME request from them, which hardly bothered me, but it did bother Easter Seals since they relied on the income from these IMEs to help support their other programs. IMES do pay well, if you are into that kind of thing; however, as always, there is a catch. Insurance companies only refer to you if you are willing to walk on their side of the line between right and wrong.

Sometime later, I was asked to testify on behalf of another patient who, I felt, was being poorly treated by his insurance company. I saw this as an opportunity to set the record straight and help someone in need. In preparation, I met with the patient's attorney, who cared only that I say "the right thing," that is, what he wanted me to say. Even though he was paying me as an expert witness, I considered myself an independent agent with the responsibility to be honest and say what I believed needed to be said. The day I testified, any faith I had in the American court system evaporated. Both lawyers spent their energies trying to manipulate both the medical record and my thoughts. Each strove to alter the truth to satisfy the goals of the person they represented.

Through experiences like these, I learned that there are three types of medical-legal experts. The first type have thoroughly researched their fields, learned from the school of hard knocks, and willingly share what they know, as well as what they don't, with others. Second are the experts who really believe they know their field. But rather than thoroughly exploring it, they cut intellectual corners and profess a knowledge they really don't possess, often relying on the expertise of others who are equally ignorant. They fear any threat to the sense of power and the feeling of being admired that go along with being considered an expert, and they ignore or feebly refute any information that may expose this façade and threaten these second-ary gains. Yes, the phenomenon of secondary gain is quite alive, not only in patients but also in their providers. Third are the experts who deploy knowledge they may or may not have, not to help anyone else but to enrich themselves. In my experience, most medical-legal "experts" in the field of chronic pain fall into the second and third categories. I put that term in quotes because in my opinion a person who is knowingly or unknowingly blind to the facts, or uses his knowledge only to enrich himself, is no expert.

In 1989, while running an outpatient pain clinic, I began to notice a symptom complex of memory impairment, fatigue, diffuse pain, depression, anxiety, and cognitive decline in patients who had suffered single or mul-tiple episodes of supposedly minor head trauma. Their MRIS did not show any damage. The medical "experts" who published on this phenomenon and represented insurers in court told me it could be readily explained by "malingering" or "conversion hysteria." After I saw ten patients, all medically unsophisticated and unknown to each other, with these same symptoms, several without any sign of secondary gain resulting from their symptoms and many with significant secondary loss, I started to question this conclusion. Still, the experts insisted on calling this entity "litiga-tion neurosis." Over the next decade, an epidemic of the same symptom complex hit the sports world, and it became clear that even head injury not sufficient to produce unconsciousness could create microscopic brain injury that an MRI could not detect, often with profound and permanent neuropsychological-physical ramifications. This entity was termed "minor head injury" or "postconcussive syndrome." Suddenly "litigation neurosis" had a name and a cause. We no longer needed to name-call those who had the nerve to have a problem we didn't understand. Minor head injury was now worthy of respect, treatment, and prevention. Stock in helmet manufacturing companies soared as it became illegal to do virtually anything without their product. One expert who previously had blamed these patients for their condition became a convert and in a national publication encouraged us to treat them with respect, oblivious to the carnage he had inflicted on those he had previously mislabeled. Too bad he didn't feel that way before.

Being an expert is not fun. You must take time off from a busy day at the office, often on short notice, to be subjected to an interrogation by an opposing attorney whose role is to confuse you and make you doubt yourself. Sometimes you can be on the stand for hours. Why would anyone want to do this? Some feel a moral obligation to stand up for their patients. Others have strong opinions about pain that they feel must be defended.

There are other, less admirable reasons, though. First, being an expert pays well! An effective expert can pocket thousands of dollars. I have actually heard the following statements from "experts":

"I'll say anything they want as long as they pay the bill!"

"They paid me $10,000 up front. Of course I would see things their way."

"I get paid so much from testifying, I really don't need to practice medicine anymore. However, it makes me look better on the stand if I do, so I still see patients two days a week."

I have a vivid memory of a rather shady character who came up to me once after I had testified and offered me a regular position as his expert:

"You were great up there. You should do this more often. That's where all the bucks are!" I politely declined his offer.

Another less-than-exemplary reason experts testify is to exact retribution on pain patients. This motivation may be conscious or unconscious, but either way it is cruel. As I have explained, pain patients require time and energy and frequently cost more to treat than they pay. They challenge our sense of omnipotence, our self-esteem, and our view of medicine. The mature response would be to try to understand pain better and seek more effective means of managing it. An immature response would be to get angry at the patient. It is not unusual for an expert to use the witness stand as a means of exacting retribution from all pain patients.

Being viewed as an expert creates a real, addictive feeling of power, even if the expertise is an illusion. When I was first sought out as an expert, I must admit, my nose rose a bit higher in the air. However, attorneys often hire experts for less complimentary reasons, as "balance shifters." Typically, a court decides that the truth lies somewhere along a continuum, not at the extremes. In this scenario, the opposing attorneys fight a legal tug-of-war to drag the rope of justice closer to their side. Like a tug-of-war team, they try to get a heavy guy, who may not be much of an athlete or move well, but just by leaning can drag the rope their way. The heavy guy has to be an expert they can count on, who will give an extreme opinion in favor of their side. Often the attorney knows that the judge or jury won't totally buy what this expert says—and often enough she doesn't believe it herself—but his net effect is to shift the balance of the judgment her way.

When I was first asked to be an expert, I had been in practice for less than a month and there was little basis to view me as one, but I actually started to believe I was an expert. Little did I know that the insurance company was merely feeling me out. They were not interested in my great medical knowledge; they wanted to find out what side of the medical-legal fence I was on and how easy it might be to manipulate me onto their side. When I insisted on trying to help the patient, I ceased overnight to be an "expert." The resulting loss of faith in medicine, business, and the legal system was devastating, and I swore that from that day on I would never be manipulated in court again and would never do another IME.

This lesson in reality fueled a growing cynicism about the practice of medicine. I found it ironic that I had spent much of my life hoping to use my skills and knowledge to help patients in need. Then, during one trial, an attorney struggling to refute my testimony gasped in desperation, "Everyone knows Dr. Nagel is a patient's doctor!" He meant that I stood up for my patients. Although his tone of voice made it sound like an insult, I felt pride in knowing that I was being seen in the way I wanted to be.

As I have noted, few experts who testify in chronic pain cases actually have much expertise in this field. For example, few surgeons have any expertise in chronic pain management. It is not taught in medical school, surgical residencies, or at surgical meetings. Yet just because surgeons are generally seen as occupying the upper echelon of medicine, they often are assumed to be experts on pain, and their word carries great weight in court. I vividly remember a local "expert," an orthopedist with "thirty-five years of experience," who was widely sought as an expert witness by insurance companies. Having reviewed many of his reports, both medical and legal, I concluded that he had no expertise in pain. His legal reports typically were one page long, all said basically the same thing, too often included the words "in my thirty-five years of practice," and interestingly, always supported the insurance company's position. One day I challenged one of my patient's attorneys to find out how much this gentleman was paid per year to serve as an expert. The answer was $350,000. He was retired, yet making as much money as any actively practicing orthopedist in town, and all he had to do was say what the insurance company wanted him to say. He was clearly and *deliberately* harming pain patients to serve his own purposes. It would be inappropriate for me to say what his motivations may have been, but he was clearly being rewarded well.

Experts often judge without ever seeing the patient. They rely on only a review of the chart to develop sometimes sweeping opinions. One reason for this is to prevent the expert who evaluates a case from developing a relationship with the patient, so that she can remain objective. The expert relies on the completeness of the chart and her knowledge of what is considered standard medical care to make a decision about the appropriateness of care. However, the information in the chart has been filtered through the eyes and mind of the treating physician and, too often, the insurance company, which may have labeled the patient a "drug addict" or "hypochondriac." The chart lacks color and details and does not depict reality. Details can be added only by talking to and examining the patient. This is especially true with complex cases; I may see the patient in a totally different manner than the treating physician. This is why physicians seek consultations. When we are stumped, we hope that another person can look at a problem differently and find a better solution. I believe it should be mandatory that the expert actually examine the patient. If the patient wishes to audio- or videotape the interaction, that should be allowed. As I have said, 90 percent of any diagnosis comes from the patient's own telling of his or her history. Moreover, chronic problems present complex issues that are outliers and regress from the mean. Standard treatments are insufficient to resolve them and should not be used as the criteria for managing them.

Some insurance companies actually prohibit an expert from ever treating the patient. It is amazing how smart we become when we have no responsibility for providing treatment or observing its outcome. Yet the accuracy of our observations and recommendations must be compromised under these circumstances. A doctor only truly comes to understand a complex patient when he sees her multiple times. It may be true that the more a doctor meets with a patient, the less objective his view may be. But I contend that the less we know the patient, the more erroneous our conclusions may be. Because we lack sufficient data, we rely on preconceived notions, even if such notions do not apply to this particular person. Experts often assume the patient is malingering (fabricating symptoms to obtain some secondary gain). There is no question that this does happen, and certainly I have been duped by such individuals, since I always choose to believe in my patients until they prove unworthy of my trust. As we have seen, secondary loss and the associated problems it creates are a much bigger problem. However, those in the insurance industry exaggerate the role that malingering plays and use it as a means to deny patients care. If the expert never meets the patient, or sees her only in a one-visit, adversarial role, it is much easier to do this.

When I did IMEs, I would review the chart only after I met with the patient. Similarly, I look at a diagnostic study only after I have examined the patient and created my own hypotheses. It is amazing how often I come to totally different conclusions from those suggested by the chart or the x-ray. In my opinion, a chart review is lazy and unethical, but physicians do them because they are quick and easy and allow us to avoid confronting our ignorance when we don't understand the patient's problems, as well as the fears evoked by being in the presence of a suffering human. And they pay so well!

Another disadvantage is that the expert assessment rarely includes follow-up, so the expert never finds out how her recommendations affected the patient. When I treat a challenging patient, especially if the treatment carries no small risk, I do fear the potential ramifications; and this fear is heightened when I take a nighttime call or see the patient at follow-up. The fear is eliminated when there is no follow-up. But expert opinions have ramifications for the assessed, and sometimes these can be devastating. The patient suffers from actions taken by the insurance company based on what may have been an unreliable observation. The expert loses because he never sees the results of his actions. If we never observe outcomes, we don't learn and are destined to keep screwing up.

I was recently sickened when I heard a taped lecturer in a pain review course admit that the main reason to serve as an expert is because it pays well. He left unspoken the reality that it only pays well if you say what your payer wants to hear, at least on a fairly regular basis. By its nature, this system eliminates those who are objective and honest. I regularly receive invitations to attend meetings that, for large sums of money, promise to help me become a better expert witness or a better independent medical evaluator. They promise that I will be more than amply rewarded for this investment. In this light it is ironic that experts love to accuse pain patients of obtaining "secondary gain." I believe that the patient more often suffers secondary loss, while the expert is the one who obtains the secondary gain.

In my opinion the expert's role is to be honest, which means that reform begins with fixing the system to promote honesty. I believe that eliminating the practice of using experts hired by each side, as in the panel system suggested in the section that follows, will do this. Such a system also will solve the problem that being an expert witness is currently so unpleasant that many ethical physicians have no interest in getting involved.

SOLUTIONS

The legal industry does not seem to care about the ramifications of this system that it is largely responsible for creating. In fact, it encourages the status quo. But perhaps the attorneys aren't totally to blame. I remember Doug Louellen's prophetic encouragement at the end of each *People's Court* episode: "Take 'em to court!" In a "me-first" world in which we are more likely to find someone to blame than to take responsibility for our own actions, and where we are unwilling to accept the misfortunes fate bestows upon us or to forgive others for their transgressions, perhaps the status quo is inevitable and the lawyers are merely going along for the ride.

In any case, our civil court system is a mess and has a tremendous adverse effect on the practice of pain management. So what can we do?

The solution starts with the individual. Please excuse my idealism, but the first step is for each of us to look into our own heart and put the Golden Rule into action by learning to put the needs of the whole ahead of our own needs. We must realize that our current system is destructive, and it is ourselves we are destroying. The legal system locks people into a desire for vengeance, promising both a financial reward and, more important, payback. But while we seek retribution, we postpone adaptation. And as I have explained, anger is a physiologically destructive emotion that increases pain, creates depression, and intensifies the functional effects of a painful disability.

Systemic change must begin with compassionate acknowledgment of the patient's pain. We know you hurt. We know what you can't do. We need to decide what you can do, and how we can get you to that point. All involved must stress rehabilitation. The patient must be involved and have control. She has rights, but must be made aware that she also has responsibilities.

The next step is to completely rethink the process by which judgment is rendered. While judgment always will be required, there are better ways to deliver it. I would start by taking the process out of the courtroom. Judges and juries do not have the expertise to deal with medical issues and are too easily swayed by emotions to be truly objective, so I would replace them with a panel of unbiased members of the community who are knowledgeable about pain. For points of law, they would have a legal advisor, but that individual would not be directly involved in decision making. Ideally, these panelists would be health-care professionals (who preferably are actively treating patients), at least one of whom has expertise in the area of pain. Each member should have a minimum of five years of experience beyond his or her training. Panelists for each case would be selected at random from a pool.

Everyone who treats personal injury or workers' compensation patients should be required to be part of this system. They would be reimbursed for their time at a reasonable rate from a fund financed from four sources: 1) tax dollars currently being used to fund the civil court system, 2) fees paid by personal injury/workers' compensation attorneys, 3) fees paid by insurance companies, and 4) fines levied against companies with excessive injury rates relative to risk. The fees paid by insurance companies and attorneys would be a redistribution of the funds these companies are already paying their own biased experts, sometimes at extremely high rates. The fines levied against businesses would encourage them to provide safer work environments. The goal is to create an unbiased panel, serving neither with undue hardship nor for excessive pay, whose primary concern is the best interest of the injured.

Experts should be encouraged to explain to the panel what we know and what we don't know. Their key role is to educate the judicial system so an appropriate judgment can be reached. Sometimes decisions must be made based on imperfect knowledge. Failure to acknowledge what we don't know while insisting that we know more than we do harms the patient. It should be recognized that there are differences of opinion between experts, and more than one expert should assess each legal presentation. Expert selection could be conducted like jury selection, with each side having some ability to eliminate experts who may have a bias against them.

The panel should meet in a comfortable setting (not a courtroom) to minimize stress to the patient. The patient can be represented by a lawyer. After the history of the injury and its treatment is presented, the panel renders a decision regarding past, current, and future care based on the reasonableness of that treatment and creates therapeutic and rehabilitative goals. The idea is to avoid dwelling on blame and vengeance and to encourage the patient to return to a productive life. Monetary awards should be reasonable and contingent on the patient's participation in rehabilitation.

Attorneys would still play an important role. However, their incentives must change. Currently, attorneys are considered successful when they win, no matter whom they represent. Although there is no way to measure honesty, it seems to me that honesty is a better measure of a good attorney. I would strongly question the honesty of an attorney who wins all the time. Perhaps the "Nagel 80 percent rule" applies here as well. In any case, the definition of what it means to "win" must change. If two attorneys can work together with all the health-care professionals to get a patient to a higher level of function, then both sides win.

Attorneys should be paid, but not in a way that harms their client. Currently, the plaintiff's attorney's goal is to maximize her client's financial settlement; and if she wins, she is rewarded with a substantial percentage of the award. The incentive is to take on high-price cases. Attorneys know that the more cases they bring in, the more they will win and the more money they will make. The risk to them is relatively low, and the potential reward is relatively high.

I propose doing away with the contingency system since it creates a disincentive for attorneys to advise patients to do what they really need to do: forgive and move on. Instead, I suggest a fee-for-service setup that is honest and transparent. Attorneys would be encouraged to publish their rates and let the market set an equilibrium rate. Fees should be capped to discourage attorneys from milking the clock and overcharging, much as insurance companies cap what physicians charge their patients. There also should be a subsidy for attorneys who represent clients who return to a productive lifestyle in a timely manner. While this may appear unfair to those who lose their cases, it would substantially reduce the incentive to bring frivolous cases. In fact, the first decision each panel should make in a case, based on an initial legal brief, is whether the case has merit.

This system should be run at the state or local level, or both. I have little faith that the federal government could manage it efficiently with sensitivity to local variations.

The next step is tort reform, which is crucial both for the health-care system to function more cost-effectively and efficiently and to eliminate the disincentives for physicians to take on pain patients. While reform of our convoluted tort system is complicated, the following are some simple, yet encompassing suggestions to start the process:

> In the legal setting for personal injury and workers' compensation, the physician must be seen as an ally of both "sides," not an adversary whose opinion must be challenged and distorted to fit an attorney's needs.

> We must recognize that most malpractice claims do not have merit. A bad treatment outcome is not necessarily malpractice. Any malpractice claim should be shown to have merit before it can proceed.

> The whole nature of communication in the legal world must change. When two sides work together to achieve a common goal, communication is maximized. When two sides oppose each other, the incentive is to minimize or distort communication. Obviously, the former is more effective. The legal system needs to understand the limits of the medical system. Just because a physician cannot explain a particular phenomenon doesn't mean it doesn't exist. The limits of "objective tests" and "authoritative evidence" must be accepted and constantly questioned. Lawyers must become more comfortable with shades of gray, since in dealing with pain there is rarely a right or wrong but rather a continuum.

Many of these suggestions may be too much to ask of a "me-first" society in the short term, so the first step must be a baby step. Before we act, each of us should take a moment to ask ourselves whether our actions are for the good of the pain patient or our own good. We should only act when we are convinced that our actions are for the greater good. This is true of patients as well as providers. The system will not be changed much by single acts; however, it will be changed by a total of many acts.

Crime and Pain

> Killing a living being is killing one's own self; showing compassion to a living being is showing compassion to oneself. He who desires his own good should avoid causing harm to a living being.
> Saman Suttam, verse 151

> Those are rare who fall without becoming degraded; there is a point, moreover, at which the unfortunate and the infamous are associated and confounded in a single word, a fatal word, Les Misérables.
> Victor Hugo, Les Misérables

Sometimes a patient finds himself in the even less friendly world of the criminal court. Many pain sufferers are what I call "Jean Valjean" patients. Jean Valjean, as you may recall from Les Misérables, was a poor gentleman who was imprisoned merely for stealing a loaf of bread to feed his sister's starving family. Unable to tolerate his confinement, he attempted to escape over and over. With each attempt, more time was added to his sentence. He eventually served nineteen years for that one selfless act of desperation.

Many chronic pain patients become similarly desperate when their physicians fail to acknowledge or adequately treat their pain. If that physician won't provide relief, they seek another, and another, until someone helps. Sometimes this help never comes, and the patient looks for another source and finds it in drug dealers and "street doctors." Like the elderly woman described in chapter 10, many patients have told me they know they can get what they need from the street and will do so if the doctor won't help. Many use marijuana to ease their pain when other agents don't work, even though it is still illegal in much of the country. Similarly, many patients obtain their medical opioids illegally from various sources, such as a sympathetic friend willing to share a prescription for free or for a price, or the street.

This so-called "aberrant, drug-seeking behavior" is really what is known as pseudoaddiction. It is actually an expected and appropriate behavior in someone whose pain is not being effectively managed. However, it remains illegal, and if caught, the patient is imprisoned. The process of arrest and incarceration can do wonders for a sense of self-esteem that already has been challenged by the pain experience. To make matters worse, the patient faces an unsympathetic environment where her pain is further challenged by work details, poor mattresses, concrete floors, and a medical staff even less medically supportive than those outside the prison walls.

Are such people criminals or victims? Which is the greater crime, their illegal drug use or their providers' failure to believe them and treat them properly? It is up to us to look into our collective heart and answer that question.

ILLEGAL DRUG SALES

The most significant area where the criminal world intersects with the pain world is the illegal sale of addictive painkillers, usually to drug abusers but also to those suffering from poorly managed pain. Unfortunately, the public often views providing these agents for legitimate purposes as less important than curbing their illegal use, even though the legitimate demand for pain management dwarfs the illegal use. As a result, the health-care system is biased toward minimizing abuse rather than providing compassionate care for those in pain, creating a barrier to effective pain management.

A significant problem is created by drug dealers who boost their supply of prescription drugs by duping doctors. Unlike illegal drugs, dealers can obtain prescription drugs at almost no cost. One method is to fraudulently present themselves as someone in pain in order to obtain a prescription. Despite some claims to the contrary, there are no easy, tried-and-true ways for a physician to determine who is legitimately in pain, especially if the supplier, or his stooge, has a legitimate medical condition. Next, the dealer sells that prescription to a distributor or consumer. An unsuspecting insurance company pays the cost. Another method is forging prescriptions. Dealers also resort to the old-fashioned tactic of stealing the drug directly from patients or pharmacies. While physicians may be unaware of these actions, the regulatory agencies still hold them responsible for how a pre-scription is used, and they may actually deem the physician an accessory to such a crime.

A few years ago, the Federation of State Medical Boards (FSMB) created a sample law, adopted in some form by most states, that was intended to help protect physicians from such legal liability. Unfortunately, the law of unintended consequences came into play in this case. I was involved in creating the state rules for pain prescription in New Hampshire. I saw this process as a way to minimize barriers to compassionate care while also protecting both physician and patient. Reducing these barriers should have promoted more effective treatment of chronic pain. Unfortunately, the opposite happened. The rules actually created a time and paperwork nightmare for rank-and-file physicians, and if not followed to the letter, functioned as a noose to hang an unsuspecting prescriber. This outcome, combined with a dramatic increase in prescription abuse that accompanied the increased availability of pain medications, effectively stopped the pendulum swing toward compassionate care and even may have swung the pendulum back toward the restrictiveness that pervaded medicine when I first began practicing pain management. With such an increase in time commitment combined with such a risk, who in their right mind would prescribe in this setting?

To make matters worse, the regulatory agencies came down hard on popularly prescribed opioids. Companies that developed and produced these drugs were held liable for the ramifications of illicit use. Supplies diminished, costs rose, and availability for people in pain was reduced. The net result was a legitimate fear on the part of pharmacies and health-care providers regarding how a prescription would be used or abused and whether they would be labeled as dealers. They feared regulatory scrutiny and the mounds of paperwork necessary to effectively meet even the minimum requirements for what was considered safe and effective controlled-substance prescription. The impact on pain management was enormous.

TEENAGE THEFT

Teenage theft of a parent's medication is an enormous problem. More than one in ten high-school seniors have used a prescription opioid without a doctor's authorization. The leading motive for nonmedical opioid use is "to relax or relieve tension" (56.4 percent), followed by the desire "to feel good or get high" (53.5 percent), "to experiment to see what it's like" (52.4 percent), "to relieve physical pain" (44.8 percent), and "to have a good time with friends" (29.5 percent).[1] Researchers believe that for most teens abusing opioids (about 70 percent), the opioids were previously prescribed to them for a legitimate medical reason. The abused opioids often are either the teen's own leftover medication or pharmaceuticals obtained from a friend or family member.[2]

If a parent's pain prescription has been stolen, she has three options. She can go without. She can be honest, tell her doctor that the medicine has disappeared, and ask for another prescription. She can lie and say that she used extra medication because of a change in her pain and is now out of it. She can confront her child, if she suspects him or her. None of these options is very appealing. Going without means living with the pain from which she longs for relief. Asking the physician for another prescription creates shame and challenges the doctor-patient relationship, since the doctor now will view her with suspicion for having violated the medication agreement (see chapter 12). In all likelihood, that doctor will refuse to treat her further, and it will be hard to find another doctor willing to take her on. Confronting the teenager means accusing her child of a crime. Not only does this accusation leave the child open to arrest, but the child is not likely to admit stealing the drug anyway. The result is more stress that the patient does not need. Meanwhile, the teenager, often oblivious to the damage created, relishes the results. He is popular with his friends—a popularity that persists only as long as the supply of drugs holds out. It comes down to "mom" or "me." Which would a vulnerable child choose?

ADDICTION AND DESPERATION

In the case of some crimes, we have unwittingly set the stage for the deviant behavior, making it difficult to determine who actually should be punished. People commit crimes for a reason, and sometimes we need to look under the surface to see what motivates them in order to more effectively deal with their crimes. In the world of pain, addiction and acts of desperation are such "crimes."

Addiction is a disease of obsession, of compulsion, which can be situational or hereditary and needs to be understood and treated as such. There is a huge difference between possession with intent to use and possession with intent to sell. The latter is a criminal act in which an individual takes advantage of the obsession of another. The former is the act of an individual struggling to control an encoded self-destructive urge. Society's punishment may modify the dealer's behavior, but it paradoxically aggravates the user's by effectively communicating that he is what he fears: a burden to others.

Addiction is a chronic disease that the addict must acknowledge and, with the support and compassion of others, continually fight. Its destructive effects on the addict's loved ones need to be understood and managed in the same way that the needs of the family of any chronic illness sufferer must be managed. A certain percentage of our population is addiction prone. But many people are at only minimal risk for addiction and can responsibly use potentially addictive drugs such as alcohol (social drinking) as well as pain medications indefinitely. The risk of prescription addiction in this population is low, although not insignificant, and it is important to not characterize such people as "addicts" when they require pain medication for chronic pain.

Sometimes pain patients do sell their prescriptions—not to profit, but to survive. It is not unusual for a pain patient to lose everything: job, family, home, insurance. Sometimes faced with starvation, and knowing that their pain pills have a high street value, they sell to survive. Many patients of all ages, sexes, and social backgrounds have assured me that they would rather obtain their prescriptions legitimately.

SOLUTIONS

Crimes of greed and crimes of desperation both challenge our society. But they require quite different solutions. While crimes attributable to greed can be deterred through punishment, crimes of desperation must be treated with compassion. There are many strategies that may help prevent the misuse of opioids. Educating physicians on how to manage pain would be a great start. This training should include not just how to prescribe opioids for pain, but also how to identify those at risk for addiction and misuse of prescriptions and information about addiction itself. Continuing education programs have been developed to educate those already in practice. In some states, physicians must be certified before they can prescribe opioids. While this practice is beneficial in one way, it also acts as a barrier to effective pain care since many physicians are not willing to be so educated, either because of the time required or the regulation involved, and simply choose not to prescribe to those in need.

Prescription monitoring programs now exist in almost every state, providing a database that physicians and pharmacists can use to find out if patients are receiving medications from other sources. Such databases should minimize doctor shopping, the practice of obtaining medication from a variety of sources for self-use or for illegal sale to others. But because access to these databases does not cross state lines, doctor shopping can continue in border areas, especially where several states come together. A national database or cooperative interstate programs could close this loophole. It would also be helpful for health-care providers to have access to a panel of pain experts by Internet or phone when questions do arise.

Patient education is also critical. Patients must be instructed to keep medications in safe places such as lockboxes, not to tell their friends what medicines they are on, and never to share their medicines with others. I know of one situation where a man shared an 80 mg pill of Oxycontin with a friend. He was afraid the dose was too big, so he cut the pill in half, yet his friend died from an overdose. It is amazing how many patients do not realize that such drug sharing is illegal.

Patients also need to learn to clean out their medicine cabinets. One patient informed me that he had thirty-eight Oxycontin pills that he would never use because he was allergic to the drug. He had a teenager at home. Most communities now have prescription drug drop-off centers where people can get rid of all their unwanted medications. Prescription drugs are considered biohazards and should not be thrown out or flushed down the toilet.

Once I was concerned that a patient of mine was selling his prescription. I knew he had been reported to his local police. To help coordinate our efforts, I called the police officer involved. He told me he was shocked to hear from me, since physicians usually were reluctant to work with him. I told him that in my experience, police officers usually were reluctant to work with me. Over the next few weeks, we worked together to solve the problem and both learned from each other. Such learning should not only happen one on one, but also in shared symposia for law enforcement and health-care providers.

As we work toward greater control of the sources of controlled substances, we also must understand better the causes of desperate actions. We need to eliminate the motivation for such acts by better understanding the problems associated with chronic pain and addiction and treating those who suffer from such maladies with the same compassion and respect we would accord to other illnesses.

TWELVE

What It Means to "Do No Harm"

Is There a Safe Way to Medicate Pain?

The evil that is in the world almost always comes
of ignorance, and good intentions may do as much harm
as malevolence if they lack understanding.
Albert Camus, *The Plague*

I find it entertaining to hear people's thoughts about how best to medicate pain—an extremely complex subject on which passion often trumps fact, frequently to the detriment of those who suffer. I once served on a grand jury. In New Hampshire, that means being sequestered in a room for eight hours while prosecutors present a never-ending series of felony indictments for almost every crime imaginable. Our charge was not to decide guilt or innocence, but rather to determine whether the prosecutor had presented sufficient evidence to take the case to trial. It is an exhausting and educational experience, and often you are surprised to discover what your legislature has chosen to define as a felony. During my session, more than half the indictments were for drug-related offenses, many involving the possession or sale of oxycodone, a common pain medication. At some point during the proceedings, an exasperated juror cried out, "What are these doctors doing these days?"

During a break, I talked briefly with the drug task force officer who was presenting these cases. People weren't as tough as they used to be, he informed me; they needed to "learn to suck it up and deal with their pain." He also complained about "bad doctors." "We know who they are," he added ominously. I wanted to tell him that for over five thousand years, long before prescription drugs existed, people have used opium, alcohol, and cannabis to relieve pain, and that they still use these drugs today—too often without a prescription—merely because they cannot get someone to manage their pain. Only in his imagination have things changed. I also wanted to know what he meant by "bad doctors," but I was afraid the conversation would get too adversarial, so I backed off. We still had thirty indictments to go, and it was getting late.

The next day, I was back at the office where, as on most days, I heard never-ending complaints from patients upset because they could not get their doctors to treat their pain—meaning they could not get pain medicine, and no other measure had worked.

To that policeman, pain patients were all addicts and the physicians who supposedly fed their habits were bad doctors. That is what he chose to perceive because his job is to prevent illegal drug use, not encourage its legal use. His perception was also fed by the fact that 70 percent of all illegal opioid use starts with a legitimate prescription. Contrast him with the pain patient, who sees these drugs as a treatment for his pain and the doctor as bad when she puts excessive barriers in the way of getting them. So the doctor who prescribes is seen as bad by the police officer and the doctor who does not is seen as bad by the pain patient. It is no wonder doctors don't want to prescribe pain medicine.

During the grand jury session, that same exasperated juror referred to pain doctors as "pill pushers"—a comment I resent, since as I have explained, although medication is just one component of pain management, it does play a significant role. Quite a few people—who are not in pain—feel like that juror. A recent Research America study showed that 47 percent of Americans view drug addiction as a major health problem in the United States, while only 18 percent view chronic pain that way.[1] As we shall see, chronic pain is a much greater public health problem.

Perhaps it is natural that those who suffer from pain long for a pill that will heal *all* their pain. I am reminded of Huey Lewis's song "I Want a New Drug," in which he imagines a drug that will make him feel like he does when he's with his girlfriend. The pain patient wants a drug that will make her feel like she did before she had the pain. That drug does not exist, and never will, but we do have medications that can help minimize pain. In the next two chapters, I present a rational approach to the use of controlled substances: opiates (opium derivatives that occur in nature), opioids (synthetic opiates), and cannabinoids (the active ingredients in marijuana).

These drugs all have been used since the dawn of civilization to treat various ailments, including pain. For most of their history, they consisted of crude preparations from the raw plants from which they are derived.

Pharmaceutical preparations of opiates have been manufactured for 140 years and of THC, a cannabinoid, for twenty years. In the past fifty years, we have discovered that the human body makes its own opiates and cannabinoids for very specific purposes, and that exogenous (originating outside the body) preparations work on these endogenous (originating within the body) systems to achieve a pharmacological effect.

Opiates, opioids, and cannabinoids share a similar legal history. For most of human history, they were largely unregulated. Not until the late 1800s, out of concern for public health, did governments begin to intervene in the drug trade. The use of opiates and opioids (which, for simplicity, I will refer to collectively as opioids) for medical purposes has remained legal, though highly regulated, but by 1950 federal law had made cannabinoids illegal for all purposes, medical and recreational, in the United States. There are many reasons why these classes of drugs are treated differently.

While there are dozens of opioids, for the most part they have a similar function in the human body. This makes research and development of opioid products relatively simple. Each pharmacological preparation consists of only a single opioid. By contrast, there are dozens of cannabinoids present in an individual marijuana cigarette, each with different effects on the body. The net effect is the sum of all the individual effects and can be hard to predict. This makes research and development of a pharmaceutical product very difficult and opens to question the reliability and safety of a smoked plant extract for medicinal purposes. Even so, the legal status of cannabinoids is changing, and chapter 14 describes state and federal policy and discusses the implications. It also discusses my conviction that cannabinoid preparation(s) can have a significant role in pain management and lays out a rational approach to achieving this end.

Before looking at opioids and medical cannabinoids, it is important to explore the medical concept of *do no harm*, first attributed to Hippocrates (*Epidemics*, book 1), and is one of the basic principles of the practice of medicine. This phrase alone does not convey the complexity of the concept. Since virtually every medical intervention, even the simplest, has the potential to cause harm, it is important to understand what this oath actually means. For example, one of my favorite medical procedures is cleaning out someone's ears. It is one of the few "walk on water" things I do in medicine. In just seconds, I can restore hearing to the deaf, and it feels wonderful. However, it usually hurts to get impacted wax out, and occasionally the procedure results in a perforated eardrum. Usually that heals, but there can be permanent damage. Does this mean that it would be better not to do this procedure—that to avoid doing harm, we should do nothing? Unfortunately, that too can cause harm. If someone has a blocked coronary artery, there are potential complications associated with unblocking it, but not doing so will result in earlier death or greater disability.

In reality, then, "do no harm" is a relative concept. In every medical decision a doctor must look at all the risks and benefits of doing something versus doing nothing, and then explain the various options and their associated risks to the patient; this is what we call "informed consent." The final decision is based on the *likelihood* that the net benefits will exceed the net risks, though there is always the possibility that things won't turn out so well. What is more, an intervention that is net beneficial for one patient may not be for another. This is why all medical decisions must be individualized.

With these ideas in mind, it becomes clear that the decision to prescribe controlled substances to pain patients is not simple. Every patient is different and every pain is different. The doctor, patient, and family must decide together when to use these substances. They must understand that palliation is the goal, not cure. A 30 percent reduction in chronic pain is a reasonable expectation for an opioid prescription. Anything better is a bonus. And the medication must be just one of several interventions, such as exercise, functional activity, vocational rehabilitation, stress/pain management techniques, and noncontrolled medications. A maximal functional outcome requires all of these interventions, and the patient must be compliant with all.

Opioid Use, Abuse, and Misuse and the Physician's Responsibility

Like any other intervention, opioids and cannabinoids have side effects. What makes them different, however, are the risks that patients may become addicted and that some will misuse or divert these medications. That brings us to the next question: who are we actually treating? The addictive nature of these pharmaceuticals has implications not just for the patient, but also for those who seek these drugs for illegal use, creating a potential, though unintended, burden on society as a whole. So when a doctor writes a prescription for a controlled substance, the question arises of to whom she is most responsible, the pain patient or society. Such a prescription has a potential ripple effect in which many others may be harmed, even if the patient is helped. The decision to prescribe must therefore include an assessment of all these factors. Given that the DEA has placed doctors on the front lines in the "war on drugs," for good or ill, the doctor has a *legal* responsibility far beyond that which obtains in any other medical decision. It is not uncommon for the needs of the patient sitting in front of the doctor to conflict with those of the world outside the exam room. The doctor must then use the dictum of relative harm in making a clinical decision. My own standard always has been that the needs of my patient take precedence. Others feel differently. As we have seen, my decision to put the patient first has sometimes had unpleasant consequences, for example, medical board investigations. Others have faced criminal prosecution; I know of well-intentioned doctors whose licenses were taken away.

As a consequence, there is a tension between the needs of the patient and those of society. Optimally regulators, patients, and physicians would work together to maximize the ability to address the needs of each party. I think we are better at this now than in the past, but the situation is far from ideal. As I have explained, the aggressiveness of the regulatory system shapes physician behavior. When I started out in the 1980s, regulatory agencies aggressively prosecuted those who prescribed opioids for chronic pain, and physicians were afraid to prescribe. Several heroic doctors questioned both regulatory agency and physician practice; and by sheer will and willingness to take risks, they swung the pendulum toward more aggressive use of pain medications. The resulting increase in prescription abuse, misuse, diversion, and prescription-related drug deaths led the agencies to tighten control again, and the pendulum began to swing in the opposite direction, with devastating effects on many patients and some doctors. Some of these regulatory actions were appropriate, some not. At this writing it appears that physicians and regulatory agencies often are working together to reach a more suitable balance. However, this has not made the pain physician's job any easier to date, and access to medication for the pain patient still can be challenging.

It is important to understand what addiction is and what it is not. This term is often used interchangeably with others: tolerance, dependency, and pseudoaddiction. Although these concepts are not mutually exclusive, neither are they the same.

Tolerance occurs when more medication is needed to achieve the same effect.

Dependency occurs when abstinence from the drug results in a withdrawal state. Sudden withdrawal of opiates results in a symptom complex of anxiety, increased heart rate, and sweating that can last for days to weeks and, for patients with sufficient cardiac risk factors, can be fatal. Sudden withdrawal of cannabinoids does not create such a profound withdrawal state. Nor is dependency unique to controlled substances such as opiates. Many other drugs, such as antidepressants and some blood pressure medications, have predictable withdrawal effects.

Addiction occurs when someone compulsively engages in a behavior despite negative consequences to herself or those around her; in this case, compulsive use of pain medication.

Pseudoaddiction occurs when a person seeks to obtain a substance illegally or inappropriately to treat a legitimate problem that is not being properly managed by health-care professionals.

These different entities have very different ramifications for doctor and patient. Here I focus on addiction and pseudoaddiction.

It is the ramifications of addiction that affect society as a whole and bring these drugs under scrutiny. Addiction is a complex entity. Physiologically it begins with the release of dopamine from the pleasure center in the brain stem, causing a sensation of reward or pleasure resulting from some action. The pleasure center serves the important role of providing positive feedback when we do something good. If we work hard and accomplish a goal, such as achieving a good grade on a test, our pleasure center is stimulated, not by the hard work but rather by seeing the good grade. This mechanism enables us to endure hardship to accomplish something worthwhile. Having experienced the pleasure, we seek to replicate it, and seeking the reward becomes a learned behavior. In other words, achieving one goal leads us to pursue others, which makes the pleasure system a valuable mechanism of positive feedback.

We have another internal system that punishes us for harmful behavior. For example, when we touch a hot stove, we get a sensation of pain that teaches us not to touch the hot stove again. When we overindulge with alcohol, we get a hangover. In theory, that educates us not to drink to excess again.

On the surface, these mechanisms seem like simple cause and effect with predictable outcomes. Unfortunately, they are not so simple. For some individuals, the systems conflict, and pleasure may actually cause pain. For example, I am addicted to computer solitaire. I will play for hours merely to be rewarded every so often by the screen announcing that I have won. *Yippee!* I then seek to replicate that behavior. Unfortunately, I am frequently oblivious to the fact that while I play, I am ignoring my work, my family, my health, and so on. When my obsessive search for reward causes harm to myself or those around me, I am in a state of addiction. When addicted, we see only the pleasure, not the pain. In fact, we are willing to tolerate a lot of harm just to feel that pleasure. Over time, though, we find it takes more and more of the addictive behavior to stimulate our pleasure center, inevitably causing more and more collateral damage.

For twenty years, I was a triathlete. In the early years, I felt rewarded by completing short races. My reward was not just a medal, but also the accolades of those who did not compete. Over time, though, finishing short races became less rewarding. I was bored, and I wanted to be admired by other triathletes. I knew I could not win a race, but I could do longer ones. I trained harder and harder and eventually finished three Ironman races. Soon I was getting praise from nontriathletes and triathletes alike. The weirdest thing was I didn't feel good about it. I kept thinking that if I just did one more thing, perhaps a double Ironman, or climbed Mount Everest, or whatever, then I would feel good. Meanwhile, I was oblivious to the adverse effects of my behavior on my family, my job, and my body. I have come to understand that competitive athletes are, in fact, addicts. They are addicted to winning and the public adulation that comes with it, and they will do whatever they need to do to win.

The take-home message is that we can become addicted to virtually anything. Physiologically, all addictive behaviors share an overstimulation of the pleasure system. Although much attention is focused on the negative effects of drug and alcohol addiction, I would argue that from a public health standpoint, the most devastating addictions are to sugar and money. Other behaviors that can be addictive include gambling, thrill seeking, television, sex, spectator sports, participatory sports, and exercise.

Pharmacological agents cheat by stimulating the pleasure center directly, thus giving the user the perception of a rewarding feeling. In addition to opioids, tobacco, alcohol, caffeine, and nonprescription drugs (marijuana, heroin, amphetamines, etc.) are also such agents. Many of these also adversely affect the body in multiple other ways. Cigarette smoke causes cancer, cardiovascular disease, and lung disease; alcohol can harm virtually every organ in our body. Believe it or not, sugar also directly stimulates this system and probably should be thought of as an addictive drug.

To complicate matters more, the risk of addiction is relative. For example, a mouse is trained to run on a wheel by rewarding this behavior with a food pellet. With very little reward, some strains of mice will run forever, while other strains will never run no matter how great the reward. We humans are like mice in this respect. The risk of addiction varies significantly from person to person, and that risk is dependent on a number of factors. Hereditary factors are thought to explain 40 to 60 percent of the risk. Individuals with mental disorders are at higher risk. Situational addiction is also important. For example, individuals who grow up in an environment where addiction is common are more likely to develop addictive behavior that can be explained beyond heredity. Peer pressure is a major factor in schools. The more risk factors a person has, the more likely addiction will develop.[2]

In the case of situational addiction, once the situation is gone, the addictive behavior often goes away. For example, heroin addiction was a common problem among soldiers serving in Vietnam. Yet many soldiers spontaneously ceased use once they returned to a more normal environment. The same is true for addictive behaviors in college. When I was in college, the abuse of marijuana, alcohol, tobacco, and cocaine was ubiquitous. At reunions it has been entertaining to see that none of my former classmates imbibe anymore. Instead, they worry about their children engaging in the same behaviors. Addictive behavior peaks in late adolescence and early adulthood for reasons that are not clear but are probably related to the uniqueness of brain function in the eighteen- to twenty-three-year-old age group, the period of thrill seeking. Adolescents are rewarded for challenging their limits, often by their peer group, but also by their adult role models. Think of the X Games. Participants engage in very dangerous activity with the support of their parents. Personally, I would rather see my kid smoke dope than take part in those events.

Certainly some pain patients become addicted to their medications. But the question is: Are they addicted to the medication itself or to relief of their pain? Answering this question for each patient is important in managing pain, since addiction to pain relief is a positive outcome if the patient demonstrates improved function. Addiction to the medication itself is considered a bad outcome. I would argue that the former outcome is much more common; and in that scenario, what typically happens is that once the pain goes away, if the patient is so lucky, the need for medication does as well.

In pseudoaddiction, or false addiction, the individual appears to be engaging in behaviors with potentially harmful effects, such as illegally obtaining pain medication. However, he is not feeding an addiction but simply trying to control his pain when those who are caring for him are not helping. This is not aberrant behavior. It is logical. Pseudoaddiction to both opiates and cannabinoids is common.

Thus we face two competing aims: preventing addiction and controlling pain. It is often assumed that the former is a bigger issue. More specifically, we assume that the consequences of drug abuse are worse in terms of lost productivity, medical consequences, and death. In fact, that is not true. As I noted in chapter 10, chronic pain affects about one hundred million American adults, more than the total affected by heart disease, cancer, and diabetes combined, and costs the nation $635 billion each year in medical treatment and lost productivity.[3] This number does not include the effects on the individual sufferer, such as loss of vocation, loss of avocational role, depression, and sexual impairment.

Chronic pain also kills. Government data show that there was a rise in drug-related suicides between 2005 and 2009. The assumption was that these incidents were merely due to substance abuse; the government researchers made no attempt to determine how many people attempting suicide in this manner were suffering from chronic, unresolved pain.[4] However, risk factors for suicide in the pain population are high. A 2004 study found that 19 percent of pain patients studied had passive ideas about suicide, 13 percent had active thoughts, 5 percent had a plan, and 5 percent had made a previous attempt. Seventy-five percent identified drug overdose as their preferred method for suicide.[5] A systematic review of the literature found that the risk of successful suicide is doubled in chronic pain patients compared to nonpain controls.[6] In 2003 the American Psychiatric Association recognized chronic pain as an independent risk factor for suicide.[7] When one superimposes this data on the Institute of Medicine figure of one hundred million, it becomes clear that the potential risks and ramifications are huge.

By comparison, a 2012 National Institute on Drug Abuse report stated that only 4.2 million Americans met the clinical criteria for dependence on or abuse of marijuana, and 1.8 million met these criteria for prescription pain relievers.[8] The evaluators of this data made no attempt to determine how many individuals who met their criteria for abuse or dependency suffered from chronic pain. Still, it is clear that there is an almost sixty-four-fold greater incidence of chronic pain in America than of prescription drug abuse, at a substantially greater cost in both economic and human terms. This fact raises the question: Why do we invest so much money and regulatory scrutiny in preventing the abuse of opioids at the expense of treating a much greater problem—chronic pain? I believe it is because the adverse effects of drug abuse are much more visible than the adverse effects of uncontrolled chronic pain, which are frequently hidden behind other issues such as suicide, drug abuse, and depression. Death generates headlines, pain doesn't. Also, until we become the one who suffers, we see pain as something that should be endured and assume that those who can't endure it have some character flaw.

This situation creates serious implications for public policy. In 2012 New York State passed a law named I-STOP, which among other things required physicians to check a prescription-monitoring database before writing *every* controlled drug prescription. The impetus for the law was a rapid rise in prescription drug–related deaths. At the time of its passage, one of the more sympathy-provoking incidents was the death of a young man "with his whole life ahead of him" from an oxycodone overdose.[9]

Needless to say, we must do our best to control the increase in prescription drug abuse and deaths. However, this bill will seriously impair physicians' ability to manage pain efficiently, and both pharmacists and medical societies in the state are fighting it, thus far without success. I-STOP is a visceral solution, feel-good legislation based less on a well-thought-out idea than on emotion, with substantial unintended consequences for those who suffer from pain. In sheer numbers, it will create more problems than it will solve. Unfortunately, this is frequently the result of our public policies.

A similar problem was created in 2014 by the DEA's reclassification of hydrocodone combination products (such as Vicodin), the most frequently prescribed opioids and the most abused, from schedule III, which allowed a prescription or refill to be called in to a pharmacy, to schedule II, which did not. The DEA reasoned that calling it in made it too convenient to prescribe this strong opiate. However, this change created a pain management nightmare. For example, some of my patients live more than a hundred miles away. Many have jobs they cannot leave easily. In the past, if someone had an exacerbation of pain, I could talk to him and get an idea of what was going on. If he needed pain medication, I had at least one option I could call in for him. The period from his call to the moment he received the prescription from his local pharmacy could be as little as one hour, and time in pain management is critical.

Now that same patient may have to leave work, drive two hundred miles round-trip to my office, pay for an office visit, and then bring a paper prescription to his pharmacy. If I don't have time to see him, he may need to wait a few days or go to the emergency room, which is expensive and time consuming. If the patient shows up too often, he will get labeled as a drug seeker. Such delays are the worst thing you can do to someone in pain. Thus, the unintended consequence of the DEA's action is needless harm to people who need pain relief.

Controlled substances will always be a part of pain management. But we must realize that we are treating both patient and society and learn to use these drugs as efficiently as possible, minimizing harm for both parties. While opioids and cannabinoids both have a role in pain management, they also have very different implications for medical care and public policy. The next two chapters, which examine these two categories separately, speak not only to doctors. Everyone, whether patient, family member, doctor, attorney, businessman, or public policy official, needs to understand how to use these drugs and why. As I discovered during my grand jury experience, the level of ignorance in people with strong opinions about these issues is frightening, since it is so often reflected in public policy. Another time, during an informal discussion with local health-care officials about medical marijuana, I found that almost everyone had a strong opinion. As the discussion unfolded, and I shared what I had learned during my research for chapter 14, they realized how little they knew. I myself knew next to nothing about marijuana before writing that chapter. Before I went into pain management, I knew next to nothing about opioids and pain. If we are to make sound public policy and medical decisions, we need to know the facts and to understand each other's perspectives. Ultimately, to make sound policy, we all need to be on the same page.

THIRTEEN

Opiates and Opioids

If we know that severe pain and suffering can be alleviated and we do
nothing about it, then we ourselves become the tormentors.
Attributed to Primo Levi, Auschwitz survivor

Opioids have been the mainstay of pain management for over four
thousand years. This group includes all drugs related to opium, hence its
name. As science and pharmacology have exploded over the past hundred
years, the number of these agents has dramatically increased, as have the
ways they can be used. They include:

buprenorphine (Suboxone, Buprenex)

butorphanol (Stadol)

codeine

fentanyl (Duragesic)

hydrocodone (Vicodin, Lortab, Norco)

hydromorphone (Dilaudid)

meperidine (Demerol)

methadone

morphine (MS Contin)

propoxyphene (Darvon, Darvocet)

oxycodone (Percocet, Tylox, Endocet, Oxycontin)

oxymorphone

pentazocine (Talwin)

These drugs simulate endogenous opiates (opiumlike substances within
the body), including endorphins, enkephalins, and dynorphins, which play
a very important role in the body's pain-control system. Exogenous opioids
artificially stimulate this system. They vary in potency, in duration of action,

and in how they can be administered: orally, transdermally (through the skin, using a topical patch), intravenously, intramuscularly, intranasally, or sublingually (under the tongue). Here I am interested only in the topical and oral routes, since the other routes are not appropriate for chronic pain management. Nor will I discuss intraspinal routes (within the spinal column) since these are used only occasionally, as a last resort.

The most important risks of taking opioids are tolerance, dependency, and addiction. The previous chapter discussed addiction and dependency. Tolerance occurs because artificially stimulating the pain-control system challenges its set point. That is, the body seeks to maintain a stable state, or *homeostasis*. When any system is overstimulated, it will seek to "down regulate" itself, or become less sensitive to stimulation, whether endogenous or exogenous (produced by medication). When a pain system down regulates, the body's inherent defense against pain will be weakened and will require more external support. That is why you have to take more of a drug to get the same effect. Eventually, even external stimulation will be insufficient, and the paradoxical effect of *opioid-induced hyperesthesia* (OIH) occurs: that is, the more opioid you take, the worse the pain gets. Tolerance and OIH are mediated a bit differently physiologically, but the net effect is somewhat similar.

It is critical to understand that we all vary in our susceptibility to each of these risks. Some can take all the pain medication they want and never risk tolerance, addiction, dependency, or hyperesthesia. Others can become dependent with very minimal exposure. Heredity predicts these risks. I also have observed that those in pain have fewer side effects (especially euphoria) than those who take these drugs recreationally. Why this appears to be the case is not clear, but the clinical ramifications are huge. In other words, if you don't need pain medicine, you are less likely to be able to handle it than if you are in pain and do need it. I point this out because often I hear people say, "If I took that much medication, I would be on the floor!" The reality is that if that person had pain, he or she might handle the dose just fine. And that statement makes a negative, harmful, and inaccurate value judgment about the pain patient.

It is nearly impossible to discuss pain management without discussing opioid drugs. Even when I give a focused talk on some other pain topic, the issue of drugs still comes up, and it is amazing what an emotional tone the discussion takes on, whether pro or con. Everyone has a story. Everyone has strong feelings based on their own experiences that they need to share. And so it is often feelings that drive public medical policy, rather than objective discussion.

A family member suffers from unremitting pain: opioids are good.

A teenager dies of an Oxycontin overdose: opioids are bad.

In fact, these drugs can be good or bad depending on the circumstances. This chapter explores four questions about opioid use for chronic pain:

Should we prescribe opioids?

To whom should we prescribe them?

Which drugs should we use?

What should the prescribing process be?

Through these questions, the chapter looks at these agents from a broader cultural perspective. Please do your best to put your preconceived notions aside, and remember that I speak here only of chronic pain, not acute pain.[1]

Should We Prescribe?

I would answer yes, no, or maybe. It depends on the situation and the person. The decision should never be easy, and it should always be well thought out. Each individual has a right to compassionate care tailored to his or her unique needs, and opioids may be an appropriate part of the treatment regimen. It is also important to note that these needs are constantly changing. At times a prescription may be appropriate, at other times not. Therefore, both the prescriber and the prescribed should be vigilant. Many patients have told me they are ready to come off drugs and deal with their pain without pharmacologic support. That is not easy to do, and it should be applauded. At the same time, reliance on medicine is not an act of cowardice. For many patients, the medications are a security blanket insulating them from the fear of their pain, and they may shed it *when they are ready*. Meanwhile, the medications are therapeutic. For some, the pain is so severe, subjectively and objectively, that most people, physicians and nonphysicians alike, would not question the need to prescribe opioids.

To Whom Should We Prescribe?

This is often a difficult question, but several rules can help answer it.

Opioids are generally used for moderate to severe pain. This means the patient rates his or her pain on a scale of 0 (meaning no pain) to 10 (the worst pain imaginable) as a 5 or higher. In grading the pain scale, the health-care provider must take the patient's report at face value. If she says she hurts, she does. This rating has little reliability (that is, it does not produce consistent results) when one compares one patient to another, but it has great reliability in comparing a patient's status at one point in time to another. It would be helpful to have a diagnostic test that objectively measures a cause for the pain. However, for many pains objective verification is not possible, and many tests are nowhere near as accurate as we would like. One should only interpret such tests in the context of the patient's history.

Ideally, the patient should have tried and failed nonopioid interventions first. This includes both medication and nonmedication therapies. However, for severe pain, opiates may be used as a first-line treatment. The decision to initiate opiate therapy may mean that the patient could be on these drugs for the rest of his life, so it should never be taken lightly.

Assess the risk of addiction. There are various instruments to help do this. However, as a rule of thumb, if someone is addicted to one thing, he is at risk for addictions to other things. The more things he is addicted to, the higher the risk. Questions to be assessed include history of smoking, gambling, alcohol use, other drug use, and sexual behaviors. A family history of addiction is predictive. However, a history of addiction does not rule out prescribing opiates. Addicts have pain. In fact, addicts may be more likely to develop chronic pain. One can treat them, but one must do so cautiously. They may be quite tolerant and need higher doses than nonaddicted patients.

Assess how the person has tolerated opioids in the past. If there were problems in the past, there will be in the future.

Assess whether the pain is structural or neuropathic. The former basically means injury to any part of the body other than a nerve; the latter means injury to a nerve. These types of pain respond very differently to opioids and nonopioid (adjunctive) medications. Pain from nerve injury is thought to be less responsive to opioids. This does not mean nerve pain will not respond to opiates. Instead, this patient may require higher doses.

The patient must agree with the decision to prescribe the opioid. This may sound silly, but one barrier to successful pain management is patients' fear of these drugs. They fear the side effects. They fear becoming addicted. They fear what others will think of them. For example, methadone has great potential for treating pain. However, usually when I raise this drug as an option, my patients shudder and say, "Isn't that just for addicts?" They don't want to be viewed in that light.

These are the general rules that I use in deciding for whom these medications are appropriate. In making my decision, I start all interactions with trust. I believe that is therapeutic. I am vigilant, but I leave it up to the patient to prove my trust in him wrong. Most of the time, the patient proves me right. I don't think you should ever punish the masses for the actions of a few. I know others believe otherwise, and that is unfortunately often the attitude behind public policies. However, starting with suspicion strains the doctor-patient relationship. Still, I take pains to impress upon the patient how serious these medications are, and that the *right* to a prescription includes the *responsibility* to take it properly.

Which Drugs Should We Use?

If the decision is to prescribe, the physician must decide which medication options are best for the patient, based on the following considerations:

The potencies of different drugs in relation to the severity of the patient's pain and his or her previous exposure to opioids.

Whether short-acting or long-acting drugs will best provide a steady level of the drug in the patient's system, helping to keep pain levels stable and to minimize the development of tolerance and the "downs" that can occur when drug levels are low.

An appropriate dosing schedule. This may mean taking the drug after a set number of hours or on an as-needed basis. For years the dictum has been to use around-the-clock dosing, meaning the drug is prescribed on a scheduled basis, perhaps every four hours, rather than on a pain-contingent basis. There are many reasons for this, but two are most important. First, it seems that pain can be controlled better with a steady level of drug in the system. Second, it takes a half hour or more for an oral pain medicine dose to start working. If the patient waits for the pain to escalate to a certain level before taking the dose, it may escalate much higher before the dose becomes effective. Pain creates stress. Stress aggravates pain. This is called a stress-pain cycle, and the idea is that scheduled dosing can minimize its potential adverse effects. While scheduled dosing is appropriate for many patients, I have observed that others can tolerate their pain most of the time. However, at times they need a periodic vacation from it. They may take a pain pill once or twice a day, or less, and this gives them a reasonable quality of life.

Many patients hope not to decrease their pain, but to eliminate it—a goal that is not realistic, as we have seen. They keep taking more and more medications with progressively less effect. Eventually, they are on huge doses and not doing well. Together, we come to the realization that this is not working. Numerous studies have suggested that such people are better off without opioids, and for many, this is true. Detoxing is difficult; the pain may increase, and their sense of well-being worsens for months after they go off the medication. Eventually, with great patience, they do feel better. Many can later return to a lower dose taken as needed for the vacation effect and do quite well, but only when they accept the permanence of their pain and the futility of trying to eliminate it. Another option when tolerance develops is to switch to an equivalent dose of another medication. This is called *opioid rotation* and can be quite successful.

Use of adjunctive medications to supplement the opioid (known as *balanced analgesia)* can create greater pain relief and theoretically makes it possible to use lower doses of each drug and minimize the side effects (this is called *opioid sparing*). However, this approach must be used carefully, since each drug has different side effects, which can lead to an accumulation of side effects. The result can become gruesomely humorous. I recall a discussion of the combined use of adjuncts and opioids. The presenter described the side effects of each medication, and then named one or two medications that could treat each side effect—each with its own side effect. Soon, the theoretical patient was on dozens of medications and experiencing so many side effects that it was impossible to tell which drugs were causing which side effects. The more medications we add, the more challenging pain management becomes. Still, balanced analgesia can be very effective.

The Prescribing Process

This process is very complicated, and it needs to be. We need to treat pain compassionately, but the ramifications of addiction are too great to be taken lightly. Thus, I want to describe what goals we set, how we monitor outcomes, and how we stop the medications when it is apparent they are not working or side effects occur.

The process begins in the office with the patient, and if possible, a supportive person such as a family member. Since the physician has a lot of information to impart, it is easy for the patient to get overwhelmed, and two heads are better than one. We work together to develop a plan, in a compassionate manner that respects the patient's needs and feelings; the physician should listen to the patient with no preconceived notions, which unfortunately does not always happen.

Risks for addiction should be assessed as objectively as possible, using "universal precautions"—meaning that all patients are considered at risk for abuse, misuse, and diversion until proven otherwise. While this may seem cruel, remember that the physician has a social responsibility to minimize potential abuse of these substances. Moreover, a prescription is not just a right, but also a responsibility. The use of universal precautions is one way of reinforcing this responsibility to the patient. There are formal instruments for doing this, including the medication agreement described in the following section. Many other instruments can be used.[2]

Next, a prescription is generated. This should be holistic, including interventions other than opioids if these have not already been provided. The patient is expected to comply with all aspects of the overall prescription. Honesty is critical. If the patient is struggling with a part of the prescription, such as side effects of a medicine or excess pain with physical therapy, the patient should not just unilaterally stop that component. She must tell the physician about the problem immediately.

If we have agreed on an opioid as part of the prescription, we discuss the goals of therapy, and I go over the risks and benefits as outlined in the medication agreement. The goals must be concretely identified and include:

Maximal patient compliance

Maximum communication

Decreased pain

Improved function with very specific short- and long-term
    goals described and the ramifications of failure to achieve
    the goals identified

Improved quality of life

Minimal side effects

Avoidance of addiction

The goals should be assessed on a regular basis. Ideally a friend, family member, or therapist is involved. Depending on the outcome of these assessments, the dosing may be increased if the drug is not effective, and the patient's compliance is documented, decreased or changed if there are side effects, or eliminated if not effective or the patient is noncompliant. Outcome should never be assessed merely on the quantity of drug taken. If the patient is demonstrating compliance and is tolerating the medication, doses can be increased until a plateau is reached, meaning that no further pain relief or functional improvement is occurring. Total relief of pain should never be the goal. A 30 percent reduction in pain with opiate therapy is a good outcome.

Prescription monitoring program (PMP) databases should be consulted *when necessary* to find out if patients are getting medications from other providers (doctor shopping). The physician also may need to consult border-state programs when appropriate (if possible). I believe PMP programs are invaluable, not just for catching those who abuse prescriptions, but also for protecting compliant patients. It is probably a good idea to check these databases before initiating any long-term therapy, and then periodically afterward. I don't think it should ever be mandatory, though; it is time consuming and would put undue pressure on providers, making them reluctant to prescribe.

All patients should have periodic urine screens to ensure they are taking the drug prescribed and not taking controlled substances that aren't. There are few predictive data on who abuses opiate prescriptions—a seventy-six-year-old patient in my town was once arrested for selling his prescription—and again, it is best to use universal precautions. However, the provider must understand the uses and limits of urine testing. Misinterpretation may unintentionally harm the patient. For example, failure to understand that codeine can cause a false positive for morphine may lead a physician to assume the patient is noncompliant and unnecessarily withhold treatment. I have seen many patients accused of noncompliance/abuse/diversion who were taking their medications properly, but the test just didn't pick it up. Once a patient is labeled noncompliant, she is functionally adorned with a scarlet letter and her care is compromised forever.

At times, opioids must be discontinued because of side effects, failure to achieve functional improvement, noncompliance with the therapeutic program, or abuse of the medication. Doing so is never easy; see the section that follows on medication agreements.

The sheer complexity of prescribing opioids creates very real strains in the doctor-patient relationship. I hope this explanation will help both patient and physician understand the pressures each faces and not question each other's motivations inappropriately.

Medication Agreements

Never impose on others what you would not choose for yourself.
Analects of Confucius (Lún Yǔ), 15.24

I began using what I referred to as "narcotics contracts" in 1990. I got the idea from working with adolescent anorexics in medical school. We had used contracts so that the patient and medical staff could agree on parameters regarding meals and weight gain or loss. The contract provided a set of rules that the patient had to follow and outlined the repercussions if she didn't. I used this agreement as a starting point for my narcotics contract, for which I had several goals.

First, I felt it would serve as informed consent for the use of opioids. Second, I created very specific rules that both the patient *and I* had to follow, to prevent diversion. Finally, I believed my patient and I both needed a document we could refer to if we had any questions about our agreement.

I got quite creative. I made up a list of ways the agreement could be violated and rated each one by severity. When the value of the violations exceeded a certain number, those were objective grounds for discontinuing the prescription. No single violation was sufficient by itself to do this. I believed, and still do, that we all deserve a second chance, and sometimes a third one. I did tell patients that any verified illegal activity would be reported, and that would be grounds for discontinuation.

I used this contract until 1993. Then I stopped, partly because using it did not accomplish any more than did providing the patient with a copy of my initial evaluation, which had all the same information as the contract and which I gave to every patient. My other reasons were more abstract. I believe in the power of the handshake and like to take people at their word. If they can't keep their word, they are not going to keep a written contract. Besides, I don't believe in contracts. In this "overpaperitized" environment where everything must be in triplicate, we have this naïve faith in the power of the legal document. However, the doctor-patient relationship is built on trust. If the parties cannot trust each other, there can be no relationship. No signed piece of paper will change that. Beyond this, patients need to be educated to respect opiates, not fear them. They have to know that opioids may be an appropriate treatment for their pain. The contract tends to reinforce the notion that opioids are bad and dangerous, thus increasing the patient's fears.

I spend a half-hour discussing the medication with the patient. I discuss the potential risks and benefits and give the patient the opportunity to ask questions. I offer websites for more information, and I have reading materials if they are interested. I tell them that they may only receive the medication from me. They are encouraged, but not required, to use a single pharmacy and must inform my office of pharmacy changes. I tell them to keep their medication locked up, not to share it, and not to tell others what they are taking. I inform them that urine checks may be done periodically and that they will be discharged and reported to the authorities if they sell their medications. I give them some freedom to alter their doses, since pain varies in intensity, but they must inform me about any changes that last for more than a few days. Finally, I tell them not to drive for two weeks after changing a dose and encourage them to call me if they have any questions, problems, or side effects. Again, I send them a copy of the office note that describes the entire visit.

Before the Oxycontin abuse problem, about half of providers in the pain community used contracts. I took part in many enlightened discussions of their pros and cons. Subsequent to Oxycontin, the use of contracts (now referred to as *agreements*) has escalated dramatically. Some suggest that physicians who don't use them are irresponsible.

Despite my dislike of contracts in principle, I think they can serve two purposes. The first is as a mutual agreement outlining the responsibility of both patient and doctor. This is positive and constructive, a form of team building.

The other, less positive, and perhaps destructive purpose, the one that drives current use, is to avoid legal problems that may later befall the practitioner. The justification is that the agreement will prevent abuse and diversion. In my experience, it doesn't. I have seen no evidence that contracts prevent diversion, but I have observed that they discourage patients from getting treatment with opiates, thereby creating an unnecessary barrier. Most patients who divert or abuse medications are, on the surface, model patients. They don't want to bite the hand that feeds them. They know that the only way to ensure their supply is to follow the rules.

Many patients apparently violate their agreement because they don't trust their doctor to be responsive to their needs. I have seen many patients who are subject to excessively rigid agreements that are insensitive to changes in pain level take more medication than prescribed, then feel they need to cover their misdeed by making up some excuse to explain the missing medication: "It fell down the sink"; "The pharmacist cut me twenty-five short"; "Someone stole it from my car"; "The cat hid it" (no lie; I heard this one).

Are they are telling the truth? Are they selling the medication? Did they take extra medication because they are not receiving enough to cover their needs, or was their pain level higher than normal, or are they becoming tolerant and afraid to be honest about it? In my experience, usually it is the latter. The appropriate response, then, is to confront the patient and encourage honesty.

I am actually not so much against agreements as I am in favor of practicality. If something is practical and makes sense, I will consider it. I find agreements less than practical, but if a physician does use them, there are some rules that should be followed:

1. First, the agreement should be used constructively as an informed consent.

2. Second, it should not be excessively rigid. Overly rigid contracts guarantee pseudoaddiction and dishonesty. Remember, a stream blocked by a dam will find a way to the sea. A patient with pain will try to find a way to ease that pain.

3. An agreement that puts all the burden of compliance on one party is not constructive. The agreement should include rights and responsibilities on the part of the physician as well as the patient. Doing so creates trust, the cornerstone of the relationship. For example, the physician's responsibility is to listen to the patient and take his concerns seriously. She has the right to withhold prescribing if the patient violates the agreement.

4. If the patient violates the agreement, patient and physician should have a discussion addressing the issue. Too often, the physician's knee-jerk reaction—angered by the patient's apparent insolence and relieved to be rid of the trouble the patient creates— is to discharge him, often by means of a phone call from a member of the office staff. The result is that responsibility for the patient's care is transferred to someone who may barely know him. A more constructive first step is to pause and examine the situation. Perhaps it is not the patient who is at fault. Perhaps the physician has not responded appropriately to his needs. Perhaps the patient, because of previous experience, is having difficulty trusting her.

The only absolute reason I discharge a patient for opioid abuse is *confirmed* evidence that the patient is selling his medications. An anonymous report is not reliable. People with a bone to pick with the patient are more than happy to seek revenge against him. Frequently, the caller has tried to "bum some meds" off the patient and been refused; the call is nothing more than blackmail. The physician who falls prey to this technique is merely punishing the patient for following the implicit doctor-patient contract. Rather than discharge the patient, I check a random urine test. Then I discuss the issue with the patient. Frequently, it becomes obvious who the caller is and what his motives are.

In all other circumstances of abuse, it is important to sit down with the patient and discuss the reasons for the abuse. The physician must assess the extent to which pseudoaddiction is present. I have seen too many patients discharged inappropriately. It takes time to educate the patient that it is oĸ to be honest, that the physician will respond to her needs, and that she doesn't have to beg for relief. Prematurely discharging such a patient only reinforces the notion that doctors are not to be trusted. Frequently, when we get things out in the open, the patient can learn to trust me, and the abusive behaviors stop. It is at such times that I willingly use a written agreement. If the patient continues to abuse the relationship, I will discharge him, but only after informing him of my concerns and my intention. If, after all options have been expended, he still can't trust me enough to be honest with me, there can be no relationship. But I must explore the reasons for the lack of trust and make sure that I have done all I can do to allay the patient's anxieties.

Note that unless the violation of the agreement is egregious, such as diverting the well-intentioned prescription for illegal uses, it is not grounds for discharging the patient from the doctor's practice. That is abandonment. By violating the agreement, the patient forfeits the right to receive opiates, but not compassionate care.

Somewhat begrudgingly, I have come to accept the written agreement as an inevitable part of the modern pain world. At a time when you can be sued if you underprescribe, sued if you overprescribe, or arrested if you prescribe to a drug dealer, it is sheer foolishness not to do all you can to protect yourself. The real reason I use them is because my medical board told me I have to. Still, I contend that the agreement can be used as a positive tool in the management of pain. The agreement I have developed can be found at www.chronicpainsucks.net. It is unique in that it is bilateral and spells out the rights and responsibilities of both the physician and the patient.

Regulating Opioids

As we have seen, in this country the pendulum of opioid regulation has swung between the extremes of compassionate care and prevention of diversion. Whenever the pendulum has swung too far in either direction, the outcome for pain patients, their providers, addicts, and society as a whole has not been good. Instead, we should seek a middle ground.

The Status of Opioid Regulation

In the mid-1800s, opium was the single most prescribed medicine in America. Toward the end of that century, government officials began to see addiction—then usually iatrogenic—as not only a public health problem but also a threat to national security. While doctors saw a use for opium, officials saw little use, creating the classic pendulum situation. The point at which the swing reverses is determined by who is in power and what the prevailing attitudes are. At that time, the opponents of opioid prescription won. But the issue was compounded by the common, recurring problem that the supporters of opium promised significantly more than the drug could deliver. When it failed to live up to their promises, and created an overwhelming problem of addiction, the government decided to crack down. The Harrison Anti-Narcotic Act of 1915 required physicians to keep records of morphine and heroin prescriptions and placed penalties, including incarceration, on those who prescribed "indiscriminately." Opioids were considered to have a role only at end of life. Even then, these drugs were used cautiously, and as a result, insufficiently.

The pendulum remained at this extreme until the mid-twentieth century. Physicians stopped prescribing and conveniently began to see complaints of persistent pain as a weakness of personality, rather than a symptom in need of palliation. Government saw people taking opiates for chronic pain as addicts and doctors who prescribed them as criminals, subject to arrest and incarceration.

The pendulum began to reverse in the 1960s with the recognition that despite these draconian measures, the problem of illegal drug use was growing rather than shrinking. Pain patients, blocked by federal and state law from receiving drugs from physicians, found illegal sources. The tide began to change with the passage of the Controlled Substances Act in 1970, which specifically categorized abuse risks of various controlled substances, established the DEA, and created a special mandatory prescription licensure for health-care providers.[3] Schedule I drugs, such as heroin, have a high abuse potential and no medical use and cannot be prescribed. Schedule II drugs, such as opiates and opioids, and schedule III drugs, such as Valium, have abuse potential but have a medical use and are the most tightly regulated. Schedule IV drugs (all other drugs—blood pressure medications, antibiotics, etc.) have a low abuse potential and a medical role, but require medical expertise to prescribe.

For the last hundred years, physicians have been taught that there is little place for opioids in the management of sustained pain. This edict is still the norm in most sites of medical education, even though that view is not consistent with that held by the pain community. However, since the 1980s pain societies have systematically attacked the prevailing medical wisdom, with some success. They suggested that opioids had a role in the treatment of first malignant, then benign pain. The World Health Organization prepared a statement on the worldwide problem/epidemic of untreated chronic pain and created the WHO Analgesic Ladder, outlining the treatment of pain according to its severity. This model recognized the use of opioids for treating pain. It also outlined barriers to pain management, specifying the factors relating to the patient, the physician, and regulatory bodies.[4]

The pain communities, armed with data, reached out to other health-care professionals and regulatory agencies in an attempt to change the views on opioid prescription and lower these barriers. There was some improvement in the education of medical students about pain. In 2010 I was heartened to hear that a young colleague was required to spend one month of his surgical residency in the pain clinic. One month isn't much, but it is better than nothing.

Perhaps the most important event was the creation of the Federation of State Medical Boards (FSMB) guidelines for opioid prescribing, first released in 1998 and updated in 2013, which have been accepted by most states. This achievement signaled that our governing bodies recognized the need for pain control and that opiates had a role in this endeavor. To emphasize this fact, Congress formally designated 2000–2010 as the Decade of Pain Control and Research.

As professional acceptance of the problem of pain increased, pain patients became empowered and began to demand their right to treatment. Some states created a patient's "bill of rights," stating that pain patients had a right to pain control; and physicians who failed to aggressively treat pain could be held liable. Lawyers licked their chops. As we saw earlier, one could now sue a physician either for not prescribing enough or for overprescribing. Medical providers shook with fear.

The pendulum had swung as far as it could go and was about to swing in the opposite direction. Just as in the 1800s, the physician-created delusion that opioids could cure all pain led to rampant addiction, while skyrocketing opioid prescriptions in the 1990s and 2000s led to prescription drug diversion and iatrogenic addiction (that inadvertently caused by prescribed medical treatment). People began to steal and kill for an Oxycontin. As it became clear once more that opioids are not a panacea, those in power again grew skeptical. Several questions arise from this situation:

What is worse: the epidemic of untreated pain or the epidemic of prescription drug diversion and abuse?

Are we artificially creating a crisis of untreated pain by promising cures that we don't have?

Is it appropriate to let someone suffer in order to control someone else's addiction?

Are opioids really that effective for long-standing pain anyway?

It is clear that the answers to these questions are different from what they were a century ago. Thanks to the efforts of many in the pain community, we do generally regard pain as a problem worthy of attention, not just a character flaw. We accept the use of opioids for some people who suffer from chronic pain. We don't view addicts and pain sufferers as criminals. Still, the problem of diversion is growing, and regulatory bodies feel a need to do something about it. So they look to control what they view as the source—the doctors who prescribe the drugs.

It would be wrong to apply a single label to everyone in regulation enforcement. Many people in the regulatory agencies are compassionate and objective and see a need and a use for these agents. But they also have seen firsthand the problems that drug abuse creates. Such observations create strong emotions, which in turn create a desire to do something, to punish those who seem responsible. Increasingly, regulators and law enforcement see physicians as responsible, as they did a century ago; and some are willing to use any tool possible to bring the perceived perpetrators to justice. And that increasingly makes physicians unwilling to use opioids to treat pain.

The litmus test of proper professional conduct is the Federation of State Medical Boards' "Model Policy Guidelines." When we created the New Hampshire guidelines based on this model, we hoped they would be easy to use and effectively lower all barriers to the prescription of opioids. But the rules actually created an unintended barrier to effective medical pain management.

First, complying with the guidelines added a lot of extra time, effort, and hassle to an already busy physician's day—time that was not well reimbursed, if at all, which meant that many physicians could not afford it. The DEA's requirement that physicians make a reasonable attempt to determine the diversion potential for every prescription and take steps to stop it means that physicians also must document some objective measure of diversion risk. If drugs are diverted, the physician risks being prosecuted as an accomplice, a drug trafficker. After 2004, there were several high-profile arrests of physicians, some of which resulted in jail time.

The most prominent case was that of Dr. William Hurwitz, who ran a pain clinic in Virginia. He was targeted for investigation, arrested, and charged with sixty-six counts of drug trafficking. The prosecution sought life imprisonment. He initially received twenty-five years, which was later reduced to four years. The case was intensely debated within the pain community in particular, and the medical community as a whole, regarding both Dr. Hurwitz's individual behavior and that of physicians who treated large numbers of pain patients and willingly prescribed pain medication to them. It was clear that Dr. Hurwitz was liberal in his prescription practices and that his prescriptions were being diverted by several patients. It was also clear that he had acquired a name as a target in the local criminal community. However, it was not clear that he violated the intent of the guidelines, and it was questionable whether his actions constituted criminal behavior. Still, he was found guilty and sentenced. It was entertaining to watch the pain physicians who initially supported Dr. Hurwitz begin to distance themselves and their actions from his, probably out of fear and denial.

Since the guidelines were published, they have been used to punish many physicians. Punishment has ranged from loss of prescription privileges to imprisonment. No matter how often officials try to console physicians by telling them they are safe if they "document, document, document," in reality they are not safe, and they know it. You can treat a hundred patients, manage ninety-nine perfectly, miss something on one, and be held liable. At a time when we seek more physicians willing to treat pain, the excess bureaucracy involved and the risk of legal repercussions has raised, not lowered, the barriers. Physicians willing to aggressively treat pain will write many prescriptions, thereby increasing their risk.

For me, this issue is personal. As I mentioned earlier, I was investigated by my state medical board. At the time, I was managing a very busy solo pain practice, following the guidelines to the letter, as I had done since beginning my practice. I had probably managed over a thousand patients over fourteen years and never had a serious adverse medical event—a very unusual record in this type of practice, which I was very proud of. While I never learned whether any medication I had prescribed was actually involved in the death of Jane's son, I was held responsible and investigated. It was while this investigation was ongoing that Dr. Hurwitz made the headlines. I was reassured by my attorney that I was not in any danger of criminal prosecution, but it was hard to feel totally comfortable.

The medical board subpoenaed eleven records, or roughly 1 percent of the patients I had seen over the previous fourteen years. These were the most challenging patients I was managing, which significantly biased their sample of my practice. It took them a full year to conclude that I had not violated the guidelines and would not be subject to any reprimand. However, they stated that I should be more vigilant in treating instances of violations of pain contracts, and added, chillingly, that I could be subject to prosecution should I be reviewed again. They never stated what "prosecution" meant, and I never found out what drugs Jane's son had overdosed on, nor did I ask.

As that year proceeded, I found it nearly impossible to function. The knowledge that I had "documented, documented, documented" did little to ease my stress, which was made worse by the cost of copying records and hiring an attorney (fortunately covered by my insurance company) and still worse by the knowledge that one of my colleagues in the pain community would not support my management of the one patient whose case he reviewed, even though I had secured several second opinions from reputable pain physicians while I was treating this patient. Nor did he ever attempt to meet with me or the patient. If pain practitioners are going to urge our colleagues to treat pain aggressively, what does it say that when push comes to shove, they do not support those who heed this advice?

The investigation had significant repercussions. I lost trust in my colleagues, the regulatory system, and my patients. I did become more vigilant and discovered that many patients were using me. Some were selling their prescriptions, one to minors. But when I reported these patients, law enforcement seemed uninterested. One official, a friend of mine, told me they don't have the resources to follow up on such reports. Worst of all, though, I no longer trusted myself. I was no longer sure that aggressively prescribing opioids was the right thing to do. I had seen too many people live in a cloud while on the medications I had prescribed, and I had seen too many people paradoxically get better when they came off medications I had given them. I was no longer sure I wasn't harming anyone. In order to function as a physician, you must be able to trust; and when you cannot even trust yourself to do what is right, you are in crisis. Is taking a chance on a pain patient worth such a risk?

I have met many other physicians who have gone through similar trials. In fact, it seems unusual to find a pain practitioner who hasn't been investigated. It seems that your chances of being investigated go up the more often you prescribe. What happens when that is your whole practice? With every reprimand, a pain practice closes and an exodus of pain patients occurs, all looking for a new home, looking for someone to take a chance on them, to care for them. While we tell them they don't have to suffer, the number of those physicians willing to risk caring for them is dropping. What does this say to the rank-and-file physician whom the pain community has been struggling to interest in pain management for the past thirty years?

The current system fails to either curb diversion or compassionately and efficiently treat pain. It is clear to me that the regulatory bodies need to modify their actions.

SOLUTIONS

The job of the regulator is daunting, and I have utmost respect for those trying to administer the guidelines. Shortly after the first subpoena arrived, I spoke to a friend who is a police officer. He told me that every time he fires a bullet, especially if the shot results in bodily injury or death, he is de facto charged with a crime and investigated. Most often police officers are cleared of wrongdoing, but the process still engenders fear. I saw the investigation of my practice in a similar light. What I objected to was the time it took. While the process should be thorough and careful, it should be accomplished in a reasonable time frame, at a reasonable cost.

Regulation and oversight are important. They encourage practitioners to stay up to date with proper techniques and procedures, which is good for both pain practitioner and patient. Nor do I oppose the guidelines. I think they are reasonable and necessary. It is possible to adjust the structure of the office visit, perhaps with the use of nurses or paraprofessionals, so that the guidelines are not onerous to adhere to. My concern is that the guidelines have been applied in a way that goes beyond their intent, to reprimand and incarcerate many compassionate physicians who were courageously caring for those in need. The oversight system must be revised in such a way that it will encourage proper pain management, while enabling the rank-and-file physician to practice pain management without undue fear. Several changes are necessary to make this possible.

Decriminalize Pain Prescribing   First, compassion should never be misconstrued as a crime. Caring for someone in pain is emotionally challenging, especially when our palliative tools are few. Often a physician needs to take a chance on the patient, because the physical, emotional, and financial cost of untreated pain dwarfs the risk of diversion. It is crucial that physicians be encouraged to take this chance, and it should never be considered a crime to do so. Criminalizing pain prescriptions creates unnecessary fear in the physician, which impairs pain management. Inevitably some patients will misuse and abuse their prescriptions, and some well-intentioned physicians will make mistakes. Rather than resort to criminal or civil action in such cases, educational tools and increased oversight should be used to correct unsound practices. And although physicians should take reasonable precautions to make sure that prescriptions will be used appropriately, they should never be put in the position of being the front line in the war on drugs. It will only discourage them from prescribing. It should be understood that what a patient does with his prescription once he leaves the doctor's office is his responsibility, not his doctor's. The system must hold the patient liable, not the physician.

Pay Pain Management Specialists Appropriately   At the same time, physicians must follow the guidelines. They should learn to quickly assess abuse risk and take universal precautions to minimize it with all patients. These measures cost both time and money, and the medical and insurance establishments must recognize that the skill involved in managing pain and the demand for this service rival, if they do not exceed, those of procedural medicine. This skill should be reimbursed at least as well as procedural medicine. If we want to encourage physicians to manage pain, we need to pay them adequately for doing it. And I argue that we can do this without raising overall health-care costs by shifting the dollar from the overcompensated proceduralist to the pain management specialist.

Get Realistic About Opioids   Health-care providers also need to get over their irrational love affair with opioids. They are useful tools for *some* patients, not all. While they help some, they harm others. Tolerance, addiction, and opioid-induced hyperesthesia are significant iatrogenic problems. While it is nearly impossible to predict who will respond well to these medications, or which specific agent or what dose to use, and a therapeutic trial may be warranted for a particular patient, it is essential to assess whether pain is decreasing and function is increasing and to monitor this process more strictly. When the drug is not working, the physician must be willing to say so and detoxify—while also not abandoning the patient as proceduralists often do.

Better Educate Both Providers and Regulators   Learning to manage pain and addiction requires education. It is abhorrent that medical schools and postmedical education only pay lip service to these important concepts. So much of medical education is wasted on teaching physicians syndromes they will never see, yet little is spent on something they will see every day of their careers. It is relatively easy for a physician to follow the guidelines, but only when taught how to do so, and the failure to teach this is a major failing of medical education.

What is more, both health-care professionals and regulators must learn to see opioids through each other's eyes, so each can better appreciate the challenges the other faces. One helpful trend since the early 1990s is holding multidisciplinary meetings that bring pain management specialists and regulatory personnel together. Only by working together can we place the pendulum at the optimal spot for both pain patient and addict. Our State Pain Management Task Force did organize one such meeting, but these gatherings must happen regularly. Once is not enough.

We need to recognize that there is no uniformly accurate test or survey that predicts diversion and that excess scrutiny will only result in care being withheld from patients who need it—some of whom happen to be addicts or criminals. The compassionate physician will err on the side of compassion. In my experience, overly suspicious physicians do not treat pain aggressively, and overly compassionate physicians are taken advantage of. But this is a risk the pain management physician must take—and should be encouraged to take, provided that the cost in time and money of following the guidelines is adequately compensated and that the physician can feel safe from prosecution.

Health-care providers and regulators need to work together to educate other health-care providers, regulators, and lay people about what opioids can and cannot do, what their risks are, and how to use them safely. This education should extend to all who create public policy pertaining to pain treatment.

Keep Regulatory Scrutiny Objective and Simple   As I have said, our regulatory system is in much need of reform because of its tendency to overregulate. Legislatures must understand that there is an inherent conflict between minimizing prescription pain medication abuse and maximizing pain management. It is unlikely that they will ever write a law that will completely resolve this dilemma, which means that each individual pain scenario must be judged on its own merits. Every law, such as the New York State "I-STOP" law, will have an unintended consequence, and the possible ramifications should be thought out in detail before these laws are passed. As with I-STOP, the unintended consequence is often worse than the problem the law was meant to address. To paraphrase Aristotle, *the law should be reason, free from passion.*

I suggest a more commonsense approach. While this approach, of necessity, places a premium on trusting the judgment of those who oversee, I believe that by doing so we can create a legal system that provokes less fear and costs less. It is clear that, like our tortuous legal system, our regulatory system dramatically increases the cost of practicing medicine, and this cost unnecessarily raises the barrier to medical care in general and pain management in particular.

Finally, in creating a body of laws to regulate opiates, legislatures must understand and accept that addiction and chronic pain are disease states, not character flaws. They create great suffering in themselves, and legislatures should not amplify that suffering, especially when creating punishments for violations. An eye for an eye is the best sentencing guide, meaning that the punishment should not exceed the crime.

FOURTEEN

Cannabinoids and Pain

Reefer Madness or Compassionate Care?

*Even if one takes every reefer madness allegation of the prohibition-
ists at face value, marijuana prohibition has done far more harm to
far more people than marijuana ever could.*

William F. Buckley Jr., *New York Post* (February 27, 1999)

I never really saw marijuana until I went to college. I say "really"
because once I got to college, I realized that the neat smell I had noticed
on a regular basis just outside my high school was actually marijuana.
At college, marijuana was ubiquitous. Hardly a week went by without
someone offering the drug to me. However, I was afraid to try it, my fears
fueled by misconceptions that are still prevalent. I guess I thought I would
hallucinate or kill someone, or whatever. What I really feared was getting
out of control and doing something I might regret later.

At the same time, we value alcohol. A real man holds his liquor. We
admire people who know their wine, beer, or liquor and refer to them as
connoisseurs. It is a rare social event that does not involve alcohol, including
White House dinners. When there is a toast, it is often considered an insult
when someone does not imbibe. But people who know their marijuana are
called *dopes,* a substantially less complimentary term.

When I did try marijuana, I was disappointed. I got a buzz and that was
about it. It wasn't a huge amount different from a few beers. However, in
contrast to my experience with alcohol, after smoking a little pot, I had
no interest in beating anyone up or in having sex with the next female
who walked by. Instead, I just mellowed out and got introspective, not
undesirable effects.

In any case, as long as I have practiced pain management, I have implicitly supported legalization of marijuana for the medical treatment of pain. I
discovered that many of my patients used it as an adjunct and functioned

better with it. I still have mixed feelings about legalizing it for recreational use—and I should note that with respect to public policy, medical use and recreational use should be mutually exclusive. They are totally different. While I believe marijuana has potential medicinal value, I do not support the existing state laws that legalize the drug for medical purposes.

Armed with newfound knowledge from researching the topic to write this chapter, I struggle to figure out why our society is so eager to restrain marijuana use, especially when alcohol is so openly promoted and imbibed. In fact, 81 percent of Americans favor legalization of marijuana for medicinal purposes[1] and 52 percent for recreational purposes.[2] As of this writing, twenty-three states and the District of Columbia have openly challenged federal authority by passing medical marijuana laws, and several more have laws in process. Four states have passed recreational marijuana laws that are being debated in the federal courts.

About 50 percent of Americans have tried marijuana. Seven percent of Americans age twelve or older use it monthly.[3] These numbers do not even begin to assess what percentage of Americans use marijuana for medical reasons. In my pain practice, it is very commonly used medically, as it has been for millennia. Yet the government's war on marijuana has ruined innumerable lives, which suggests to me that the cost of the current policies is much greater than the benefit. Seventy-two percent of Americans believe that government efforts to enforce existing marijuana laws cost more than they are worth.[4] In other words, a lot of people are asking the federal government: What's the big deal? And the government really doesn't have a great answer.

This is not a trivial debate. An estimated 693,481 arrests were made nationwide for marijuana in 2013, according to the Federal Bureau of Investigation's annual Uniform Crime Reporting statistics. More than 87 percent of these arrests were for possession, which means one person was arrested for marijuana possession approximately every fifty-one seconds on average.[5] Fifteen percent (or more) of chronic pain patients risk arrest by using marijuana to control their pain, as suggested by a limited study of random urine toxicology testing in pain patients on opioids.[6]

Marijuana causes surprisingly little organ damage, certainly less than legally obtained addictive drugs such as alcohol, caffeine, and nicotine. While the federal government claims that marijuana has no medical value, numerous studies challenge that assertion for many conditions such as pain of all sorts, posttraumatic stress disorder, social anxiety, other forms of anxiety, glaucoma, and chemotherapy-related nausea and anorexia—conditions that are often refractory to current modes of treatment.

I believe that opinions about this issue—including those of the federal government—are based more on passion than on sound reason. As with opioid drugs, the naïveté of those with often very strong opinions about this subject is striking. Even more interesting, the lines between "medical" use and "recreational" use are so blurred that it is often difficult to determine what the intentions are of those who seek to control public policy. Public policy reflects this conundrum.

In this chapter, I will review what we know about marijuana as objectively as possible and explain how I came to feel as I do. I will explore the history of the medical, recreational, and spiritual use of marijuana and how it came to be illegal in much of the world and then describe what cannabinoids, the active ingredients in marijuana, are, both exogenous and endogenous (yes, our body makes its own cannabinoids), and what they do in our bodies. I will explain what the concept of medical marijuana really means and that, while the federal government has a better understanding of this than the states, it does not mean that its public policy is correct. I will look at the barriers to successful use of cannabinoids for treating a whole variety of illnesses. Finally, I will propose a more rational public policy for the use of these agents.

Marijuana Through the Ages

The history of marijuana use dates back 8,500 years or more.[7] The plants from which marijuana is derived, *Cannabis sativa* and *Cannabis indica,* are not just imbibed. Their fibrous stems were and still are used to make a diverse array of hemp-related products, such as hemp seed foods, hemp oil, wax, resin, rope, cloth, pulp, and fuel. There is evidence that the Chinese cultivated and used the plant for many of these purposes 8,500 years ago and that its use as a medicine followed soon after.[8] There is evidence of medical use—including pain treatment—in China, Egypt, Greece, India, and Southeast Asia prior to the time of Christ.[9] Arab physicians noted its diuretic, antiemetic (preventing nausea and vomiting), antiepileptic, antiinflammatory, analgesic, and antipyretic (fever-reducing) properties and used it extensively as a medication from the eighth to the eighteenth centuries.[10] Over the years, its industrial and medical uses developed in a somewhat parallel fashion. THC is one of many cannabinoids found in these plants, and it is thought that the THC content gives the smoked plant its intoxicating qualities. While both medical marijuana and hemp are derived from *Cannabis*, there are many subspecies of this plant, and those used for industrial purposes have a high fiber and low THC content.[11]

Cannabis was first introduced into Western medicine by William Brook O'Shaughnessy, an Irish physician who began conducting experiments with the drug in the 1830s while serving as assistant surgeon and professor of chemistry at the Medical College of Calcutta. He first tested the drug on animals, then humans, in order to treat muscle spasms, stomach cramps, and general pain.[12] The drug became common throughout the Western world by the end of the nineteenth century and was used as the primary pain reliever until the invention of aspirin. By 1937 over 280 manufacturers made at least two thousand cannabis medicines.[13]

At the same time, cannabis was used for recreational and spiritual purposes. In the late 1800s, recreational cannabis was listed as a "fashionable narcotic," and oriental-style hashish parlors flourished in major U.S. cities.[14] This use began to attract the attention of regulators, and by the mid-1800s, state efforts to regulate the sale of pharmaceuticals began. By the end of the nineteenth century, many pharmaceutical boards listed cannabis as a narcotic, and concerns about recreational use and abuse of the drug influenced individual state antinarcotics legislation in the early twentieth century, which aimed to control the use of all narcotics, including cannabis, by limiting the sale of the drugs to pharmacies and for purchase only with a doctor's prescription. All states had some form of regulation. Between 1925 and 1932, the Uniform State Narcotic Act was created to recommend policy that would make safeguards and regulations uniform among the states. By 1937 thirty-five states had adopted its policies.[15]

In 1930 the Federal Bureau of Narcotics (FBN) was created, headed by Harry Anslinger, who sought to outlaw all recreational drugs, including marijuana. The FBN produced propaganda films promoting Anslinger's claims that it caused people to commit violent crimes and act irrationally and hypersexually. One result was the Marijuana Tax Act of 1937, which made possession or transfer of cannabis illegal under federal law, except for medical and industrial uses. The act was championed by Anslinger and by William Randolph Hearst, who used his empire of newspapers to run "yellow" stories demonizing the cannabis plant. While their motivations were different, they teamed up to pass this act. Anslinger believed that marijuana had an adverse effect on society; but several scholars argue that Hearst's goal was to destroy the hemp industry, which he saw as a threat to his extensive timber holdings as a cheaper source of pulp for newspaper. The bill also was championed by the Mellon and Dupont families, in order to destroy the hemp industry for the sake of Dupont's new product, nylon. Based on their efforts and the misinformation disseminated in Hearst's newspapers, the U.S. Congress passed the act in 1937.[16] More legislation passed in the 1950s created a minimum incarceration of two to ten years with a fine of up to $20,000 for a first-time cannabis possession offense. [17]

In 1970 the Comprehensive Drug Abuse Prevention and Control Act repealed previous legislation. One part of this act, the Controlled Substances Act (CSA), listed marijuana as a schedule I drug, meaning that it had high abuse potential with no proven medical benefit; that is, the CSA has zero tolerance for any THC. Therefore, since 1970, according to federal law, it has been illegal to grow hemp in the United States, even though hemp is one of the most versatile, environmentally friendly, and important crops in the world. All hemp products are imported and must demonstrate 0 percent THC content. Only twenty-six years earlier, during World War II, the U.S. government had produced a short film, *Hemp for Victory*, promoting hemp as a necessary crop to win the war. [18]

In 1973 Oregon decriminalized marijuana. Over the next forty years, other states followed suit. Despite this trend, all use of cannabinoids remains illegal under federal law, which overrules state law. Therefore, until Congress passes a new law, all uses of marijuana remain a federal crime. However, on October 19, 2009, the U.S. deputy attorney general issued a memorandum to all U.S. attorneys in the Department of Justice, providing seven criteria for ascertaining whether a patient's use, or her caregiver's provision, of medical cannabis represents part of a recommended treatment regimen consistent with applicable state law and recommending against prosecuting patients who use medical cannabis products according to state laws. Not applying these criteria, the memo concludes, "would likely be an inefficient use of limited federal resources."[19]

Four states took this debate a step further. In 2012 Washington and Colorado passed laws legalizing the use of cannabinoids for "recreational" purposes similar to the use of alcohol or tobacco. Alaska and Oregon followed in 2014. These laws are currently being challenged by the federal government.

The take-home message is that for most of the past ten thousand years, humans have legally used hemp and cannabis for myriad purposes, including medical and recreational ones. It has only been in the past 140 years that government has sought to control them. The current questions are:

Do the potential benefits of cannabis outweigh the harm it may cause?

Are the problems created by governmental control of cannabis use worse than the problems it creates?

These are not easy questions to answer. In talking with others about this subject, I have been struck by how little most people know about what cannabis actually is and what it does in the body. So I will begin by explaining this, in order to help us understand how it can be safely used.

What Are Cannabis and Cannabinoids?

Cannabis is considered the same as marijuana, and so far I have used these terms interchangeably. The active ingredients in these plants are cannabinoids, substances found in a variety of plants in addition to *Cannabis,* including several Echinacea species, *Helichrysum umbraculigerum* (a yellow-flowering species native to Africa) and *Radula marginata* (a type of liverwort). There are three different classes of cannabinoids: phytocannabinoids, endocannabinoids, and synthetic cannabinoids. All activate cannabinoid receptors in the human body.[20]

Phytocannabinoids are found in plants. At least eighty-five cannabinoids have been isolated from the cannabis plant, all with differing biological activities. Of these, delta 9 tetrahydrocannabinol (THC) and cannabidiol (CBD) are the ones that medical use studies have focused on.[21]

Endocannabinoids are substances produced within the body.

Synthetic cannabinoids are manufactured drugs. Two have FDA approval and are available by prescription in the United States: Dronabinol (Marinol) and Nabilone (Cesamet). Dronabinol is a CSA schedule III drug, meaning that it has a moderate abuse potential and is available by prescription. It is used as an appetite stimulant, antiemetic, and analgesic. Nabilone is a schedule II drug, meaning that its abuse potential is higher. Both are THC analogues.[22]

All cannabinoids bind to cannabinoid receptors in the human body. To date, two types of receptors have been identified, CB1 and CB2. More will no doubt be discovered. CB1 receptors are found in several brainstem structures, but not in the medulla, where cardiovascular and respiratory functions are controlled. Thus, unlike opioids, cannabinoids do not impair respiratory or cardiovascular function. This type of receptor is thought to be responsible for the euphoric and anticonvulsive effects of cannabis.[23]

CB2 receptors are found in the immune system and immune-derived cells. We know relatively little about the effects of cannabinoids on immune cells, though their net effect appears to be stimulatory. CB2 receptors also are found in the peripheral nervous system. They are thought to be responsible for the antiinflammatory effects of cannabinoids.[24]

Endocannabinoids are released by one cell and act on cannabinoid receptors on nearby cells; they can travel only short distances. They are not stored in fat cells like smoked or ingested cannabinoids, but synthesized when needed. They work in a reverse direction in the nervous system. Normally a nerve cell (the presynaptic neuron) transmits an electrical impulse to another nerve cell (the postsynaptic neuron) across a space called a synapse. The signal triggers the release of a chemical called a neurotransmitter that crosses the synapse and either inhibits or stimulates the second neuron. What happens in the postsynaptic neuron depends on the additive effect of all the presynaptic neurons acting on it. Endocannabinoids, by contrast, are produced by the postsynaptic neuron, travel to the presynaptic neuron, and bind to receptors there that inhibit the release of other neurotransmitters from the presynaptic cell. If the neurotransmitter being affected is inhibitory, the effect on the postsynaptic neuron will be excitatory. If a presynaptic neurotransmitter is excitatory, the effect on the postsynaptic cell will be inhibitory. This mechanism enables the postsynaptic cell to control the input it receives.[25]

Smoking phytocannabinoids or ingesting them orally creates an extremely complex reaction. A typical marijuana preparation contains dozens of cannabinoids, all with varying actions on different cannabinoid receptors. To complicate matters even more, many of these cannabinoids can stimulate noncannabinoid receptors. The net effect of the preparation is the sum of all of these activities and can be difficult to predict in an individual, thus making it difficult, if not impossible, to create a reliable pharmaceutical preparation from the plant.

Often the effects of a marijuana preparation are predicted by looking at the THC/CBD ratio of the preparation. This is too simplistic. It ignores the contribution of the dozens of other cannabinoids. We use this ratio because we know what THC and CBD do in the body. THC has an equal affinity for both CB1 and CB2 receptors. It is thought to be the primary psychoactive component of the plant, to ease moderate pain, and to be neuroprotective.[26] This latter effect may be huge in chronic pain, since we know that persistent pain leads to nerve cell death, which may exacerbate chronic pain. CBD is not psychoactive and may minimize the pschoactivity of THC.[27] It also has antidepressant, antianxiety, and neuroprotective effects.[28] Preparations from *Cannabis indica* have a four to five times higher CBD/THC ratio than preparations from *Cannabis sativa*. Thus, the primary effect of sativa preparations is stimulation; it should be used during the day. It affects mostly mind and emotions and can be used to treat the psychological aspects of many illnesses, giving the patient a greater sense of well-being. Indica preparations are more sedating and anxiety reducing and should be used at night.[29]

Medical Marijuana: Benefits Versus Risks

In order to weigh risks and benefits, one must understand the FDA's three main criteria for approving a drug:

The exact chemical it contains and the amount present in the drug must be specified.

The drug must be shown to be efficacious for a specific condition(s).

Its potential benefits must outweigh the risks, and the risks must be specified.

It is not clear that marijuana itself will ever meet these criteria. The two cannabinoid preparations that have been approved for use in the United States are both THC derivatives. Each is a single, specific cannabinoid, in a specified amount taken orally. But a 2011 report from the National Institute on Drug Abuse stated: "Marijuana itself is an unlikely medication candidate for several reasons: 1) it is an unpurified plant containing numerous chemicals with unknown health effects; 2) it is typically consumed by smoking, further contributing to potential adverse effects; and 3) its cognitive-impairing effects may limit its utility."

Reliability and specificity. The first major problem with medical marijuana is that a typical preparation contains dozens of cannabinoids, each with different effects and potencies. At this time, we don't even know what the effects of many of them are, and we don't know if the net effect of a preparation is due to the actions of one or two of these drugs alone, or a synergistic effect of all of them acting together. In addition, we rarely know how much of each cannabinoid is present in a particular preparation with any great certainty.

FDA-approved preparations of two drugs mixed together are not unusual. Percocet, for example, is a mixture of Tylenol and oxycodone in specified and predictable amounts. No currently approved drug is similar to marijuana. By this criterion alone, approval of marijuana as a legitimate drug would require either a shift of FDA policy or an exception to the rule. While the former is possible, the latter is unlikely.

Efficacy. Proponents of medical marijuana cite studies that support its use in a number of conditions, including pain, spasticity (multiple sclerosis), Alzheimer's, breast cancer, anorexia in cancer and AIDS patients, brain cancer, opioid dependence, posttraumatic stress disorder, glaucoma, and ALS. Here I will discuss its use to treat pain.

There are substantial barriers to studying marijuana (see the next section). In the United States, much of the research comes from California, which established the Center for Medicinal Cannabis Research in 1999 to determine whether marijuana has therapeutic value. As of 2010, four studies of the effects of medical marijuana on neuropathic pain had been completed and published. All demonstrated a greater than 30 percent decrease in pain. The number thirty is important because a reduction equal to or greater than this is associated with a meaningful quality of life. Patients enrolled in these studies continued any opioids they had been taking. Side effects were few and consisted of mild anxiety, sedation, and dizziness. No mood changes were noted. Three observations are significant:

One study used both low (3.5 percent) and high (7.0 percent) THC-dose marijuana and found no difference in analgesia between the two doses. This is important because the goal of any drug is to maximize effects and minimize side effects. The effect is analgesia. The side effect is euphoria. In effect, then, by minimizing THC content, one can maximize analgesia while minimizing euphoria.

Although these four studies used smoked cannabis, an unrelated
study that compared drug levels using vaporized versus smoked
marijuana found the levels to be similar. This observation is
important because of the concern over the risks of a smoked
product and the search for an alternative mode of delivery.[30]

All these studies were short term and involved just a few exposures
to the drug. Such a limited exposure cannot answer the
questions of safety and efficacy for what would certainly be a
long-term use in treating chronic pain.

In 2012 the Center ran out of funding, and studies in progress at that
time were discontinued. At this writing the Center was not involved in
further research. At this point, the studies described above comprise the
best evidence available. However, it is not sufficient to meet FDA requirements, and it is unlikely that the FDA would be swayed by this limited data.
Long-term studies are needed (see the following section).

Safety. There are five specific safety concerns: cancer and pulmonary risk
from smoking the drug, adverse effects on the brain, the addiction-gateway
phenomenon, development of mental disorders (specifically, schizophrenia), and death.

CANCER AND PULMONARY RISK

Cannabis smoke contains over fifty known carcinogens. However, a large
2006 study showed no causative link to oral, laryngeal, pharyngeal, esoph-
ageal, or lung cancer, or to chronic obstructive pulmonary disease (COPD)
when adjusting for cigarette smoking and alcohol use.[31] These results were
confirmed by researchers at the University of British Columbia. However,
they found that smoking cannabis and tobacco together tripled the risk of
developing COPD over just smoking tobacco alone.[32] Many other studies
have confirmed this data.

NEUROPSYCHOLOGICAL RISK

There are concerns about permanent adverse effects on brain function,
especially in those under age twenty-three. Studying this issue, of necessity, requires an assessment prior to the onset of drug use and long-term
follow-up. This is logistically difficult to do. In 2012, Meier and others
published a study of the neuropsychological effects of cannabis use for

1,037 individuals from birth to age thirty-eight. They found that heavy marijuana use in adolescence did result in decline in all neuropsychological domains studied, and that cessation did not fully restore neuropsychological functioning. Specifically, they found an average eight-point drop in IQ scores in these individuals. They did not find a significant effect in those who had mild to moderate exposures or in individuals who began smoking after age twenty-three. The authors concluded that their findings suggested that cannabis had a toxic effect on the adolescent brain.[33] Their data were reanalyzed by Rogeberg, who believed there was a methodological flaw in the Meier study. He corrected the data and concluded that marijuana had no adverse long-term effects on the brain function of any study participants, no matter the age of onset of cannabis use or the intensity of use.[34] The take-home message is that current scientific evidence does not clearly support the causation of permanent neurological damage in adults who smoke cannabis or adolescents who smoke mild to moderate amounts, but it does suggest a neurotoxic effect in adolescents with heavy usage.

It is also true that a number of studies have shown similar changes in neuropsychological functioning in adolescents and adults whose risk factor is heading a soccer ball. One study of young adult American soccer players found that attention and concentration deficits were common among those who headed the ball often.[35] Another study found that nearly 50 percent of soccer players aged twelve to seventeen who sustained head injuries had had symptoms of a concussion during the season, and half of those individuals experienced more than one concussion *during one season.* The point is that the young brain is susceptible to both physical and chemical trauma. Yet we encourage our kids to engage in sports with high risk for head trauma. These issues need to be considered when making policy for all sorts of exposures for young adults.

ADDICTION RISK

There is no question that cannabis use carries a risk of addiction. As I noted in chapter 11, the risk of any addiction is relative and depends on a number of factors, an important one being age of onset of use. We also know that some substances are inherently more addictive than others, and cannabis carries a relatively low risk. Some have questioned whether marijuana is addictive at all.[36] Jack E. Henningfield of the National Institute on Drug Abuse and Neal L. Benowitz of the University of California at San

Francisco ranked the addictiveness of six substances (cannabis, caffeine, cocaine, nicotine, alcohol, and heroin). Both found marijuana to be the least addictive in their initial assessment, although in 1997 Henningfield adjusted his ratings, listing marijuana ahead of caffeine.[37]

While marijuana may not be excessively addictive in and of itself relative to other legal drugs, there are concerns that its use leads to the use of other drugs that are much more addictive. This is called the gateway drug theory, and it has guided U.S. drug policy since the 1950s. To date, this theory is unproven, and there is much to suggest that it is not valid. In 2010 researchers from the University of New Hampshire found that whether teenagers who smoke pot go on to use other illicit drugs as young adults has more to do with life factors such as employment status and stress. The strongest predictor of illicit drug use was race/ethnicity, not whether someone used marijuana. Employment in young adulthood was protective, and any gateway effect subsided entirely after age twenty-one.[38]

Note that all addictive behaviors have a gateway behavior of some sort. Most of those who engage in the gateway behavior will not develop an addiction. We all engage in sex. Most of us are not sex addicts. Most of us have imbibed alcohol at some point. Most of us are not alcoholics. Most of us have smoked marijuana at some point in our lives. Most of us are not addicted to marijuana, nor have we progressed to other more dangerous drugs.

DEVELOPMENT OF MENTAL DISORDERS

At one time, it was thought that marijuana might cause schizophrenia or other psychoses. Two studies supported this conclusion. One was questionable because the exposure to cannabis was minimal. The other, though, was a ten-year study of 1,923 individuals aged fourteen to twenty-four which concluded that cannabis use in this age group was a risk factor for development of later psychotic symptoms.[39] Of these 1,923 individuals, 247 had used cannabis. Of this 247, roughly 75 percent were heavy users. Unlike the Meier study mentioned earlier, no attempt was made to determine if the amount of exposure made a difference. Still, the results should be taken into account when constructing public policy for the young. However, although the incidence of marijuana use has increased in the U.S. population, the incidence of schizophrenia has not. That observation is used to suggest that marijuana use does not lead to psychosis.

RISK OF DEATH

Death is always a feared outcome of any addictive substance. I have already discussed the problem of prescription drug deaths from opioids. This is not a problem with marijuana. As cannabis researcher Paul Hornby noted, "You have to smoke something like 15,000 joints in 20 minutes to get a toxic amount of THC." In evaluating a 1988 petition to reschedule marijuana, U.S. DEA chief administrative law judge Francis Young, after reviewing considerable evidence on the subject, stated: "There is no record in the extensive medical literature describing a proven, documented cannabis-induced fatality. . . . Despite [a] long history of use and the extraordinarily high numbers of social smokers, there are simply no credible medical reports to suggest that consuming marijuana has caused a single death. . . . Marijuana, in its natural form, is one of the safest therapeutically active substances known to man."[40]

Barriers to Legalization of Medicinal Marijuana

In terms of the FDA's criteria, then, marijuana certainly appears safe relative to other pharmaceutical preparations. Problems of efficacy and appropriate drug formulations are surmountable, at least in theory. However, substantial, unnecessary barriers stand in the way of FDA approval. The following discussion applies only to the medical use of marijuana. However, medical and recreational uses, in practice, are not mutually exclusive, so some of the following statements apply to both.

THE NATURE OF THE DRUG

As I have said, marijuana is a conglomeration of dozens of drugs, each with its own potential medicinal effects and side effects, each present in variable absolute and relative amounts in each preparation. Thus the net effect of a smoked cigarette of unpurified plant matter is unpredictable. This issue alone is enough to create an insurmountable barrier to achieving FDA approval for smoked marijuana.

However, there are other ways to deliver cannabinoids. One option is to vaporize the preparation. The unpurified substance is heated to the point where the active ingredients evaporate into a vapor without burning the plant material. This vapor is then inhaled. The process extracts the harmful substances, providing the user with a purer, safer product. The marijuana also may be ingested orally, either directly or mixed into something else, for example, brownies. While each of these methods may eliminate the potential adverse effects of smoked material on the lungs or cardiovascular system, neither solves the problem of inconsistency of dosing of the active ingredients.

The two FDA-approved preparations were an attempt to get around this problem. However, we really don't know which constituents of marijuana are responsible for its different net therapeutic effects. This makes creating an effective pharmaceutical product difficult. Should it contain one or more cannabinoids? If more than one is present, which is likely, how many should there be and in what relative amounts? How does one even begin to research this? What conditions are we creating the product to treat?

Another problem is that the main side effect of effective medical marijuana is the one that is actually desired in recreational use: the buzz, or what researchers call the psychomimetic effect, which is not acceptable in a medicinal product. How does one create a pharmaceutical product that does not give a buzz but is still effective? Does it matter? As I noted, patients who use opioids for pain control are less likely to experience a high. I also have noticed that within a few days to two weeks of starting opioids, any high that is experienced goes away, while the medication remains effective for pain control. Is the same true for marijuana? If the psychomimetic effect is short-lived but the pharmacological effect is sustained long term, then this barrier is substantially lower, possibly moot. I don't have an answer based on personal experience, since I rarely know which of my patients use the drug. Nor am I aware of any studies that address this issue.

This question is complicated by the specifics of the situation in which the drug is used. For example, for end-of-life care, there probably is nothing wrong with the patient experiencing a buzz if the drug provides useful analgesia. However, in treating pain in a nonterminal setting, any adverse effect on a patient's function is important. For example, if the buzz impairs someone's ability to perform a job or raise a child, then it is a problem.

A related question is how long cannabinoids can remain effective for pain. Is there tolerance? How quickly does it occur? These are huge issues in treating chronic pain. Virtually all the studies are short term, some with only one exposure to the drug. We know that the data regarding opioids used for acute pain cannot be generalized to treating chronic pain. It is likely that the same is true for cannabinoids. To date, the studies show that cannabinoids are a useful adjunct for acute pain, but not a stand-alone drug. They are opioid sparing, meaning using both drugs together allows one to use lower doses of each, hopefully with fewer side effects. While that outcome would be acceptable for treating chronic pain, there is no data at this point to suggest that is true.

We also don't know how long the drug stays effective in the body. When taken in, cannabinoids are stored in fat throughout the body, and then slowly released for up to a month from a single dose. Is a slowly released drug clinically useful? Is it clinically harmful? Are all cannabinoids released at similar rates? In other words, if a specific effect requires a specific formulation of cannabinoids in specific relative amounts, are the amounts released from fat stores in the same relative amounts over the month? The answers to these questions are unknown, but have huge implications for dosing and questions of efficacy and safety.

The final question is: do cannabinoids actually reduce pain or do they only allow the patient to tolerate it better? Does it really matter? In other words, if a medication allows someone to endure pain better, is that an effective use? Some say yes, others no. If the drug improves function, I would say that it is an effective use. As Michael Lee, lead researcher of Oxford University's Centre for Functional Magnetic Resonance Imaging of the Brain, has noted, "Cannabis does not seem to act like a conventional pain medicine. Some people respond really well, others not at all, or even poorly. Brain imaging shows little reduction in the brain regions that code for the sensation of pain, which is what we tend to see with drugs like opiates. Instead cannabis appears to mainly affect the emotional reaction to pain in a highly variable way." Researchers studying the effects of cannabis on specific brain functioning in pain patients found that an oral tablet of THC tended to make the experience of pain more bearable, instead of actually reducing the pain's intensity.[41] In making policy, we need to decide whether this effect is clinically meaningful. Not all believe it is, but I do. The goal of holistic management of pain is not to eliminate pain, but rather to help the patient adapt to it. Using various psychological techniques, we ask patients to learn not to focus on their pain, but rather to "put it to the side." We know that as pain is processed in the brain, an emotional signal is attached which greatly affects how the patient reacts to it. In the chronic pain state this reaction can be quite destructive. Cannabinoids seem to have the ability to dissociate this emotional response, which is the goal of therapy. In cases of refractory pain, this ability can be very helpful.

These questions must be resolved before cannabinoids or marijuana can be considered acceptable for medicinal use—assuming that the regulatory paradigms remain unchanged, an assumption which may turn out to be wrong if public opinion is taken into account.

FEDERAL POLICY

The collective point of view of the Executive Office of the President, the DEA, and the FDA is articulated in a 2013 statement from the Office of National Drug Control Policy:

> Marijuana itself is not an approved medicine under the Food and Drug Administration's (FDA) scientific review process. . . . To date, the FDA has not found smoked marijuana to be either safe or effective medicine for any condition. . . .
>
> No major medical association has come out in favor of smoked marijuana for widespread use. . . . The American Medical Association has called for more research on the subject with the caveat that this "should not be viewed as an endorsement of state-based cannabis programs, the legalization of marijuana, or that scientific evidence on the therapeutic use of cannabis meets the current standards for a prescription drug product."
>
> This Administration joins major medical societies in supporting increased research into marijuana's many components, delivered in a safe (non-smoked) manner, in the hopes they can be available for medical professionals to legally prescribe if proven safe and effective.[42]

On the surface, this policy would not seem to represent a substantial barrier. Like the policies of several states and most medical associations, it endorses research into the development of a uniform product that is safe and effective for well-defined conditions. While many would argue that the product's safety already has been demonstrated, few if any studies meet the FDA requirements for proving efficacy; and as we have seen, the drug cannot be considered reliable.[43]

Moreover, while the statement suggests that the federal government endorses research on this topic, in reality public policy creates significant barriers to it. Federal agencies have preferred to support studies of marijuana as a drug of abuse, not as a potential medical benefit. AIDS researcher Donald Abrams of the University of California at San Francisco said, "I don't think science drives the train here. . . . It's a difficult environment at the current time to get funding."[44]

Cannabis research is challenging because marijuana is a schedule I drug. The only legal marijuana in the United States is controlled by the National Institute on Drug Abuse (NIDA) of the National Institutes of Health. Most drugs in the United States are produced by private-sector businesses, often in partnership with the government or public or private universities. Drug companies require that such research result in a product they can bring to market and make a profit from. Current federal policy creates several significant barriers to achieving such an outcome with medicinal marijuana. First, any research involving marijuana first must be approved by the FDA. Second, once approved, the marijuana must be obtained from NIDA, which does not always provide it even for FDA-approved projects.[45] Finally, even if a product does overcome these hurdles, it may have no meaningful market because it will likely be labeled a schedule I drug. So in effect government policies discourage research. While many states currently allow medical marijuana, the product they are providing is not truly medicinal; and although at this writing the Obama administration Department of Justice was not enforcing federal law in these states, there is no reason to believe that a different administration will be so kind. This situation creates even more uncertainty for a potential medicinal marijuana product.

Igor Grant, director of California's Center for Medicinal Cannabis Research, has said, "The convergence of evidence makes me convinced there is a medical benefit here, and there may be a niche for cannabis." He added that the listing of marijuana as a schedule I drug—on a par with heroin and LSD—"is completely at odds with the existing science. It is intellectually dishonest to say it has no value whatsoever, because it's just not true."

STATE POLICY

As I noted, as of 2015 twenty-three states had legislation allowing medical marijuana, many others were in the process of creating such legislation, and four states have legalized marijuana for recreational purposes. While

I applaud their passion, there are many problems with their reasoning, and that creates another barrier.

The states have made an end run around federal policy by allowing unrefined marijuana to be smoked, eaten, or vaporized for a whole host of conditions. They have thus removed the incentives for developing safe and effective products. At the same time, after spending several months researching this topic, I have concluded that current federal policy is anti-intellectual and unreasonable, and that it has, in effect, forced the states to take the stance they have. Still, what the states have done is not right from a medical standpoint.

My greatest experience is with Colorado's law, since both of my sons attended college there. In Colorado, medical marijuana can be obtained with a doctor's prescription for a variety of conditions from a state-licensed dispensary, not a pharmacy. There is very little monitoring of the process or tracking of where the drugs are going.

The outcomes are predictable. In the beginning, there were very few dispensaries, and those who ran them had a certain passion for what they did. Once the Department of Justice chose not to challenge state laws, the number of dispensaries increased dramatically. Then a whole cottage industry of doctors arose to take advantage of some easy bucks. For a couple of hundred dollars, you can see one of these doctors, claim you have some condition, and he or she will sign your marijuana registry card, allowing you access to two ounces of marijuana. Within two weeks of their arrival in Colorado, my sons were educated on how to get "legal" marijuana. What was striking to me as a parent was the number of dispensaries located around the perimeter of their college campuses. I was not aware colleges were home to so many with intractable illnesses.

I participated in an American Pain Society subgroup that discussed this issue and noted that in the states which allow medical marijuana there is no good tracking of the marijuana or the physicians who prescribe it, nor is there is good data on what it is really being used for. In a BBC news story about Colorado's law, one grower said, "Ninety percent of the users probably do it for recreation."[46] Ed Gogek, an addiction psychiatrist, told the *New York Times* that the marijuana laws "were sold to more than a dozen states with promises that they're only for serious illnesses like cancer. But that's not how they work in practice. Almost all marijuana cardholders claim they need it for various kinds of pain, but pain is easy to fake and almost impossible to disprove. In Oregon and Colorado, 94 percent of cardholders get their pot for pain. In Arizona, it's 90 percent. Serious illnesses barely register."[47]

Most experts would agree that medical marijuana should most often be used as an adjunct to care and only rarely as a primary agent. Like opioids, it should be used as a part of an organized, comprehensive treatment approach, carried out by an experienced professional, that is documented and available for review. That is not what is happening. Too often there is no significant clinical assessment. There are no trials of alternative therapies. The patient wants pot, and the professional wants the revenue stream that comes with giving it to her.

In proving the clinical utility of new therapies, it is critical to do things right from the start. It is clear to me that what the states are doing now is not right and will forever harm the development of any potential uses of marijuana.

ORGANIZED HEALTH-CARE POLICY

Although I am an expert in pain management, before I wrote this chapter I knew next to nothing about marijuana. Since I began researching the subject, I have had a lot of informal conversations about it with colleagues. Usually they make giddy comments about past college experiences, and that is the limit of their knowledge. In fact, there is a marked discrepancy between the passion with which even experts approach this subject and their knowledge. Too often it is the passion that creates public policy, not sound reasoning. Misperceptions about medicinal marijuana and its risk-benefit ratio—especially the underestimating of that ratio—drive policy and create an unnecessary barrier for its potential use.

Before I began writing this chapter, I was a vocal opponent of medical marijuana. Now, armed with a lot more objective knowledge, I am an advocate, albeit a cautious one. What bothers me most is that in medical education, physicians are taught about marijuana only as a drug of abuse, not as a potential therapeutic agent. To compound the problem, those who wish to prescribe it as a pharmaceutical in the states where it is legal are never taught what to use it for or how to prescribe it. Sad to say, I have learned more from my patients about this. Is that not the tail wagging the dog?

PUBLIC MISPERCEPTION

It is dispiriting to know that marijuana policy is still driven by the misperceptions of the Hearst, Anslinger, and Dupont smear campaign. In the novel *I, Michael Bennett*, by James Patterson and Michael Ledwidge, Bennett is a New York City detective battling Mexican drug cartels and their infiltrates in the United States. To celebrate their successful drug busts, the men in blue hit the bars or go on picnics and have a few (too many) drinks. Michael Bennett is too good a guy to drink and drive, so he finds a ride. It is never specified how the others get home.

Alcohol is part of our culture. When we're happy, we celebrate by "having a few." When we're sad, we "drown our sorrows." Imagine that you're ready to celebrate something. Instead of handing your friend a beer, you hand him a joint. What do you think he would say? Most likely he would freak out. That seems odd considering that marijuana is less toxic than alcohol and probably less addictive. I like to ask people: suppose you were going to start a new society and could make all the rules. If you could choose only one vice—either alcohol or marijuana—which would you choose? The answer is almost always marijuana. When I ask why, the answer is always that the buzz is about the same and the side effects of alcohol are much worse.

While marijuana clearly has toxicity, we choose to look at that only in an absolute sense, not relative to the vices we prefer and protect. To protect us from this evil substance, we incarcerate millions and fight a drug war against it that probably causes much more harm than it prevents. It seems to me almost comical that the drug we seek to eliminate is substantially less toxic than those we use to celebrate. But until there is a more vocal majority in favor of marijuana, the status quo remains, and that is another barrier.

Solutions

All available evidence suggests that cannabinoids are safe relative to other pharmaceutical preparations and that they have potential benefits. I believe it is reasonable to develop appropriate pharmaceutical options, especially for pain management. But for this to be possible, a number of things must happen.

RECLASSIFY MARIJUANA AS A SCHEDULE II DRUG

While making marijuana and cannabinoids schedule II drugs would continue to acknowledge their potentially abusive nature, it also would acknowledge their potential safe, medicinal use *under appropriate medical supervision.* Such a change is reasonable at this time with respect to both efficacy and safety. This change would not legalize the medical use of marijuana, nor would it reconcile the incompatibility between state and federal laws. But it would dramatically increase the incentive for government, the pharmaceutical industry, and the scientific community to study and create potential safe uses of these drugs.

It must be recognized that safety is a relative concept; that is, marijuana must be judged in comparison to other pharmaceuticals. The individual needs of the patient also should be considered. For example, while marijuana may be inappropriate as the first drug of choice and a solo agent for treating an adolescent with back pain, it may be a great adjunctive agent for a patient suffering from pain from end-stage cancer. It is politically and medically unethical to fail to acknowledge this relativity. And as I noted, all the current scientific data suggest that cannabinoids are safe relative to other FDA-approved products such as opioids. Nevertheless, even with a change in DEA classification, marijuana should remain illegal under federal law until a product meets FDA standards.

RECONSIDER FDA STANDARDS

Given the substantial research obstacles marijuana faces in meeting FDA approval, plus the fact that current data suggest the raw product may be medicinally useful and safe, especially for end-of-life care, the FDA may need to consider a paradigm shift in the criteria it uses to judge potential pharmaceutical products. Such a shift would dramatically lower the barriers to bringing a product to market.

ALLOW RESEARCHERS TO GROW MARIJUANA FOR STUDY

Changing the classification will mean something only if the product is more readily available to pharmaceutical companies for study. It is not reasonable that the product is available from only a single government source and a single grower. For research to be productive, researchers must be given licenses to grow and develop their own product. This process can be regulated similarly to the way the government oversees the production of alcohol, tobacco, and opioid products.

IMMEDIATELY DEVELOP A MARIJUANA PROGRAM
FOR INTRACTABLE CONDITIONS

Concomitant with a change in DEA classification, I would recommend the immediate approval and development of a medical marijuana program for intractable conditions such as pain and end-of-life care, either as an adjunct or a first-line treatment for defined conditions. For such patients, the therapeutic risk-benefit ratio is favorable.

EXTEND FEDERAL TOLERATION
OF STATE PROGRAMS FOR TEN YEARS

Assuming the above changes are made at the federal level, it is imperative that the Department of Justice formally extend the current policy of not contesting any individual state's medicinal marijuana programs for a minimum of ten years. Any state that wishes to create such a policy in that ten-year period would be free to do so without federal interference. First, although it is apparent that many individuals are abusing current state policies, many patients are using these agents for appropriate medical reasons. It makes more sense to strengthen state policies than to deny these patients their right to compassionate care. Leaving future federal policy uncertain is not fair to them. Second, the pharmaceutical industry would have a sufficient period of time to develop more appropriate and specific cannabinoid preparations.

EDUCATE HEALTH-CARE PROFESSIONALS
ABOUT MEDICAL MARIJUANA

Medical education at all levels must be developed to teach health-care professionals about the risks, benefits, uses, misuses, and abuses of medical marijuana and how to prescribe it. Again, I am struck by how ignorant most health-care professionals are about this topic, including those who do prescribe it or look the other way when they learn that their patients are using it. You cannot effectively prescribe any therapy or counsel any patients on its use unless you understand it yourself.

IMPROVE STATE POLICIES

It is critical that state policies, which are not working now, be dramatically improved. I don't believe this is a challenging problem, and it can be done in three ways:

1. First, a separate license should be required to prescribe marijuana, as is currently the case for methadone and buprenorphine for opioid detoxification and in some states for opioid prescription for pain. In order to be licensed, health-care providers take an online or in-person course and pass an examination.

2. Second, there must be some sort of oversight. I recommend adopting a set of guidelines similar to the Federation of State Medical Boards guidelines for responsible opioid prescribing referred to in chapter 13.[48] Among other requirements, these guidelines provide for a comprehensive diagnostic and treatment plan, obtaining informed consent, periodic assessments of advancement toward therapeutic goals, and referrals to specialists when necessary.

3. Appropriate oversight of health-care providers by the state medical board and of patients by appropriate regulatory agencies is also necessary, with compliance with these guidelines as the litmus test, the same as for opioids. Prescriptions must be tracked just as opioids are. Minimal specific information should include who is prescribing, who is the patient, what condition is being treated, and what doses and amounts of the drugs are being used. Currently none of this occurs, which almost ensures that these drugs will be used inappropriately.

These simple changes—already in place for opioids—would guarantee that those who prescribe are motivated more by a genuine compassion born of knowledge of therapeutic options than by ignorant passion or greed. Morgan Kier, cofounder of Top Shelf Dispensary in Boulder, Colorado, remarked, "Colorado will be the standard that states all over the country will follow. It's important to get it right the first time."[49] They didn't, and as a result, too many are abusing the privilege of medicinal marijuana.

SCRUTINIZE MARIJUANA SUPPLIERS

Currently, many states license dispensaries. While there are standards, they seem to be minimal. I am not opposed to dispensaries, but I believe they must be held to the same standards as pharmacies. It makes more sense for pharmacies to be the distributors since they already are licensed to distribute pharmaceuticals, track prescriptions, and report irregularities.

LIMIT PRESCRIPTIONS TO ADULTS

Except in the case of end-stage disease, medicinal marijuana prescription should be limited to those over the age of twenty-one. There is sufficient evidence to raise concern about the adverse long-term effects of marijuana on brain function in adolescents. In reality, we know that brain function probably does not fully mature until age twenty-three, so one would be safer in using that age as more appropriate.

DECRIMINALIZE MEDICAL USE WITHOUT A PRESCRIPTION

It is inappropriate to punish those who use marijuana medicinally without a prescription for one of its many indications, such as pain. These users should no longer be punished merely for trying to survive. Often, they are not addicted, but rather pseudoaddicted, which is frequently the result of a health-care provider's unwillingness to listen to these individuals and take them seriously. The patient should not be punished for the ignorance of the caregivers.

Recreational Marijuana

Medical marijuana and recreational marijuana are not the same thing. As a final note, I want to add that my research and observations have convinced me that recreational marijuana, in moderation, is certainly no more dangerous than alcohol, and probably less so. I do believe it is hypocritical for a culture so wedded to alcohol to continue to prohibit marijuana, especially given that the prohibition is based largely on myth and that the carnage current marijuana laws have inflicted is disgraceful. Millions have been incarcerated, their records scarred permanently. The war on this particular drug has created far more harm than it has prevented.

A majority of Americans believe the drug should be legalized. At the very minimum, it should be decriminalized. If legalized, it should be regulated in the same manner as alcohol. Certainly there will be problems, but it is extremely difficult to argue that these will be worse than the problems created by alcohol.

At the same time, we should not lose sight of the fact that the recreational drug is functionally not the same as the medical drug, and we still need to research the drug to identify products that are safe and effective medicinally, with a minimum of psychomimetic effects.

At a meeting in the mid-2000s, an investigator proudly announced that a cure for pain was around the corner. A chemical isolated from the venom of a frog found in the rain forests of South America was exponentially more powerful than morphine and had fewer side effects, he explained, and it was only a matter of time before it was available. We are still waiting. While we spend millions, if not billions, of dollars on research on all the wonderful drugs that surely await us in the rain forest, I find it odd that we limit our study of the potential medical uses of one of the most plentiful plants in the world, one that is right under our nose at almost every college party in the country. Perhaps it is time.

FIFTEEN

Health-Care Reform and Chronic Pain

We All Have a Role to Play

You're either part of the solution or you're part of the problem.
Charles Rosner, VISTA recruitment slogan (1967)

Chapter 10 described the history of health insurance in the United States and the various attempts at reforming a system that is in financial trouble, most recently via the PP/ACA. I emphasized specifically how this system affects the person with a chronic disability, such as chronic pain. Throughout, the focus was on the role government and private insurers have played in this process. But nothing is ever that simple, and I do not believe we should assume that reform is purely the prerogative of the government. We all have a role to play.

Imagine you and a friend are going out to dinner. The bill will be paid by someone you don't know, nor does your benefactor know either of you. You have the freedom to pick any restaurant and order whatever you want. Would you order responsibly, or spend lavishly?

This scenario (which has been called the "three-party system") is exactly what has been going on in the American health-care system since the inception of medical insurance. The benefactor paying the bill is the insurer: either the government (Medicare and Medicaid) or an insurance company. The diners are the health-care provider and the patient. With limited responsibility for paying the bill, they spend too lavishly, each arguing that it is in the patient's best interest to do so. That is often not true, especially with regard to pain. Even though the patient's condition cannot be cured, he demands a cure, including access to any therapy that may provide even a glimmer of hope. As we have seen, the physician, increasingly under the control of a corporate manager, profits greatly from providing what are often heavily reimbursed procedures. Yet this very profitable care is fragmented and inefficient, and does not provide the best care for the patient.

Insurers are increasingly trying to find ways to control this wasteful and expensive patient and physician behavior. Government insurers impose expensive, challenging regulations. Private insurers examine every treatment decision, often denying care—in effect, rationing care—and transferring the cost of care to the patient through high deductibles and co-pays. Although the goal is to lower costs, the result is the opposite. Regulations cost time and money. Challenging denials also costs time and money, two things that are lacking in pain management. High costs encourage patients to defer or avoid care until they are desperate and the problem less treatable. In theory, the PP/ACA has increased access to insurance for all patients, including those with chronic pain. However, I contend that in reality, access to care for these patients has decreased.

As I noted, the history of health-care reform is marked by unintended consequences. Our futile attempts at reform have made health care worse, although it is not always the attempt at reform that creates the problem. Often the problem is caused by the circling of the wagons that occurs in response by those with a stake in the status quo. Each party wants change, but is only willing to accept it if someone else pays the price. Each seeks to protect its own interest. Much work is done, at great cost. The powerful control the discussion and take advantage of the weak. In the end, nothing changes; or worse, the powerful further increase their control of the system, while the weak, the functionally oppressed, sink further into despair. I believe health-care reform can occur only if all parties are willing to give up something. It is sad that our excessively competitive society sees compromise as a weakness, a loss. It is only when we come to the table willing to give and take openly and honestly that real progress can occur.

When I went into private practice, I quickly saw how inefficient our system was. Patients waited weeks to get in to see a doctor, then more weeks between tests and treatments. The system was far more frustrating for patients than for doctors, since doctors were busy and the dollars flowed in. Pain patients had virtually no clout. They were not organized. Most got better despite our ministrations, and when their condition improved, they had little or no incentive to come together as a cohesive group to create a more powerful voice. I learned that chronic pain patients, ridiculed as they are, are often too embarrassed to come together. For example, we now know that fibromyalgia is a legitimate, debilitating problem. There is objective evidence to support it. Yet I still counsel patients not to mention the word *fibromyalgia* when seeing a new doctor because many physicians do not accept the diagnosis as real and assume the patient has a psychiatric condition, not worthy of the physician's time. You only get one chance to make a first impression. If you are not believed, you have no voice. Chronic pain patients have no voice.

In those early days, I believed we could change how we did things, at least in my town. We had all the pieces of the pain management puzzle in place: doctors, surgeons, physical therapists, vocational rehabilitation specialists, emergency personnel, rehabilitation managers, and so on. I had a vision that we could all come together to create an efficient system. I spent hours diagramming that system. Patients would flow into a central triage setting staffed by various doctors. Their problem would be assessed. These doctors would manage the system and distribute referrals to the various therapists and specialists in our community.

I discussed my plans with many, including the local hospital administration. We organized a meeting. I was surprised by how many people came. I later learned that if you threaten someone's place in the status quo, she will show up, more to defend her own position than to promote the cause. As a colleague and I traveled to the meeting, he said he wanted to brief me, since he felt he understood the pulse of the community better. He looked at my notes and suggested that he should present the plan. I very reluctantly agreed.

Listening to his presentation, I realized the plan was dead. He had every intention of killing it, since he saw it as affecting his income stream. His personal needs and those of many around the table took precedence, and I lacked the power to overcome that.

If we cannot work together at a local level, how can we do so at a national level?

The Patient Protection/Affordable Care Act: A Starting Point

The PP/ACA, or "Obamacare," tries to balance the free market, with its tendency toward self-interest, with government control. I think the act does this to some extent, but it also puts too much control in the hands of the federal government. The question is whether the law improves access, decreases cost (or at least slows the rate of growth), and improves quality. My concern is specifically how it improves care for people in pain.

Chapter 10 discussed how the PP/ACA addresses (or does not address) issues of cost and access. Here I would like to discuss how its unintended consequences actually increase cost and decrease real access, especially for those with complicated medical problems such as chronic pain.

A significant issue is that the law does not even address the factors that accelerate costs: that is, malpractice costs, overregulation, and excess use of electronic technology. In fact, the law dramatically increases regulatory and information-technology requirements such as billing procedures and electronic health records (EHR), all of which greatly increase the complexity of practice, divert money from care, and do nothing to improve quality of care.

To take one example, the current EHR used throughout the country is nothing short of a joke. It does virtually nothing to actually communicate medical information. Its structure is set up to comply with Medicare billing requirements, such as the concept of "meaningful use" (meaning that the provider needs to show he is using technology in ways specified by the government), and to minimize medical-legal risk. In other words, what should be the primary tool physicians use to think about medical problems and communicate their thoughts to patients and other doctors gets hijacked by the needs of the business and its bottom line and the regulatory requirements of the government.

To comply with all these new requirements, offices need to train more staff, buy expensive software, and hire consultants to help them be compliant. The result is an acceleration of the process of corporatization, with all its problems. Technology pools may help by allowing several practices to share resources, just as they shared on-call responsibilities in the past. However, I have seen nothing in the law that proposes help for such a solution.

An even bigger question is: who will take care of all these patients? We already have a shortage of primary care providers and a substantial shortage of health-care professionals trained to treat physical and psychological disabilities. When the PP/ACA's individual mandate (the requirement that most people have health insurance) came into effect, Gallup Poll numbers indicated that 17.1 percent of the *adult* U.S. population, or 41.5 million people, were uninsured. This figure does not include those under eighteen, who make up roughly 23 percent of the population. As of March 2015, the number of uninsured had decreased to 11.9 percent of adults, or twenty-nine million.[1] In theory, if the ACA were to be fully effective, all these individuals would be insured and would enter the health-care market.

In order to stay financially viable, physicians are already forced to see more patients per unit time. Will they be forced to see even more per unit time, as they are in socialized medicine programs? The act greatly expands Medicare and Medicaid and promises to decrease Medicare expenditures. But these two programs are not financially viable now and do not reimburse physicians sufficiently to cover costs and deliver a reasonable rate of return (Medicaid being worse). Because of this, many physicians do not accept either insurance now. If these programs are expanded, who will take care of those patients? Since most disabled patients are covered by these insurances, who will spend the time with them that they need? To offset this inevitable trend, some experts involved in the initial planning of Obamacare suggested that physicians who did not accept these insurances receive draconian punishments such as fines or criminal prosecution. They did not say who would be there to help when medical offices went bankrupt. Fortunately, this measure was not included in the final bill, and it is likely that someone (probably not physicians, who are often not good at business) will find a way to make practices that accept Medicare and Medicaid financially viable. This means that the PP/ACA will actually accelerate the trends toward corporatization, specialization, and bottom-line medicine.

What concerns me more is that the law does not rebalance the medical pyramid. It does not provide incentives for physicians to manage complex problems or care for people with chronic illness. It does not give young physicians incentives to go into what I have called tier I (primary) or tier II (management of complex psychological and physical disability) care. In fact, it actually deters them from doing so, and the result is increased fragmentation of care for people with complex problems. Those who suffer from chronic illness will continue to suffer.

At least for my patients, the PP/ACA's creation of state exchanges has not been beneficial. I really thought that opening state borders to outside insurers would promote competition, lower costs, and increase portability, which is a good thing. I don't believe that any more. Competition was supposed to lower consumer costs. That did not happen. Instead, there is an increasing trend toward national health-care oligopolies replacing local oligopolies. Our local hospital recently hired a consultant to advise on steps it should take to fit into the changing health-care environment. He explained that within ten years, health care would be dominated by fifty to sixty conglomerates and claimed that one such conglomerate now controls 125 hospitals "and still has not reached its economy of scale." However, economy of scale is not the appropriate measure here. The greater the economy of scale, the less personal decision making becomes. When you cannot see the face of the person your decisions affect, your decisions will be flawed. There is nothing good about this trend, and it needs to be stopped. I fear the consequences for those who cost the most, those in pain.

By its sheer weight, its burdensome regulations, its adverse effects on small practices, its failure to solve the inefficiencies of our current frag-mented model of medicine, and its overemphasis on expensive medical information technologies, the PP/ACA will most certainly increase cost in both human and dollar terms. Nevertheless, I see it as a start, a first step. But there are many more steps to take.

Solutions: All Parties Play a Role

Solutions begin with teamwork, and the key to teamwork is the willingness to put the needs of the whole above the needs of the self. So the solution begins with the individual, which is to say all of us. I recall attending a speech Hillary Clinton gave to a group of physicians in 1993 at Dartmouth College as she began her attempt to sell "Hillary-Care." In her closing re-marks, she admonished us to provide only services we felt were necessary and charge a fee that was reasonable. Every time I circle a charge on a billing form, I think of those words and ask: "What would I be willing to pay for that service?"

From this perspective, it seems almost comical to see all the characters in our national health-care debate point the finger at others to assign blame and responsibility. We argue whether the solution should be provided by the government or by the private market. Democrats and Republicans choose sides and refuse to budge. I recall a dear old friend, Jo Adcock, who ran a district committee I sat on. Every time someone whined or complained about her committee or another, she would say: "If you don't like it, stop whining and join the committee and fix it. If you aren't going to, stop whining and support those who will do it!"

Instead of asking who is responsible, we should ask, "What can I do to help?" Relevant parties include all the players I have described. But I focus here on doctors, corporate health-care providers, patients, insurance companies, and the government. Each has a hand in resolving this dilemma. The following discussion does not define specific policy proposals. I will leave that to those more gifted than I. Instead, I will outline what I see as the responsibilities of those involved in reforming our health-care system.

PHYSICIANS

Responsibility begins with honesty, and physicians must honestly acknowledge what they can offer a patient, what action will realistically help, and when no further therapy is likely to be helpful. They also must realize that they offer care, not product lines. Market share and the bottom line should be secondary considerations.

Physicians need to be more educated about the costs of their services. I am amazed at how often doctors offer a high-priced therapy when a lower-priced one would work as well if not better. Often they are oblivious to the relative costs of each. Frequently, a patient is referred to me for an expensive procedure when a simple prescription was not tried first.

Physicians can behave responsibly only when they better understand the problem they are treating. Medical schools need to step up to the plate here. The misguided care that results from physicians' ignorance about pain—the symptom that 75 percent of patients present with—not only costs many excess dollars but also dooms patients to receive fragmented, ineffective care. In this respect I am concerned by the trends in medical education. For example, in 2013 the physical medicine and rehabilitation residency program in which I received my training and first learned how to care for people with complex disabilities was closed by the university so that residency positions could be reallocated to more lucrative specialties. This is penny-wise and pound-foolish and should not be tolerated, especially when age and disability are increasing in our population.

It is quite clear that change in medical education will not occur without incentives, a fact emphasized by the 2011 Institute of Medicine report, *Relieving Pain in America*. Based on this report, grants were awarded to several universities to create programs to teach pain management to doctors and other health-care professionals. Education is also one of the pillars of the National Pain Strategy which, as of February 2016, is in the final stages of development. These actions represent only a start, though. The education component also must include postgraduate education (continuing medical education, or CME). While making CME mandatory for a specific topic, such as pain, is unusual, physicians already in practice and denied access to this important area of training need to catch up, and this may be the only way to do it. I believe positive incentives, such as tax breaks or grants to cover the cost of this training, are always better. However, if these measures do not inspire physicians to educate themselves about pain, negative reinforcement may be needed. In New Hampshire, physicians were required to sign up for the prescription monitoring program. If they did not, they could not renew their medical licenses. States could use a similar tactic for pain management. All health-care providers would need to demonstrate a baseline level of competency, which online educational technology has made easier to achieve than in the past. Similarly, positive and negative incentives can be used to ensure that CME programs such as national meetings allocate a bare minimum of time on pain-related issues pertinent to a given specialty.

CORPORATE HEALTH-CARE PROVIDERS

As I have explained, many physicians are now employed by corporations, whose primary goal is not the welfare of the patient but that of the bottom line. Physicians are judged on "productivity," that is, money generation; and the number of patients they must see per unit time and what they can do in that time is controlled. Poorly remunerative specialties such as psychiatry, psychology, and pain management are either eliminated or minimized. Often they are left to less well-trained allied health-care professionals, frequently with little oversight.

These trends must change. I recognize that given the dramatic increase in the cost and complexity of practicing medicine, corporatization is a necessary evil. But these corporate employers do not need to behave like traditional businesses. The first change must be to recognize the importance of specialties such as mental health, addiction, and pain management. Next, the corporate provider needs to include these areas within its health-care framework. I hope that, in the long term, insurers will reimburse these services more appropriately. In the short term, however, the revenue from more lucrative specialties, such as surgery, can be used to offset losses from these other important specialties.

Corporate providers also must recognize that assessment and management of complicated problems, such as chronic pain, cannot be limited to a ten-minute time slot. Providers treating such patients must be given time to do what is needed.

Finally, corporate providers must create a more meaningful electronic health record. It is not difficult. My medical group has done it. The primary focus remains the purpose of the patient visit, the communication engendered, the thought process in patient management, the recommendations made, and the results. While I believe that "meaningful use" should be abolished as an excessive invasion by government into the private medical market, it is also possible to achieve compliance without making it the focus of the record as it is now.

PATIENTS

Patients do not play a passive role in controlling health-care access and cost. Because they are consumers who vote with their dollars, they play a very big role. But they must be willing to accept the realities of health care today.

First, patients must recognize that we cannot solve every medical problem. They must have realistic expectations and take more responsibility for their use of the health-care system. It is not an "all you can eat" buffet of unlimited therapies. It can be a challenge to encourage such responsibility without creating a disincentive to seek care when necessary, but it can be done by rewarding responsible behavior such as exercise, preventive health-care checks, smoking cessation, and alcohol avoidance. Insurance companies are already doing this by lowering premiums for those who engage in healthy habits, paying a percentage of health club fees, lowering the costs of routine physicals, and so forth. To the argument that giving individuals an economic stake in their health-care decisions by requiring that they pay a certain percentage of their medical bills will discourage them from seeking care when sick, and their untreated illness will cost more in the long run, I respond that the system can be structured so as to eliminate such disincentives. For example, we can limit deductibles for preventive and minor illness care and provide a safety net for catastrophic care. Nonemergency care for less-disabling conditions should be rationed.

It amazes me how many patients could afford health insurance if they used the money they now waste on alcohol, cigarettes, and junk food to pay for it. Health and medical savings accounts may be helpful, but policies with high deductibles are not, since they make patients reluctant to seek help until a problem gets out of control or they have sufficient funds in their account. Lower deductibles for preventive and catastrophic care would help minimize this effect.

Second, patients must realize that everyone benefits when all citizens insure their health. Public education commercials are already used in all media to explain that uninsured people who need care create substantial costs not only for the health-care system, but also in lost productivity, which must be borne by the rest of us. We need to encourage people in all age groups to think not just microeconomically (the self), but also macroeconomically (the big picture). For example, while going uninsured may make sense microeconomically in the short run, in the long run, as we have seen, when lots of young people do this, insurance premiums rise for all; and the young will find themselves facing this cost when they are no longer so young. Paying in when we are healthy and don't need services will be offset in the years when we are not so healthy. In fact, most health-care costs occur in the last two years of life, when we are the least productive. While some political conservatives argue that requiring individuals to pay into the system is not consistent with capitalism, many states require car owners to have auto insurance. Why should health insurance not be the same?

Despite the saying "your lack of preparation is not my emergency," few in our country would be willing to completely remove the safety net for these uninsured. However, those who can afford to should pay for health insurance. Costs are lowered when everyone pays in to the collective risk pool, and it is the rare individual who will never utilize health insurance. Is it fair to the system for someone not to pay in when he does not require care, and then later use excessive resources?

Schools can include personal management/responsibility courses to teach the young not only how to manage money and insure themselves, but also why it is important—not just for themselves, but for all of us. I have heard that a message must be given seven times before the average person retains it. Considering the importance of the health-care message, it should be repeated regularly, from junior high through college. But education alone is not enough. People need an incentive such as imposing meaningful fines on those who go uninsured. Over the first fifteen months of Obamacare, this incentive had some success in decreasing the number of uninsured, as the previous figures indicate, but the effect was modest and there is a long way to go.

INSURERS

Although the government has played an increasing role in health-care insurance over the past decades, we still function in a market-driven economy where each corporate entity is free to maximize its bottom line, subject to governmental regulation where appropriate. Our version of the market economy has long since abandoned the edict "Let the buyer beware." Rather, we seek to protect the consumer from the excesses of the free market through a mix of government regulation and private consumer advocacy.

Given this situation, it is reasonable to expect that the health insurance industry provide coverage for as many patients as possible at the lowest possible cost. Companies have the right to make a reasonable return on their investment, but they also have the responsibility not to let their self-interest harm the customer. However, the further the boardroom is from the front lines of health care, the less likely it is that high-risk patients, such as pain patients, will be adequately covered.

With respect to cost and access, which are not mutually exclusive, the insurance industry must address four issues: rapidly rising deductibles and co-pays, the increasing use of prior approval for care, portability of care, and inclusion of preexisting conditions.

Rising Deductibles and Co-pays   While the PP/ACA does increase access to health insurance, rapidly rising deductibles and co-pays prevent patients from using it, in effect blocking access to health care. In the not-too-distant past, a $1,000 deductible was considered high. Now it is the norm. According to a 2014 study from the Kaiser Family Foundation, in 2006 fewer than 10 percent of workers had deductibles of $1,000. As of 2014, the number was 41 percent and rising; the average deductible was $2,000 or more for single coverage and $2,000–$4,500 for families.[2] "A recent Commonwealth Fund survey found that four in ten working-age adults skipped some kind of care because of the cost, and other surveys have found much the same. The portion of workers with annual deductibles—what consumers must pay before insurance kicks in—rose from 55 percent eight years ago to 80 percent today."[3] The causes of this disturbing trend are multifactorial and beyond the scope of this discussion. But I see its consequences every day in the form of insured patients forgoing medical treatments because they cannot afford them. Prompt, interdisciplinary care, so important in preventing and treating chronic pain, is more and more difficult to provide because of cost. The insurance industry must work in collaboration with business and the government to find solutions to reverse this trend.

Prior Approval   Prior approval (PA) means that an insurer reviews any or all treatment plans before agreeing to cover them, usually with stipulations. Private insurers are increasingly using PAS to control health-care costs. I work with two companies that do this. One is a private company that runs a managed Medicaid fund for our state. The other is a commercial insurer. The former uses PAS to place seemingly insurmountable barriers in patients' way, and many are too faint of heart to persevere. Often they give up without ever receiving care. The latter uses PAS more rationally, but often supports its decisions with a questionable evidence base. Both companies' approval processes require excessive physician or staff time and cost to implement.

   I am not opposed to PAS as a means of controlling cost. I do think it is incumbent on me, as a doctor, to explain the potential cost-effectiveness of my treatment decisions, and a PA forces me to think before I act. However, to prevent it from being a barrier to care, the approval process must be quick, convenient for the user, and rational. There is nothing quick about the Medicaid process I mentioned above. Decisions take weeks, sometimes months. The commercial company makes a decision in hours. If I disagree, I can appeal to a live physician within days. That is the way the process should work. The problem there is that the representatives must use an evidence base that is advantageous to the insurer. As chapter 6 explained, there are significant limits to evidence-based medicine, and the criteria the insurance company relies on must respect these limits and be reasonable. For example, a friend of mine has a chronic condition that includes chronic pain. He has been in physical therapy more often than not over the past few years. When he had a severe exacerbation that made him unable to work, his doctor wanted to get an MRI to find out what was going on. The insurer required my friend to go through another six weeks of PT before it would approve the MRI. Why? Because that is what the evidence-based algorithm required. But in my friend's case this made no sense, and he suffered needlessly until they made their decision. In order for PAS to be adaptive and responsive, the reviewing physician must be given the ability to "think outside the box" when necessary, and this does not happen in either of these plans.

Portability of Care   The PP/ACA provides for portability, so that if you relocate, your insurance is supposed to come with you. But it is not so simple. Few private insurance companies have a national presence, so when you move, you must find new coverage; and if you have chronic pain or another expensive health problem, that may not be so easy (see the following section). This is interregional portability. However, portability may be a local issue as well, which I call intraregional portability. President Obama, when promoting the PP/ACA, promised numerous times that if you liked your doctor, you could keep her. But that has turned out not to be true. Changing insurance plans is still a yearly burden for many individuals who do not move. Often their physician is not included in the new plan, and they must find a new doctor. This is especially a problem for people with complex medical problems, for whom continuity of care is so crucial. I doubt that the creators of the PP/ACA envisioned these difficulties.

The ACA's requirement that all citizens be insured and its provision of a way to obtain insurance did address the problem of interregional portability. However, intraregional portability remains a problem, which can only be solved if all local physicians are included in all plans within a given region—a solution that may challenge some insurers' desire to control physician behavior. For intraregional portability to be effective, all local physicians must participate, and that requires the terms of the agreement between the physician and the insurer to be reasonable. Often, however, physicians decide not to participate in a plan because they consider the terms of an agreement unreasonable. For example, our group does not participate with one insurer because it requires that providers outside its network send a written office note within twenty minutes of a visit. The norm for sending such a note is twenty-four to forty-eight hours. Even in the most efficient medical office, it is nearly impossible to see a patient, dictate a report, get it to a typist, get the report back to the doctor for review, fix any changes, and send it back to the secretary for faxing in one day, much less in twenty minutes. Significantly, this insurer does not impose this requirement on its in-network providers. By making an impossible demand on the out-of-network provider, the insurer effectively controls its provider network. This practice should not be allowed. I believe the health-care system is strongest when all providers belong to it, which means that for this model to work, insurers must give up some control.

Removal of Preexisting Conditions   To make portability effective, the PP/ACA prohibits insurance companies from discriminating based on preexisting conditions. On paper, that is a win for those with chronic and expensive health problems, such as chronic pain. But it is not always so in practice. You can let a person in the door, but you don't have to let him eat. Through creative use of PAS and other limitations, insurers can control what services an individual may receive. The PP/ACA requires that the insurer provide only certain services, such as preventive services, without a co-pay or deductible. Anything else is fair game for manipulation by the insurer. Even though the patient is insured, he or she may not be able to afford certain services or may have important services denied, such as my friend's MRI. The health-care system only works when all patients are treated equally and with respect, and the insurance companies must take responsibility for doing so.

In the end, I accept insurance companies' need to be profitable. If we took that away, they would cease to exist, and I have no faith that government, state or federal, could fill the void left behind. However, insurers have a responsibility not just to stockholders and policyholders, but also to our society, and it is incumbent on them to resolve the issues I have outlined if we are to keep our health-care system solvent for the long term.

GOVERNMENT

I believe that all sectors of our economy should be involved in solving this problem. It seems silly to me to totally dismantle the market-driven health-care system merely to solve our cost and access issues. It would make more sense to modify the system we have. Even in a market-driven economy, there is much government can do to lower cost and improve access.

Reduce Regulations   First, as I have said, health care is drastically overregulated. The excess cost created by making these regulations, informing the populace of them, and enforcing them is staggering. Excess regulation creates a climate of fear among medical practitioners, especially given the threat of jail time or large fines for noncompliance. Most regulations are created out of a shortsighted need to solve a specific issue, with little thought to the long-term ramifications. As a result, physicians have no incentive to care for challenging patients such as pain patients, who "reimburse" poorly and take up too much time.

While we would like our legal and regulatory systems to have an answer for every question, that is clearly not possible. The costs associated with unintended consequences, in both financial and human terms, are staggering. I am concerned about the federal government's increasing involvement in the health-care sector. Its micromanagement with a strangling, ever-growing network of regulations seems to me inefficient and not responsive to the needs of individual localities. Micromanaging assumes that supervisors do not trust "supervisees" and creates great resentment. It also limits innovation and self-initiative. The health-care sector, as well as other sectors, works better when we give individuals the ball and let them run with it. That is the beauty of a market-based approach. Thus I believe that responsibility for health care should be returned to the individual states and individual providers, who are also in a much better position to assess the needs of their citizens.

Take the concept of "meaningful use," referred to previously. The public health system, a part of the federal government, decided to create a computerized network to gather public health information for various purposes, to be obtained from individual health-care providers. In order to make this system work, all providers had to computerize their practice and create an electronic health record that included a number of "meaningful use" criteria intended to satisfy the needs of the public health community. None of these criteria had anything to do with providing high-quality, efficient care. On the contrary, they actually made it harder to do so. The incentive was that Medicare reimbursement would be withheld from anyone not in compliance. It is not at all clear to me that the excessive cost of complying is worth the information being collected. But given that medical practices are increasingly struggling financially, doctors cannot afford not to comply, and most do. I know of a few brave souls who aren't.

Unfortunately, "meaningful use" criteria are only the beginning. I attended a public policy meeting on the National Pain Strategy, where many participants were academicians and federal policy bureaucrats. In response to the need for more data, their knee-jerk response was to add a few more "meaningful use" questions for clinicians to assess at each visit, again adding great cost to the health-care provider and distracting from the doctor-patient relationship.

There is nothing sensible about this process, and it ends up costing way more than is reasonable for questionable ends. The commonsense solution would be for bureaucrats to sit down with providers in the trenches, give them a wish list of what they need, decide what is reasonable in terms of time and cost, and create a policy that would be doable. Instead, government actions such as these threaten the existence of private practice, accelerate the cost of practicing medicine, increase the trends toward corporatization and fragmentation of medicine, and reduce the efficiency and quality of health care.

Balance Private Insurance and Government-Provided Services   Regulation is only one way the government gets involved in health care. Government also provides services. This arrangement raises the question of what level of government can most efficiently provide care. Currently, the federal government administers Medicare and the state governments administer Medicaid. Local governments also provide some assistance.

I do not know exactly what the most effective combination of public and private forms of health care should be; but as I have said, I believe that regional problems such as health care are best handled by state and local governments with support from the federal government. When large systems become too big and impersonal, they become expensive; when the right hand doesn't know what the left hand is doing, they replicate unnecessarily. More important, the farther the locus of control of the system is from those served, the less responsive it is to each individual's needs. Therefore, health issues should be delegated to the states—or to regions of the more populous states—much as we currently manage education and Medicaid.

What is more, overhauling the American health-care system is in effect an enormous experiment that could explode in our faces at great cost. To me it makes more sense to experiment on a smaller scale at the state level, with incentives provided by federal funding. While an error at this level still has a cost, it creates substantially less harm. States and local governments could learn from each other by sharing their experiences.

I referred previously to the danger that creating insurance exchanges and lowering interstate barriers to out-of-state insurers in order to increase intrastate competition (which in many states does not exist) would lead to the development of national oligopolies controlling the private health-care market. Yet state regulation of private insurance companies already has created virtual monopolies in many states because only a few companies can meet the state's requirements. A competitive, market-driven system is supposed to allow consumers to control price by purchasing products based on cost and quality. In a monopoly there is no competition, and the supplier can control cost and quality. I do appreciate that the ACA allows the states to set up an insurance environment which respects the wishes of the residents of each state, and I do think each state should oversee its own system. I also think, in theory, that allowing interstate competition could be a good thing. However, it is quite clear to me that the system, as it is evolving, is not working in the manner intended, and that it needs to be tweaked by both state and federal governments to maximize competition.

Reform the Tort System   Finally, it is imperative that all levels of government address the excesses of an out-of-control tort system, which as I have said creates excess costs through burdensome regulations and risk management behaviors. While much attention has been paid to the crises the tort system has created in the fields of obstetrics and neurosurgery, a similar, though less apparent, crisis exists in pain management. Because pain patients pose both a tort risk and a criminal risk for health-care providers, they struggle to find providers willing to care for them. How does one measure the cost that a lack of care creates?

One such cost is that patients file civil suits against their doctors for lack of care or insufficient pain management. This trend creates a frightening dynamic. The possibility of being sued for overtreating *or* undertreating puts the rank-and-file doctor in a perilous position that often requires the assistance of a pain specialist—but such practitioners are frequently not available. I have often asked myself, who in their right mind would choose such a specialty? I must be insane.

Perhaps we could divert a small portion of the funds devoted to defensive medicine to educating patients so they are in a better position to make their own health-care decisions. We can do this in a variety of ways; for example, by distributing state and federal money as grants to public and private entities that would create educational programs in various media. This money would have two sources. First, it would be diverted from the current state and federal budgets allocated to court costs. An ounce of prevention in the form of education would eliminate a pound of court cases. Second, insurers pay user or registration fees for the right to operate in any area. A portion of these fees could be dedicated for this purpose. Such education would enable people to recognize that all medical decisions entail risk. This empowerment of the patient should be considered a necessary part of the doctor-patient relationship. It could substantially reduce error, adverse outcomes, and medical expenditures.

Should We Ration Care?

In addition to deciding who should pay for care, we need to decide whether we should ration care to limit costs. Some advocates support a single-payer health plan similar to those in other countries. To provide universal access, many of those countries not only levy high taxes but also ration care. All must pay into the system, but no one has unlimited access to services. I believe that we must do the same, although perhaps with a more market-driven approach. In certain ways we are already doing so. For example, the PP/ACA provides for no deductible for preventive services, but standard deductibles for optional treatments. Prior approval is another way of rationing care. Many insurance companies list in their fine print what they will and will not cover. For example, most will not cover cosmetic surgery, but many will allow breast reduction if there is a demonstrated health problem such as back pain. I believe we need to build on these approaches. The challenge is to ration effectively without creating barriers to needed care. This is particularly challenging in pain management, since the evidence base (used as the tool for rationing in other fields) is lacking and the concept of "medically reasonable and necessary" is murky.

It might be argued that rationing is draconian. But in fact it is part and parcel of any economic system. An economic system is simply the way a society chooses to allocate scarce resources. Our refusal to make tough choices and our irresponsible funding of our excesses through selling debt are creating a national deficit that will destroy us, and our health-care excesses are part of the problem. Health care accounted for 17.16 percent of our gross domestic product in 2013, or $2.87 trillion,[4] and the total increases every year. This trajectory cannot continue. Controlling our spending is a national emergency, perhaps more pressing than the challenges posed after Pearl Harbor was bombed and after the September 11 attacks. Osama Bin Laden likened the United States economy to a stack of cards that would collapse with a mere flick of a finger. I worry that he was right and that our wasteful, excessive spending will destroy us.

Righting the Inverted Pyramid

Our current overspecialization has provided an inefficient system—the inverted pyramid of health care—in which no one provider takes on the responsibility of caring for the whole person. The system can be righted only by creating incentives for doctors to go into primary care and by giving primary care doctors more control over the care of their patients.

Providing incentives for young physicians to go into tiers I and II and for older tier I and II physicians to stay in those fields, empowering those physicians to manage care, and limiting referrals to expensive specialists to cases when they are really necessary will lower costs, decrease fragmentation, and improve efficiency of care. We can achieve these reforms by increasing medical students' exposure to these important fields, subsidizing the education of those who make a commitment to enter them, and empowering these providers to be gatekeepers.

I believe that the gatekeeper model created by the HMOs has merit. However, because consumers demanded access to specialists, even for problems that could easily be handled by a primary care doctor, this approach fell out of favor. But consumers must be educated to accept that in the name of cost and quality, access to specialty care must be limited. Once the demand for these services is reduced, there will be an inevitable shift to primary care.

With respect to pain management in particular, government can help by easing regulatory scrutiny of pain doctors—whose primary focus is opioid prescription—so that physicians will no longer be frightened away from taking on the responsibility of managing pain. We can achieve this by a more balanced approach to the "opioid abuse/compassionate prescribing pendulum" I described previously. It will require an acknowledgment by legislative bodies and law enforcement agencies such as the DEA that physicians have the responsibility to ease suffering, that untreated or poorly treated pain represents a health-care crisis far greater in scope than prescription drug abuse, and that physicians need to be supported by these entities in this aspect of their job. While physicians do need to take reasonable steps to minimize prescription drug abuse, they should not have to experience law enforcement as an adversary. I have been able to do my job much more effectively when I could work with law enforcement on the mutual, though sometimes conflicting, problems we face. My impression was that law enforcement officers who chose to work with me felt the same way. Creating such supportive relationships can be done through regular dialogue between law enforcement officials and medical groups at the grassroots level.

I have met two people who were fortunate enough to spend time with Mother Teresa in Calcutta. Both said they had expressed remorse upon leaving her mission, feeling guilty that they were no longer able to care for the "poorest of the poor." Mother Teresa admonished them to see the poor who exist in their own backyard. She reminded them that they didn't need to go to India to find such people.

The poor of the medical world are in our backyard. Do we have the courage to make the sacrifices needed to change our system to provide care for them? I look forward to the challenge, but based on past performance, I fear the outcome.

Living in the Forest

Each person has inside a basic decency and goodness. If he listens to it and acts on it, he is giving a great deal of what it is the world needs most. It is not complicated but it takes courage. It takes courage for a person to listen to his own goodness and act on it.

Pablo Casals, *Saturday Review* (December 12, 1959)

The opposite of courage in our society is not cowardice, it is conformity.

Rollo May, *The Courage to Create*

Am I a Coward?

By now you are aware that I adored my mother. She was a wonderful woman, and she is still my guiding light. Most people knew her as the woman with the smile she lavished freely on everyone around her, making them feel better about themselves.

There was another side to my mother, though, one few had an opportunity to see, and I once had the misfortune of it being directed at me. Where we lived, the drinking age was eighteen; and when I turned eighteen, I took advantage of that law. On the morning of that glorious day my friends and I went to the convenience store. Proudly brandishing my ID, I purchased a few cases of Genesee Cream Ale, the favored local brew. We proceeded to the park, where we consumed the entire purchase in relatively short order. Fortunately, one of us chose not to indulge, and he inherited the job of designated driver.

I had consumed way more than my fill, and my stomach rejected much of what I had put in it. Out of concern for my well-being, my friend drove me home. I thought it was nearly midnight, but it was actually closer to 6:00 PM. As I walked into the house, I expected to find my parents in bed. Rather, they were at the dinner table. There was no hiding the state I was in. My mother came up and slapped me in the face. It was the only time that I remember her hitting me. I can still feel that slap and the shame it created. My mother believed in rules, based on a stern sense of morality. The only actions that would stir such a reaction in her were violations of those rules. She was averse to drunkenness, and I had committed the ultimate sin.

Whenever she sensed an injustice due to a violation of morality, she spoke her mind. I swear the local television station had its own private line for her, knowing that whenever they dared speak a curse, or display an exposed "private part," or run a violent children's show, my mother would call, in effect slapping them. We laughed at her, but down deep I admired her for her courage to stand up for her convictions. I always prayed for such courage, born of virtue.

Opportunities to be courageous only come along so often. Such moments must be seized without hesitation, or the opportunity disappears. One such opportunity presented itself to me in 2003; it tested my soul. Others applauded my actions, but I truly believe I flunked this test of my convictions; and I have been haunted by my choice ever since. There is no right or wrong answer to most of the important questions in life. In the end, the one important judge of our actions is ourself. My self did not and does not think I reacted courageously; and I am left to deal with the aftermath, forever wondering if I did the "right" thing.

When my patient Jane's son died of an overdose, and the police suspected that some of the medications I had prescribed for her had contributed, the medical board investigated me, as I have described. They subpoenaed the records of my most challenging patients—people who represented the outliers among my practice.

Before this happened, I had publicly stood up for the rights of pain patients to have adequate treatment and of physicians to prescribe for them. I had served on the task force that drafted rules for opiate prescription that were accepted by the medical board and our state legislature. I was proud of these actions. I had a practice of over 350 pain patients for whom I was prescribing pain medication. I worked long hours to meet their needs, being remunerated barely enough to cover my costs to my medical group. Yet my work gave me a satisfaction that money never could.

As the investigation unfolded, I was being challenged to stand up for my beliefs. I lived in constant anxiety, fear, and panic. I feared losing my license and going to jail. Other physicians had suffered this fate. I wondered if I had the courage of a Gandhi, a Jesus, or a Martin Luther King to accept incarceration or chastisement rather than betray my beliefs. My patients were counting on me.

Pietro Aretino (1492–1556), an Italian author, playwright, poet, satirist, and blackmailer, who wielded immense influence on art and politics in his time, said, "A high heart ought to bear calamities and not flee them, since in bearing them appears the grandeur of the mind and in fleeing them the cowardice of the heart."

I was not looking for an out, but two were offered to me, one by my partners and one by the DEA. For reasons unrelated to the investigation, the members of my medical group wanted me to change my practice. They were concerned about the waiting list for procedures I performed, and the effect of the resulting delays on their ability to treat the patients I cared for. They asked me to close my pain management practice and focus on my interventional (procedural) practice. They had a job to do, and my waiting list was adversely affecting their ability to do that job. I was enticed by the prospect of more money, less stress, and shorter hours.

I have every reason to assume that their offer was honorable. I, a nonorthopedist, had been hired by an orthopedic group to help meet their needs. I was not hired to manage pain; but as I practiced, I came to understand the plight of those in chronic pain as I have described it in this book. I saw that the medical world was largely ignoring them and believed I could do something about that. As the years passed, the scope of my practice diverged dramatically from what my group had envisioned when I was hired. I was not meeting their needs, and something needed to change. It was also quite clear to me that this offer was not a suggestion. I never asked what would happen if I refused to close my practice, but I had every reason to believe I would need to find another place of employment.

The DEA's motivation was less honorable. Around that time, they were prosecuting the Hurwitz case I referred to in chapter 13. Not long before, pain physicians had been struggling to figure out how to refill schedule II opiates in a manner that would not be too onerous for pain patients, especially those on high doses who often needed refills once a week. Our leaders met with the DEA to craft a policy. This level of cooperation was unprecedented, and it was very important for the development of a balanced public policy on opioid medications. The agreed-on policy was published on the DEA website and served as guide for all physicians who prescribed opiates. I used it daily. But when Dr. Hurwitz's lawyers relied on it in their defense, it miraculously disappeared from the DEA website. When pressed about this, the DEA claimed that they had never accepted the agreement as policy. Any doctor who now followed it was in violation of the Controlled Substance Act, in effect guilty of a felony. The result was that when I was out of the office, someone had to write prescriptions for me, which most of my untrained orthopedic partners were unwilling to do, and I cannot blame them.

I now faced a dilemma. Should I put the needs of my 350 patients first— needs that strained my life, my family, my marriage, my emotions? It would be very easy to leave my group and open a new office, although I would have a substantially lower income. However, the DEA's removal of the policy meant that as a solo practitioner, I could never go away. Should I instead put my family's needs first? To meet my patients' needs I worked fourteen-hour days and took calls 24/7. I brought work home, mentally more than physically. This put a great strain on our family. Should I put my group's needs first? In hiring me, they had offered me a previously unimagined opportunity, and I felt that I did owe them something. Yet if I took this option, I would create a huge diaspora of patients who would need to find someone else to care for them in a world where few were willing to prescribe or even care for the poorest of the medical world.

I had long sought to be part of the solution to the problem of untreated pain, and had encouraged others to take up this charge. If I discharged my patients, would I not be a hypocrite? Would I not be a coward? If I stayed with my group, would I not become part of the problem society creates in ignoring the plight of those in chronic pain? At the same time, if I stayed, would I not still be providing a valuable service for those who suffered? Was it fair to let the people on my procedural waiting list suffer while they waited for treatment? In this sense, choosing my group would be a "win" for them, as well as for my family and for me. Imagine a "win-win-win" scenario. How often does that occur?

But it still would be a "lose" for my pain patients, as well as for the local community and the local medical community, which needed someone to take on this task. Like an experienced politician, I sought a middle ground. Perhaps I could still care for some of my patients? The answer was no. I had to make a choice, and it was mine alone to make.

I would love to say I languished over the decision, sweating blood. But in fact any thoughts of altruism succumbed to fear. I feared the repercussions if I continued to practice pain management as I had been doing, and I was willing to stand up for my beliefs only up to a point. The problem was magnified by the realization that I was no longer sure I was doing the right thing. Was I helping my pain patients, or enabling them? Were the medications I prescribed helping or harming? I was no longer sure. I had been pondering these questions at some level for quite some time, but once the investigation began, they rose to the forefront of my thoughts.

I chose what felt like the cowardly way out and closed my practice. The only honorable thing I did do was give my patients six months to find new doctors, substantially more than the customary one month prescribed by the medical ethicists. Over the next few years, my choice of an interventional practice over a management practice doubled my income, while my hours were cut nearly in half. Though on paper I was on call 24/7, the actual burden lightened considerably. I spent more hours with my family than ever before and got to experience firsthand their successes and failures.

Many people would trade anything to be in my shoes. I live a comfortable life with no financial worries. I have everything money could ever buy, at least that I would want. Still I feel an emptiness that will never go away. There is a reward in being willing to stand up for those in need, to be there for them in their time of desperation, to get to know them and be a part of their lives. While many patients still thank me for what I do, that special aspect of my life, my job, is gone.

I had a chance to be courageous and choose meaning in life. Instead, I chose my own needs over those I cared for, to follow the path of least resistance. I chose to be a slave to money, to security, to fear. Does that make me a coward? A hypocrite? About a year after I closed my practice, I learned that a former patient of mine had shot himself. He never could come to grips with his inabilities or his pain, and he could find no one willing to care for him. Out of despair, he took his own life.

Sometimes, to save someone else, you need to put yourself at risk. You need to suffer, even if the suffering is only financial; for as Gandhi said, "The truth may turn out in terms of the current moods and trends of a blind society to be supremely unprofitable."[1]

I had a chance to be courageous. If I could not be, how can I expect others to? I had a chance to seize the moment. I pray the moment has not passed me by and that I will have another opportunity. While I believe my actions fall considerably short of cowardice, they fall substantially short of the heroism I desire.

The choice I had to make is increasingly being forced on physicians who manage complex medical problems such as pain, and many wind up doing what I did. The consequences for medical care are immense, as physicians effectively transfer authority over the medical ship to the businessman, the lawyer, and the regulator.

How we treat those who suffer from pain is a measure of how we stand in relation to our ideals. I think we can do a lot better—me included. In the end, I have come to understand that I am not a hero. Nor am I a coward. I am merely someone who seeks every day to do unto others as I would have them do to me. In doing so, I seek to live in the forest. Criticize me if you will, but I like the view much better there.

NOTES

PART ONE *Poor Man, Pained Man*

1. Institute of Medicine, *Relieving Pain in America: A Blueprint for Transforming Prevention, Care, Education, and Research* (Washington, DC: National Academies Press, 2011), http://www.nap.edu/read/13172/chapter/1.

TWO What Is Pain? Its Neurophysiology and Psychology: Chasing Two Moving Targets

1. S. Tyrer, *British Journal of Psychiatry* 188 (2006): 91–93.
2. Ibid.
3. American Psychiatric Association, *Diagnostic and Statistical Manual of Mental Disorders*, 5th ed. (DSM-5) (Arlington, VA: American Psychiatric Publishing, 2013), 271–80.

THREE You *Do* Have to Suffer . . . Just Not as Much as We Make You

1. J. Kuch, S. Schuman, and H. Curry, "The Problem Patient and the Problem Doctor or Do Quacks Make Crocks," *Journal of Family Practice* 5, no. 4 (1977): 647–53.
2. "2001 to 2010: The Decade of Pain Control and Research," *LIFE in Pain* (blog), Feb. 22, 2001, accessed on Oct. 27, 2015, http://lifeinpain.org/node/141.
3. D. M. Goldenbaum et al., "Physicians Charged with Opiate Analgesic-Prescribing Offenses," *Pain Medicine* 9, no. 6 (Sept. 2008): 737–47. doi: 10.1111/j.1526-4637.2008.00482.x.

FIVE Family, Friends, and Community

1. Rev. G. W. Kosicki, *Faustina: Saint for Our Times* (Stockbridge, MA: Marian Press, 2011), 32.
2. *Diary of Saint Maria Faustina Kowalska: Divine Mercy in My Soul,* (Stockbridge, MA: Marian Press, 2013), 67.
3. Ibid., 117.
4. Ibid., 342.
5. Ibid., 163.

SIX The Physician and the Pain Patient: Poorly Equipped for the Role?

Epigraph source: The Oath of Maimonides is a traditional oath for physicians often substituted for the Oath of Hippocrates, attributed to Rabbi Moshe Ben Maimon (1135–1204 AD), a prominent Jewish scholar.

1. L. Mezei, B. Murinson et al., "Pain Education in North American Medical Schools," *Journal of Pain* 12, no. 12 (Dec. 2011): 1199–1208.

2. D. L. Sacket et al., "Evidence-Based Medicine: What It Is and What It Isn't," *British Medical Journal* 312 (1996): 71–72.

3. R. P. El Dib, A. N. Atallah, and R. B. Andriolo, "Mapping the Cochrane Evidence for Decision Making in Health Care," *Journal of Evaluation in Clinical Practice* 13, no. 4 (2007): 689–92.

4. Thought to have been written by Hippocrates or one of his students in the fifth century BC. "Hippocratic Oath, Modern Version," Sheridan Libraries, Johns Hopkins University, September 24, 2015, accessed on Nov. 11, 2015, http://guides.library.jhu .edu/c.php?g=202502&p=1335759.

SEVEN Regulatory Agencies and Pain Management:
Overregulation Breeds Underregulation

1. United States Drug Enforcement Agency, "DEA Mission Statement," DEA.gov, accessed on Nov. 11, 2015, http://www.dea.gov/about/mission.shtml.

2. U.S. Food and Drug Administration, "What Does FDA Do?" FDA.gov, May 6, 2013, accessed on Nov. 15, 2015, http://www.fda.gov/AboutFDA/Transparency /Basics/ucm194877.htm.

3. U.S. Food and Drug Administration, "Don't Be Fooled by Health Fraud Scams," FDA.gov, accessed on Nov. 15, 2015, http://www.fda.gov/ForConsumers/Consumer Updates/ucm278980.htm.

4. N. Reuter, "Scheduling of Drugs under the Controlled Substances Act," U.S. Food and Drug Administration, March 11, 1999, accessed on Oct. 27, 2015, http:// www.fda.gov/NewsEvents/Testimony/ucm115087.htm.

EIGHT The Business of Health Care: Whose Bottom Line Are We Treating?

1. A. Young, "Unmasking the People Behind Risky Pills," *USA Today*, Dec. 20, 2013.

2. "Miracle Health Claims," Federal Trade Commission, Consumer Information, accessed on Oct. 27, 2015, http://www.consumer.ftc.gov/articles/0167-miracle -health-claims.

3. P. L. Gildenberg, "History of Neuromodulation for Chronic Pain," *Pain Medicine* 7, no. S1 (2006): 7–13.

4. Center for Devices and Radiological Health, U.S. Food and Drug Administration, "The New 510(k) Paradigm—Alternate Approaches to Demonstrating Substantial Equivalence in Premarket Notifications—Final Guidance," FDA.gov, March 20, 1998, accessed on Oct. 27, 2015, http://www.fda.gov/MedicalDevices /DeviceRegulationandGuidance/GuidanceDocuments/ucm080187.htm#.

5. U.S. Food and Drug Administration, "What Is the Approval Process for a New Prescription Drug?" FDA.gov, Oct. 19, 2015, accessed on Nov. 15, 2015, http://www .fda.gov/AboutFDA/Transparency/Basics/ucm194949.htm.

6. "New Approval Drug Process," Drugs.com, Sept. 1, 2015, accessed on Nov. 11, 2015, http://www.drugs.com/fda-approval-process.html.

7. U.S. Food and Drug Administration, "Is It Really FDA Approved?" FDA Consumer Health Information, FDA.gov, Feb. 20, 2009, accessed on Nov. 15, 2015, www.fda.gov/consumer/updates/approvals093008.pdf.

8. J. Akre, "FDA-101-What Does FDA Approval Mean? (Part One)," Injury Board National News Desk, October 6, 2008, accessed on Nov. 15, 2015, http://news .legalexaminer.com/fda---01---what-does-it-do-part-one.aspx?googleid=248938.

9. G. Koleva, "Loophole in FDA's Approval Process for Medical Devices Prompts Letter from Congress," *Forbes*, August 17, 2012, http://www.forbes.com/sites /gerganakoleva/2012/08/17/loophole-in-fdas-approval-process-for-medical -devices-prompts-letter-from-congress/.

10. Ibid.

NINE The Workplace and Entitlements: Creating "Inability" out of "Disability"

1. Centers for Disease Control, "Prevalence and Most Common Causes of Disability Among Adults—United States, 2005," *MMWR Weekly* 58, no. 16 (May 2009): 421-26, www.cdc.gov/mmwr/preview/mmwrhtml/mm5816a2.htm.

2. Chances of Disability, "Disability Statistics," Council for Disability Awareness, July 3, 2013, accessed on Nov. 15, 2015, http://www.disabilitycanhappen.org /chances_disability/disability_stats.asp.

3. "Americans with Disabilities Act of 1990," http://en.wikipedia.org/wiki /Americans_with_Disabilites _Act_of_1990.

4. Disability.gov, https://www.disability.gov.

5. Ibid.

6. F. Guyton, "A Brief History of Workers' Compensation," *Iowa Orthopaedic Journal* 19 (1999): 106-10.

7. Ibid.

8. Ibid.

9. Ibid.

10. Ibid.

11. Ibid.

12. Ibid.

13. Ibid.

14. B. Kolodiejchuk, *Mother Teresa: Come Be My Light* (New York: Doubleday, 2007), 144-45.

TEN Health and Disability Insurance: The Law of Unintended Consequences

Epigraph source: As quoted in R. Norton, "Unintended Consequences," Library of Economics and Liberty, 2002, accessed on Nov. 11, 2015, http://www.econlib.org.

1. A. Flexner, *Medical Education in the United States and Canada* (New York: Carnegie Foundation for the Advancement of Teaching, 1910).

2. A 2008 study by the Texas Medical Association found that only 38 percent of the state's primary care doctors accepted Medicare. Also, a 2008 study by the Medicare Payment Advisory Commission found that 29 percent of the Medicare beneficiaries it surveyed had trouble finding a primary care doctor (http://www.nytimes.com/2009/04/02/business/retirementspecial/02health.html?_r=0). A 2006 study by the Center for Studying Health System Change showed that almost half of all physicians polled said they had stopped accepting or were limiting the number of new Medicaid beneficiaries they will see (http://www.medicalnewstoday.com/releases/77387.php).

3. G. Harris, "More Doctors Giving Up Primary Practice," *New York Times,* March 25, 2010.

4. D. Beaulieu-Volk "Physician Employment Could Hit 75%, Eclipsing Private Practice," July 18, 2012, accessed on Nov. 15, 2015, http://www.fiercepracticemanagement.com/story/survey-hospital-employment-eclipse-private-practice/2012-07-18.

5. J. Kennedy, J. Roll, T. Schraudner, S. Murphy, and S. McPherson, "Prevalence of Persistent Pain in the U.S. Adult Population: New Data from the 2010 National Health Interview," *Journal of Pain* 15, no. 10 (October 2014): 979–84. In this book I follow most experts and use the one hundred million figure.

6. S. Cohen and W. Yu, "The Concentration and Persistence in the Level of Health Expenditures over Time: Estimates for the U.S. Population, 2008-2009," Medical Expenditure Panel Survey, Agency for Health Care Research and Quality, Jan. 2012, accessed on Nov. 11, 2015, http:/meps.ahrq.gov/mepsweb/data_files/publications/st354/stat354.pdf.

7. J. Tozzi, "Losing Patience, and Patients, with Medicaid," *Bloomberg Business,* April 10, 2014, http://www.businessweek.com/articles/2014-04-10/doctors-shun-patients-who-pay-with-medicaid.

8. The following historical discussion is adapted from "Disability Insurance," Myceisonline, 2000-2007, http://myceisonline.com/courses/disabilityIns/Book/description.html.

ELEVEN The Legal System: Disorder in the Court!

1. P. Anderson, "Nonprescription Opioid Use Prevalent among Older Teens," *Medscape Multispecialty,* Aug. 6, 2009, accessed on Nov. 11, 2015, http://www.medscape.com/viewarticle/707082. http://www.medscape.com/viewarticle/707082.

2. S. Ogozaly, "Teen Opioid Abuse Occurring at a Younger Age," *MD All Specialties,* May 8, 2012, accessed on Nov. 17, 2015, http://www.hcplive.com/web-exclusive/Teen-Opioid-Abuse-Occurring-at-Younger-Age.

TWELVE What It Means to "Do No Harm": Is There a Safe Way to Medicate Pain?

1. Zogby Analytics, "National Poll: Chronic Pain and Drug Addiction," Research America: An Alliance for Discoveries in Health, April 2013, accessed on Nov. 11, 2015,

http://www.researchamerica.org/ . . . /files/uploads/March2013painaddiction
.pdf.

2. National Institute on Drug Abuse, "Drugs, Brains, and Behavior: The Science of
Addiction," July 2014, accessed on Nov. 11, 2015, National Institutes of Health (NIH),
http://www.drugabuse.gov/publications/drugs-brains-behavior-science-addiction
/drug-abuse-addiction.

3. Committee on Advancing Pain Research, Care, and Education, Institute of
Medicine of the National Academies, *Relieving Pain in America: A Blueprint for
Transforming Prevention, Care, Education, and Research* (Washington, DC: National
Academies Press, 2011).

4. S. Leavitt, "More about Chronic Pain, Opioids, and Suicide," *Pain-Topics News/
Research Updates,* July 1, 2011, accessed on Nov. 15, 2015, http://updates.pain-topics
.org/2011/07/more_about_chronic_pain_opioids_suicide.html.

5. M. T. Smith, R. R. Edwards, R. C. Robinson, and R. H. Dworkin, "Suicidal
Ideation, Plans, and Attempts in Chronic Pain Patients: Factors Associated with
Increased Risk," *Pain* 111, nos. 1–2 (2004): 201–8.

6. N. K. Tang and C. Crane, "Suicidality in Chronic Pain: A Review of the
Prevalence, Risk Factors, and Psychological Links," *Psychological Medicine* 36, no. 5
(2006): 575–86.

7. D. G. Jacobs, R. J. Baldessarini, Y. Conwell et al., "Practice Guideline for
the Assessment and Treatment of Patients With Suicidal Behaviors," American
Psychiatric Association, Nov. 2003, accessed Nov. 29, 2015, http://psychiatryonline
.org/pb/assets/raw/sitewide/practice_guidelines/guidelines/suicide.pdf.

8. National Institute on Drug Abuse, "Drug Facts: Nationwide Trends," National
Institutes of Health, December 2012, accessed on Nov. 17, 2015, http://www
.drugabuse.gov/publications/drugfacts/nationwide-trends.

9. G. Koleva, "Plan to Stem Prescription Drug Crisis in New York Fuels Disagree-
ment," *Forbes,* March 2, 2012, http://www.forbes.com/sites/gerganakoleva/2012
/03/02/plan-to-stem-prescription-drug-crisis-in-new-york-fuels-disagreement/.

THIRTEEN Opiates and Opioids

1. This is not intended to be an exhaustive medical discussion. For physicians
interested in exploring this issue further, I recommend Dr. Scott Fishman's
Responsible Opioid Prescribing: A Physician's Guide (Washington, DC: Waterford Life
Sciences, 2007).

2. New Hampshire Medical Society, "New Hampshire Opioid Prescribing
Resource," accessed on Nov. 11, 2015, http://www.nhms.org/resources/opioid.

3. J. Duncan, "Law Enforcement and Regulatory Issues," in *Weiner's Pain
Management: A Practical Guide for Clinicians,* ed. M. Boswell and B. Cole (Boca
Raton, FL: CRC Press, 2006), 1407–14.

4. A. Jacox, D. B. Carr, and R. Payne et al., *Management of Cancer Pain, Clinical*

Practice Guideline Number 9 (Rockville, MD: Agency for Health Care Policy and Research, U.S. Department of Health and Human Services, Public Health Service, March 1994), 12–19. AHCPR Publication No. 94–0593.

FOURTEEN   Cannabinoids and Pain: Reefer Madness or Compassionate Care?

1. B. Langer, "High Support for Medical Marijuana," ABC News, January 18, 2010, http://abcnews.go.com/PollingUnit/Politics/medical-marijuana-abc-news-poll -analysis/story?id=9586503.

2. B. Bratu, "Survey: 52% of Americans in Favor of Legalizing Marijuana," NBC News, April 4, 2013, http://usnews.nbcnews.com/_news/2013/04/04/17603170 -survey-52-percent-of-americans-in-favor-of-legalizing-marijuana?lite.

3. Ibid.

4. Ibid.

5. Uniform Crime Reports, "Crime in the United States 2013," Federal Bureau of Investigation, accessed on Nov. 15, 2015, https://www.fbi.gov/about-us/cjis/ucr /crime-in-the-u.s/2013/crime-in-the-u.s.-2013/persons-arrested/persons-arrested.

6. Katz et al., "Behavioral Monitoring and Urine Toxicology Testing in Patients Receiving Long-Term Opioid Therapy," *Anesthesia and Analgesia* 97, no. 4 (Oct. 2003): 1097–1102.

7. E. Small and D. Marcus, *Hemp: A New Crop with New Uses for North America* (Alexandria, VA: ASHS Press, 2002), 284, http://www.hort.purdue.edu/newcrop /ncnu02/v5-284.html.

8. Ibid.

9. K. Webley, "Brief History: Medical Marijuana," *Time*, June 21, 2010, http:// content.time.com/time/magazine/article/0,9171,1995849,00.html.

10. I. Lozano, "The Therapeutic Use of Cannabis Sativa (L.) in Arabic Medicine," *Journal of Cannabis Therapeutics* 1 (2001): 63. doi:10.1300/J175v01n01_05.

11. Small, *Hemp*.

12. A. Mack and J. Joy, *Marijuana as Medicine?: The Science Beyond the Controversy* (Washington, DC: National Academy Press, 2000), 15.

13. *The Antique Cannabis Book,* 3rd ed., January 2014, accessed on Nov. 12, 2015, http://www.antiquecannabisbook.com/.

14. "Our Fashionable Narcotics," *New York Times,* January 10, 1854.

15. R. J. Bonnie and C. H. Whitebread II, "The Forbidden Fruit and the Tree of Knowledge: An Inquiry into the Legal History of American Marijuana Prohibition," Schaffer Library of Drug Policy, http://druglibrary.org/schaffer/library/studies/vlr /vlr3.htm.

16. L. French and M. Manzanárez, *Nafta and Neocolonialism: Comparative Criminal, Human and Social Justice* (Lanham, MD: University Press of America, 2004), 129.

17. Frontline, "Marijuana Timeline," Public Broadcasting Service, accessed on

Nov. 12, 2015, http://www.pbs.org/wgbh/pages/frontline/shows/dope/etc/cron .html.

18. Ibid.

19. David W. Ogden, "Investigations and Prosecutions in States Authorizing the Medical Use of Marijuana," Office of the Deputy Attorney General, U.S. Department of Justice, Washington, DC, October 19, 2009, http://www.justice.gov/opa /documents/medical-marijuana.pdf.

20. P. Pacher, S. Bátkai, and G. Kunos, "The Endocannabinoid System as an Emerging Target of Pharmacotherapy," *Pharmacological Reviews* 58, no. 3 (2006): 389–462. doi:10.1124/pr.58.3.2. PMC 2241751. PMID 16968947.

21. A. El-Alfy, "Antidepressant-like Effect of Δ9-Tetrahydrocannabinol and Other Cannabinoids Isolated from Cannabis sativa L.," *Pharmacology Biochemistry and Behavior* 95, no. 4 (June 2010): 434–42. Published online March 21, 2010. doi: 10.1016/j.pbb.2010.03.004.

22. R. Meyer, "Potential Merits of Cannabinoids for Medical Uses," U.S. Food and Drug Administration, News and Events, April 1, 2004, accessed on Nov. 12, 2015, http://www.fda.gov/NewsEvents/Testimony/ucm114741.htm.

23. Pacher, Bátkai, and Kunos, "The Endocannabinoid System."

24. Ibid.

25. Ibid.

26. J. Huffman, "The Search for Selective Ligands for the CB2 Receptor," *Current Pharmaceutical Design* 6, no. 13 (2000): 1323–37. doi:10.2174/1381612003399347. PMID 10903395.

27. T. Iseger and M. Bossong, "A Systematic Review of the Antipsychotic Properties of Cannabidiol in Humans," *Schizophrenia Research* 162, nos. 1–3 (March 2015): 153–61. doi:10.1016/j.schres.2015.01.033. PMID 25667194.

28. R. Mechoulam, M. Peters, E. Murillo-Rodriguez, and L. Hanuš, "Cannabidiol: Recent Advances," *Chemistry and Biodiversity* 4, no. 8 (2007): 1678–92. doi:10.1002 /cbdv.200790147. PMID 17712814.

29. "Cannabis Sativa vs. Cannabis Indica," Patient's Marijuana Caregiver Services, February 28, 2013, accessed on Nov. 11, 2015, http://patientsmarijuana.org/Sativa _or_Indica.html.

30. I. Grant, J. Hampton Atkinson, and A. Mattison, "Report to the Legislature and Governor of the State of California Presenting Findings Pursuant to SB847 Which Created the CMCR and Provided State Funding," Center for Medicinal Cannabis Research, University of California, February 11, 2010, http://www.cmcr .ucsd.edu/images/pdfs/CMCR_REPORT_FEB17.pdf.

31. M. Hashibe, H. Morgenstern, Y. Cui, D. P. Tashkin, Z.-F. Zhang, W. Cozen, T. M. Mack, and S. Greenland, "Marijuana Use and the Risk of Lung and Upper Aerodigestive Tract Cancers: Results of a Population-Based Case-Control Study," *Cancer Epidemiology Biomarkers and Prevention* 15, no. 10 (2006): 1829–34.

32. W. C. Tan, C. Lo, A. Jong, L. Xing, M. J. Fitzgerald, W. M. Vollmer, S. A. Buist, and D. D. Sin et al., "Marijuana and Chronic Obstructive Lung Disease: A Population-Based Study" (PDF), *CMAJ* (Toronto: Canadian Medical Association) 180, no. 8 (April 14, 2009): 814-20.

33. M. H. Meier et al., "Persistent Cannabis Users Show Neuropsychological Decline from Childhood to Midlife," *Proceedings of the National Academy of Sciences* 109, no. 40 (Aug. 27, 2012): E2657-E2664, www.pnas.org/cgi/doi/10.1073/pnas.1206820109.

34. O. Rogeberg, "Correlations between Cannabis Use and IQ Change in the Dunedin Cohort Are Consistent with Confounding from Socioeconomic Status," *Proceedings of the National Academy of Sciences* 110, no. 11 (Jan. 14, 2013): 4251-54, www.pnas.org/cgi/doi/10.1073/pnas.1215678110.

35. Brain Injury Resource Center, "Pediatric Committee Issues Warning on Youth Soccer," Headline News Archive, Dec. 1998, http://www.headinjury.com/newsltr.htm.

36. American Cancer Society, "Marijuana and Cancer," March 4, 2015, accessed on Nov. 12, 2015, http://www.cancer.org/treatment/treatmentsandsideeffects/physicalsideeffects/chemotherapyeffects/marijuana-and-cancer.

37. P. Hilts, "Relative Addictiveness of Drugs," *New York Times,* August 2, 1994.

38. University of New Hampshire, "Risk of Marijuana's 'Gateway Effect' Overblown, New Research Shows," ScienceDaily, September 2, 2010, http://www.sciencedaily.com/releases/2010/09/100902073507.htm.

39. R. Kuepper et al., "Continued Cannabis Use and Risk of Incidence and Persistence of Psychotic Symptoms: 10 Year Follow-up Cohort Study," *British Medical Journal* (online), no. 342 (March 1, 2011): d738. doi: 10.1136/bmj.d738.

40. Drug Enforcement Administration, United States Department of Justice, "In the Matter of Marijuana Rescheduling Petition Docket no 86-22, Opinion and Recommended Ruling, Findings of Fact, Conclusions of Law and Decision of Administrative Law Judge, Francis Young," Schaffer Library of Drug Policy, Sept. 6, 1988, http://www.druglibrary.org/schaffer/library/studies/YOUNG/index.html.

41. T. Pedersen, "Marijuana Pain Relief Varies among Users," PsychCentral, Dec. 29, 2012, http://psychcentral.com/news/2012/12/29/marijuana-pain-relief-varies-among-users/49770.html.

42. Office of National Drug Control Policy, "Marijuana," WhiteHouse.gov, accessed on April 14, 2013, http://www.whitehouse.gov/ondcp/marijuana.

43. American Cancer Society, "Marijuana and Cancer."

44. P. Hecht, "California Pot Research Backs Therapeutic Claims," *Sacramento Bee,* July 12, 2012, http://www.sacbee.com/2012/07/12/4625608/california-pot-research-backs.html.

45. Ibid.

46. P. Adams, "Colorado Medical Marijuana—Sellers Aim High," BBC News, http://www.bbc.co.uk/news/mobile/world-us+canada-10623493.

47. E. Gogek, "A Bad Trip for Democrats," *New York Times,* Nov. 7, 2012, http://www.nytimes.com/2012/11/08/opinion/a-bad-trip-for-democrats.html?_r=0.

48. S. Fishman, *Responsible Opioid Prescribing: A Physician's Guide* (Washington, DC: Federation of State Medical Boards, 2007).

49. Adams, "Colorado Medical Marijuana."

FIFTEEN   Health-Care Reform and Chronic Pain: We All Have a Role to Play

1. J. Levy, "In U.S., Uninsured Rate Dips to 11.9% in First Quarter," Gallup, April 13, 2015, http://www.gallup.com/poll/182348/uninsured-rate-dips-first-quarter.aspx.

2. L. Ungar and O. Donnell, "Dilemma over Deductibles: Costs Crippling Middle Class," *USA Today,* Jan. 1, 2015, http://www.usatoday.com/story/news/nation/2015/01/01/middle-class-workers-struggle-to-pay-for-care-despite-insurance/19841235/.

3. Ibid.

4. World Bank, "Data: Health Care Expenditure, Total % (of GDP)," 2015, http://data.worldbank.org/indicator/SH.XPD.TOTL.ZS/.

EPILOGUE   Living in the Forest

1. T. Merton, *Ghandi on Non-Violence* (New York: New Directions, 1965), 18.

INDEX